Baillière's
CLINICAL
OBSTETRICS
AND
GYNAECOLOGY
INTERNATIONAL PRACTICE AND RESEARCH

SOUTHERN HEMISPHERE WINES

Blaauwklippen Pinot Noir 1985 - Dry medium bodied Pinot with flavour	£	80.00
Blaauwklippen Cabernet Sauvignon 1980 - Aging beautifully - full in style	£	94.00
Blaauwklippen Zinfandel 1984 - An outstanding year - light Oak with good fruit	£	67.00
Blaauwklippen International Auction Cabernet Sauvignon 1983 - Vintners Reserve	£	106.00
Blaauwklippen Chardonnay 1988 - Full round flavour and depth of taste	£	126.00
Vriesenhof Estate 1983 - Firm and prominent Cabernet flavour	£	78.50
Vriesenhof Cabernet Sauvignon 1983 (6 x 150 cl) - Magnum - as 1983 Estate	£	78.50
Vriesenhof Kalista 1985 - Mature and well founded. Cabernet Sauvignon	£	78.50
Vriesenhof Kalista 1986 - as 1985 to be released Sept 1989	£	78.50
Vriesenhof Kalista 1983 - Firm and prominent Cabernet flavour and longevity	£	78.50
Vriesenhof Chardonnay 1987 - Stylish, well made and developing well	£	90.00
Rozendal Estate Cabernet 1983 - Exceptional wine, complex and full flavoured	£	106.00
Hamilton Russel Hemel en Aarde Blanc de Blanc - Oak aged Burgundian style	£	75.00
Hamilton Russel Grand Vin Noir - Pure Pinot Noir. Very Fine	£	89.00
Hamilton Russel Chardonnay - Classic; Balance flavour and great length	£	172.50
Delheim Blanc Fume 1987/88 - First Class Sauvignon Blanc flavour and finish	£	62.00
Delheim Special Late Harvest 1987 - Chenin Blanc. Beautiful full taste	£	65.00
Delheim Pinotage 1986 - Traditional full flavour and lasting fruit	£	75.00
Delheim Cabernet Sauvignon 1985 - Honest Cabernet with character and style	£	78.50

Baillière's

CLINICAL OBSTETRICS AND GYNAECOLOGY

INTERNATIONAL PRACTICE AND RESEARCH

Volume 4/Number 1
March 1990

Antenatal Care

M. H. HALL MB ChB, MD, FRCOG
Guest Editor

Baillière Tindall
London Philadelphia Sydney Tokyo Toronto

This book is printed on acid-free paper. ∞

Baillière Tindall 24–28 Oval Road,
W.B. Saunders London NW1 7DX

The Curtis Center, Independence Square West,
Philadelphia, PA 19106–3399, USA

55 Horner Avenue
Toronto, Ontario M8Z 4X6, Canada

Harcourt Brace Jovanovich Group (Australia) Pty Ltd,
30–52 Smidmore Street, Marrickville, NSW 2204, Australia

Harcourt Brace Jovanovich Japan, Inc,
Ichibancho Central Building,
22-1 Ichibancho, Chiyoda-ku, Tokyo 102, Japan

ISSN 0950–3552

ISBN 0–7020–1476–1 (single copy)

Baillière's Clinical Obstetrics and Gynaecology is published four times each year by Baillière Tindall. Annual subscription prices are:

TERRITORY	ANNUAL SUBSCRIPTION	SINGLE ISSUE
1. UK	£49.00 post free	£22.50 post free
2. Europe	£57.00 post free	£22.50 post free
3. All other countries	Consult your local Harcourt Brace Jovanovich office for dollar price	

The editor of this publication is Margaret Macdonald, Baillière Tindall, 24–28 Oval Road, London NW1 7DX.

Baillière's Clinical Obstetrics and Gynaecology was published from 1983 to 1986 as *Clinics in Obstetrics and Gynaecology*.

Typeset by Phoenix Photosetting, Chatham.
Printed and bound in Great Britain by Mackays of Chatham PLC, Chatham, Kent.

Contributors to this issue

ADEYEMI O. ADEKUNLE MB, BS, FWACS, FMCOG, Lecturer in Obstetrics and Gynaecology, University of Ibadan; Consultant Obstetrician and Gynaecologist to the University College Hospital, Ibadan, Nigeria.

GERARD BREART MD, MSc, Directeur, INSERM (U149), 123, bd de Port Royal, 75014 Paris, France.

ROBERT LEIGH BRYCE MB BS, MSc, MRCOG, FRACOG, Senior Staff Specialist in Obstetrics, Gynaecology and Perinatal Medicine and Senior Lecturer, Flinders Medical Centre, Bedford Park, South Australia 5042.

PIERRE BUEKENS MD, MPH, PhD, Research Associate of the Belgian National Research Fund, Department of Epidemiology and Social Medicine, School of Public Health, Free University of Brussels, Route de Lennik, 808 (CP 590), 1070 Brussels, Belgium.

DORIS M. CAMPBELL MD, MBChB, MRCOG, Senior Lecturer in Obstetrics and Gynaecology and Reproductive Physiology, University of Aberdeen, Aberdeen Maternity Hospital, Aberdeen AB9 2ZA, UK.

KATHARINE A. GUTHRIE BSc(Hons), MBChB, Senior Registrar, Department of Obstetrics and Gynaecology, St. James's University Hospital, Leeds LS9 7TF, UK.

MARION H. HALL MBChB, MD, FRCOG, Consultant Obstetrician/Gynaecologist (Honorary Clinical Senior Lecturer in the University of Aberdeen), Aberdeen Maternity Hospital/Aberdeen Royal Infirmary, Cornhill Road, Aberdeen AB9 2ZA, UK.

MARY HEPBURN BSc, MD, MRCGP, MRCOG, Senior Lecturer in Women's Reproductive Health, Departments of Obstetrics and Gynaecology/Social Administration, University of Glasgow, Royal Maternity Hospital, Glasgow G4 0NA, UK.

DAVID JEWELL MA, MB, BChir, MRCGP, Consultant Senior Lecturer in General Practice, Department of Epidemiology and Public Health Medicine, University of Bristol, Canynge Hall, Whiteladies Road, Bristol BS8 2PR, UK.

M. KELLY BTech(Hons), PhD, Department of Obstetrics and Gynaecology, St. James's University Hospital, Leeds LS9 7TF, UK.

R. J. LILFORD MRCOG, MRCP, PhD, Professor, Department of Obstetrics and Gynaecology, St. James's University Hospital, Leeds LS9, 7TF, UK.

M. J. A. MARESH BSc, MB, BS, MRCOG, Consultant Obstetrician, St. Mary's Hospital for Women and Children, Whitworth Park, Manchester M13 0JH, UK.

PERCY P. S. NYLANDER MD, FRCPE, FMCOG, FRCOG, Emeritus Professor of Obstetrics and Gynaecology at University of Ibadan, Ibadan and University College Hospital, Ibadan, Nigeria.

VIRGINIE RINGA MD, MSc, Epidemiologist, INSERM (U149), Unité de Recherches Epidemiologiques sur la Mère et l'enfant, 123, bd de Port Royal, 75014 Paris, France.

KATHRYN ROSENBERG BA, PhD, Epidemiologist, Department of Community Medicine, Glasgow Royal Maternity Hospital, Rottenrow, Glasgow G4 0NA, UK.

PETER B. TERRY MBChB, MD, FRCSEd, MRCOG, Consultant Obstetrician and Gynaecologist, Aberdeen Maternity Hospital, Aberdeen AB9 2ZA, UK.

SARA TWADDLE BA(Hons), MSc, Health Economist, Department of Community Medicine, Royal Maternity Hospital, Rottenrow, Glasgow G4 0NA, UK.

Table of contents

PREVIOUS ISSUES

FORTHCOMING ISSUES

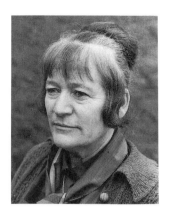

Foreword

Current practice of antenatal care in the developed world usually involves frequent surveillance of all pregnant women by different combinations of midwives, family doctors and specialist obstetricians. Because normal pregnancies last longer than complicated ones, and because healthy, well-educated urban women attend clinics assiduously, most antenatal care is actually received by women without risk factors or complications. In addition to routine clinical observations, many investigations and interventions initially developed for the benefit of women with complicated pregnancies have been applied to all women. With the exception of screening for fetal malformation, economic analysis of the benefits of antenatal care has rarely been attempted, perhaps not surprisingly in view of the lack of a clear scientific basis for much of the care provided, and the lack of knowledge of the psychological costs of screening.

A number of questions arise. Which elements of testing or care should be offered to all women and which should be offered selectively? How can risk be identified? What extra care do high risk women need? How often should women be seen? What is the appropriate ratio of in-patient to out-patient care? By whom should care be provided—do all women need to see a specialist? How can care be made more accessible for women with social problems? Would social interventions be more effective than enhanced medical input? Is Western traditional antenatal care appropriate in developing countries? How should care be recorded and audited?

I am grateful to the contributors to this book who have addressed some of these problems from different perspectives and have critically evaluated current and future practice.

MARION H. HALL

1

Prepregnancy and early pregnancy care

DAVID JEWELL

GENERAL PREGNANCY ADVICE

Pregnancy is seen by both health care professionals and pregnant women as a time when healthy behaviour can have a significant effect on outcome, and when there is therefore a need for appropriate information and advice. There is a wealth of scientific evidence on the effects of, for instance, alcohol and cigarette smoking on the developing fetus. However, simple links between knowledge, attitudes and behaviour cannot be assumed (Ajzen and Fishbein, 1980); the processes of passing on evidence to pregnant women and their families in a style that is easy to accept and assimilate and of helping them to act on it both require particular consideration. In this section the evidence for the various influences on fetal development is discussed first, and at the end the practical problems of giving advice are considered.

Nutrition

The action of starvation or severe undernutrition (including anorexia) in delaying menarche or suppressing menstruation is well known (Frisch and McArthur, 1974). The birth rate falls in times of famine, although whether this operates through the mechanism of malnutrition or psychological effects is not clear (Bongaarts, 1980). With lesser degrees of chronic maternal malnutrition the fetus is very well protected, becoming thinner but not stunted in growth. This empirical observation is supported by theoretical evolutionary considerations: man has evolved under probably very unfavourable conditions and it is doubtful if the species could have survived without being able to procreate while chronically short of food (Hytten, 1980).

However, proven benefits of supplementing the diets of undernourished women during pregnancy are meagre. In one study of women in Bogota with poor nutritional intake who had older children and of whom at least 50% were undernourished, dietary supplementation improved perinatal mortality rate slightly, and also the birthweight, but only of male fetuses (Herrera et al, 1980). Rush et al (1980) studied 770 women who were all underweight and had at least one other index of undernutrition, in the setting of a municipal hospital clinic serving a poor black community in New York. Groups were assigned to receive a high-protein supplement, a high-calorie supplement or nothing. There was no overall difference in weight gain or birthweight of infants between all three groups. Comparing the result of this study with data from babies born at times of famine led the authors to suggest that the effects of nutritional deprivation on birthweight were found only below some threshold level of intake, and that the effect was one of calorie and not protein deficiency. A similar study has recently been reported from a semi-arid area of East Java known to be nutritionally vulnerable (Kardjati et al, 1988). In this area the usual diet was very low in energy and marginal in protein; the women mostly worked as housewives and productive farm labourers. Women were randomly given high- or low-energy supplements from 26–28 weeks' gestation. Supplementation had no effect on birthweight, although there was some benefit for those most in need. The authors concluded that in areas such as this, with chronic but moderate undernutrition, supplementation should be targeted to lean seasons or to women with low prepregnant weight.

Claims have been made for a more specific effect of diet in the familiar controversy of the association between neural tube defects and vitamin intake. Laurence et al (1980) interviewed women who had previously had babies affected by neural tube defects in South Wales in order to assess their diets in the index, other and current pregnancies. All babies affected by neural tube defects in the current pregnancy were born to women with a poor diet. In two subsequent papers (Smithells et al, 1980, 1983) women who had had one or more previous babies affected by neural tube defects were invited to receive supplementary iron and multivitamin tablets at least 28 days before conception. Supplementation appeared to bring about a striking reduction in the rate of neural tube defect: rates of 0.6% and 0.9% in the supplemented group compared with 11.5% and 5.1% in the unsupplemented group for the two reports respectively. Problems of interpretation arise in this study because allocation to supplemented or unsupplemented group was not random. Those in the unsupplemented group either declined to receive treatment or were already pregnant when they were recruited to the trial. The result of this policy was that women not receiving supplements were more heavily drawn from the centres in Northern Ireland, and from social classes III, IV and V. Two recent studies have reported that multivitamin and folic acid supplementation does (Milunsky et al, 1989) and does not (Mills et al, 1989) reduce the prevalence of neural tube defects. A strictly controlled trial of periconceptual vitamin supplements is now taking place, and will report in due course. It is thought unlikely that the trial will support a simple relationship between neural tube defects and vitamin and folic acid intake, given the marked geographical variation in incidence of the condition.

Smoking

The first account of the adverse effects of smoking in pregnancy was the observation of an increase in the number of preterm deliveries to smoking women in a disadvantaged population attending maternity hospital in New

York (Simpson, 1957). Analyses of data from the British Perinatal Mortality Survey showed that smoking more than ten cigarettes daily during pregnancy was associated with a mean reduction in birthweight of 170 g and a 28% increase in late fetal and neonatal mortality. The association with birthweight was found to persist after allowing for maternal age, parity, height and social class. It was seen to disappear if the women gave up smoking by the end of the fourth month of pregnancy, which gave weight to the idea that the association was causal (Butler et al, 1972). A later analysis confirmed the association between maternal smoking and preterm delivery independent of birthweight (Fedrick and Anderson, 1976). Meyer et al (1976) examined the incidence of placental abnormalities in order to explain the increase in the perinatal mortality rate of babies born to smoking mothers: they found an increase in placenta praevia and abruptio. Naeye (1978) examined the effect of smoking in 53 518 births from 1959 to 1966. He concluded that the increase in perinatal mortality rate was due to congenital malformations, which increased at all stages of gestation. Others have failed to confirm such a teratogenic effect for smoking. Golding and Butler (1983) found an increased risk of anencephaly in babies born to smoking mothers, but the difference disappeared after correcting for social class. Similarly Hemminki et al (1983) found no effect in a multivariate analysis of smoking and oral clefts and malformations of the central nervous and musculoskeletal systems. Some effects of maternal smoking may be persistent; Butler and Goldstein (1973) found that height and reading ability at the age of seven years were reduced by maternal smoking in pregnancy, and general ability, reading ability and mathematical ability were all reduced at the age of 11 years. This persisted after allowing for maternal height, age, social class and the number of older and younger children in the household. However, the effect was small, much smaller, for instance, than that of having three or more older children in the household. After so long an interval there could also be other confounding variables operating, not least the possible influence of passive smoking by children after birth.

There is a tendency for women to smoke less during pregnancy. A survey of 5100 pregnancies in Tasmania in 1981 found that 2.7% women reported giving up smoking during pregnancy, and 36.3% smoked throughout pregnancy (Kwok et al, 1983). MacArthur and Knox (1988) studied 1235 women smoking at the outset of their pregnancy: 85 stopped in the first six weeks of pregnancy, 119 between 6 and 16 weeks, 56 after 16 weeks, 51 stopped and restarted before delivery, and 924 carried on smoking throughout. This study also showed the benefits of stopping smoking: those who stopped smoking before the end of 16 weeks' gestation had heavier babies than those smoking throughout pregnancy. Those who stopped after 16 weeks' gestation were intermediate. Madeley et al (1989) studied 3483 patients attending antenatal clinics in Nottingham at all stages of pregnancy between July and August 1986. Of these 31% smoked in pregnancy, 36% had never smoked and 26% had stopped before becoming pregnant; 7% stopped on hearing they were pregnant and 21% smoked less in pregnancy than before.

Encouraging women to stop smoking after becoming pregnant has positive effects. Sexton and Hebel (1984) identified 935 women smoking prior to the eighteenth week of gestation and randomized them to a control group or one offering counselling, support and behavioural strategies to help them stop smoking. By eight months' gestation 43% of the treatment group had given up, compared with 20% of the control group; 3.9% were smoking more than 20 cigarettes a day compared with 14% of the control group, and their babies had a mean birthweight of 3.28 kg compared with 3.19 kg in the control group. No difference was found in the head circumference, Apgar scores or length of gestation in the two groups. In this study 16% of the treatment group and 17% of the control group had given up smoking before randomization at 18 weeks' gestation.

Such advice is not always offered. McKnight and Merrett (1986) studied 500 women, of whom 191 were smokers, attending 11 centres in Belfast for antenatal care. Although 19% had discussed smoking with general practitioners, and 85% had done so with midwives, 7.8% said that they had not discussed it with any professional. In the Nottingham study (see above) only 40% claimed to have heard about smoking from their general practitioners and even fewer from the hospital doctors or nursing staff (Madeley et al, 1989).

In addition to effects on the developing fetus, possible effects of smoking on fertility have been described. In a survey of women conceiving after stopping use of different contraceptive methods, smoking more than 15 cigarettes a day was reported to cause a slight impairment in fertility (Vessey et al, 1978). Cigarette smoking has been reported to be associated with sperm abnormalities, with an increase in abnormal forms in specimens from men attending an infertility clinic (Evans et al, 1981) and a decrease in motility as well as an increase in abnormal forms in men who had already fathered children (Shaarawy and Mahmoud, 1982).

Alcohol

The dangers of consuming alcohol have been recognized since ancient times, and in 1736 infants born to alcoholic mothers were noted to look starved (Newman and Correy, 1980). The fetal alcohol syndrome found in infants born to alcoholic mothers was first described in 1973 (Jones and Smith, 1973; Jones et al, 1973). The syndrome comprises growth retardation both prenatally and postnatally, microcephaly, short palpebral fissures, maxillary hypoplasia and cardiac anomalies. Persistent mental retardation has been found at the ages of one year (Olegard et al, 1979) and seven years (Jones et al, 1974). Subsequent reports have appeared which have linked lower levels of maternal alcohol intake with spontaneous abortion (Harlap and Shiono, 1980; Kline et al, 1980), reduced average birthweight, and an increase in the proportion of babies born with a birthweight less than 2.5 kg (Lumley et al, 1985). The effect is unlikely to be a result of associated factors such as malnutrition since it affects women of all social classes, and the pattern of growth retardation is different from that found in malnourished mothers (Newman and Correy, 1980).

The effect appears at an intake of two to three drinks daily; below this there does not seem to be any adverse risk (Lumley et al, 1985). This finding was confirmed by a review of 32 870 pregnancies attending a Kaiser Permanente centre over three years. Drinking less than one drink every day was not associated with any increase in malformations. Alcohol intake at levels consumed by most women in pregnancy is not a significant cause of congenital malformation (Mills and Graubard, 1987).

Medicines

The two best known examples of major side-effects from drug therapy during pregnancy have been those of limb abnormalities in children born to mothers who had taken thalidomide during pregnancy (Lenz and Knapp, 1962) and adenocarcinoma of the vagina reported in eight females between the ages of 15 and 22 whose mothers had been given stilboestrol during pregnancy (Herbst et al, 1971). These illustrate how difficult it is to identify clearly the side-effects of drugs in any context, including pregnancy. In both of these instances the background incidence of the abnormality reported was extremely low, so that clusters of drug-induced cases were easily identified. Usually when drugs are suspected of being teratogenic it is on the basis of causing a small increase in the incidence of an abnormality that may be, in terms of congenital abnormalities, less rare than those above. David (1985) has pointed out that the list of possibly teratogenic drugs has now become very long. However, while many drugs can cause malformations, most do so infrequently, and drugs only account for a small fraction of all congenital abnormalities. Observational studies bear this out. In a survey of 6837 pregnancies, Jick et al (1981) found an overall rate of 1.2% affected by congenital disorders, with no increase among those who had taken drugs during pregnancy. However, it was pointed out in this study that despite the large numbers studied, only small numbers were exposed to drugs, such as phenytoin, that were already believed to be teratogenic. Kalter and Warkany (1983) in a review article concluded that most drugs used in the first trimester are not associated with teratogenesis.

Substantial numbers of women do seem to take drugs during pregnancy, although the proportion may be declining over time. Eskes et al (1985) surveyed women attending an antenatal clinic in Nijmegen in 1974–1975 and 1978–1979 and found that the number taking any sort of drug in pregnancy had decreased from 82.7 to 71.7%. In a later study from Glasgow, between 1982 and 1984, Rubin et al (1986) found a smaller proportion of drug takers. Of 2765 women who completed the study, 93.3% had taken no drug during the first trimester, and 65.2% had taken no drug at all in the whole pregnancy. The drug groups most commonly used were non-narcotic analgesics, antibacterials, antacids and antiemetics; of these only the non-narcotic analgesics were bought directly by the patients, the rest being obtained on a prescription from the doctor. (This result may owe something to the restricted range of drugs available for purchase across the counter in the United Kingdom compared with many other countries.)

Despite uncertainty over the extent of teratogenic effect for most suspected drugs, the overall conclusion is that it is simplest to advise patients to avoid therapeutic drugs as far as possible throughout pregnancy, and certainly during the first trimester. Such advice is usually both welcomed and expected by the patients. Baric and MacArthur (1977) showed that 75% of pregnant women identified as a social norm the idea that they should not take drugs in pregnancy without consulting a doctor; a further 19% thought special care should be taken. Furthermore, the women showed a high degree of consistency between the social norm and their own behaviour, with 82% showing such 'conformist' behaviour. This finding was different from the rest of the study, where similar questions were asked about smoking, diet and alcohol, and where there was a marked divergence between the social norm and the women's own behaviour. This appears to be one area where advice to pregnant women to avoid taking medicines does not conflict with their perceived view of social norms or with their own behaviour and it should therefore be easy to follow.

However, when women with chronic conditions are pregnant it may be impossible to avoid the therapeutic use of drugs. The decisions about their use follow exactly the same principles that apply to those who are not pregnant, namely necessity, efficacy, safety, acceptability and cost; the only difference is in having to consider the safety aspects of effects on the fetus and pregnancy, both of the untreated condition and of the drugs used to treat it.

The balancing of risks and benefits of treatment is a simple matter with diabetes since the treatment is intended to reproduce normal physiology; not surprisingly there are no reports of teratogenic effects of treatment with insulin. In women with epilepsy the problem is more complex, with a dilemma between controlling seizures and protecting the fetus from unwanted effects of anticonvulsant drugs.

The details of prepregnancy and early pregnancy advice for women with diabetes and epilepsy are discussed in Chapter 8. General practitioners and obstetricians seeing women in early pregnancy should review all prescribed and non-prescribed drugs and discuss whether they should be continued.

Work

When considering the effects of work on pregnancy it is important to distinguish the general effects of doing work from effects caused by work in specific industries.

General effects of work

Studies done in the 1940s and 1950s showed a reduction in the birthweight of babies born to primigravid women who had worked late in pregnancy. This finding lent support to the original explanation for the birthweight differential between different social classes, i.e. that it was caused by heavy manual work done by those in the lower social class groups (Garcia and Elbourne, 1984). Later studies have failed to confirm this finding. In an analysis of data from the 1958 British Perinatal Mortality Survey, Peters et al (1984) found that hours worked early in pregnancy might have had a small protective effect against toxaemia, after the effect of parity had been taken into account. There was no influence on the incidence of preterm delivery or on growth retardation at term. There was an increase in perinatal deaths for mothers working in certain specified industries and an increase in some congenital abnormalities for those in others (see below). The authors thought it was difficult to conclude that working in pregnancy is harmful, except for those working in certain designated industries.

Murphy et al (1984) extracted data from the Cardiff Births Survey for the 15 years from 1964 to 1979 to examine the effect of work in 20 613 married primigravid women. They found that the non-employed group had a higher proportion of preterm deliveries and low birthweight (< 2501 g) babies, and a higher perinatal mortality rate. A higher perinatal mortality rate was found in those stopping work before 30 weeks' gestation than in those stopping after 30 weeks' gestation. After exclusion of those with an adverse medical history or a history of previous abortion, the difference in the proportion of low birthweight infants vanished, but the difference in preterm deliveries remained. Also no difference in perinatal mortality rate was found between employed and non-employed women in social classes IV and V, so that in the non-employed group overall no class-dependent difference in perinatal mortality rate was observed. Non-employed women in social classes I and II with an adverse medical history were seen to be a group at particular risk. Non-employed women were more likely to be found at the extremes of reproductive age and attended for antenatal care less frequently. The findings of this study give considerable support to the concept of a 'healthy worker effect', that employment selects a group of healthy women who are already at low risk because of their health and who are, in this instance, better able to make use of available facilities. Nevertheless the protection against preterm delivery was thought to be genuinely conferred by employment and to be independent of the 'healthy worker effect'.

These findings also support those from an earlier study of French women. Saurel and Kaminski (1983) used data from a national survey of 3218 women who delivered in 1976, of whom 61% worked during their pregnancy. Preterm delivery was less common among those who worked, and the difference persisted after correcting for maternal class, education and parity. The same finding was shown in a separate study of immigrant women who tended to have physically more demanding jobs. No relationship was found between employment and mean birthweight or intrauterine growth retardation, although after correction for differences in maternal character-istics intrauterine growth retardation was found to be less frequent among employed women.

It is, however, essential to be wary when extrapolating from such figures to other cultures. Tafari et al (1980) studied the effects of work on 130 pregnant women attending clinics in Addis Ababa. Women were classified according to the nature of their work: heavy work was defined as housework with no domestic help available or work outside the home requiring physical labour, and light work was defined as housework if domestic help was present at home or sedentary work outside the home. Housework in this culture could include carrying water long distances, grinding grain and making beer. It was also found that the women in this study, as a whole, had food intakes below WHO recommendations, and tended to restrict their food intake in the last trimester deliberately in order to limit the size of their babies. Babies born to mothers involved in hard work had a mean birthweight of 3068 g, compared with 3270 g for those born to mothers involved in light work. This difference was independent of the women's prepregnancy weights.

Such studies demonstrate the care that must be taken in their interpretation. First, as stated above, the 'healthy worker effect' must be considered. Second, for most employed women their occupation constitutes only part of their work. The housework that the majority of women do may be physically demanding, and for many women more so than their paid employment. Third, paid work for women is an extremely heterogeneous entity. For some it will mean long hours of hard physical work, standing up, with a long bus ride to and from work, and only a smoke-filled canteen serving an unhealthy diet to relax in. For others it will mean a physically undemanding job in a pleasant environment that confers a sense of self-worth and a wider circle of friends. Reviewing the available evidence, Garcia and Elbourne (1984) concluded, for these reasons, that although there was no fear in general of an adverse effect of paid employment on pregnancy, it was difficult to translate this directly into helpful advice for individual women.

Specific industrial hazards

Identifying specific industrial hazards to pregnant women is a difficult epidemiological problem, shared with identifying teratogenic effects of drugs. Both require the discovery of often small increases in frequencies of already rare events, and separating them from the many confounding factors such as age, parity, class and employment. Peters et al (1984) found an increase in perinatal mortality for women working in the chemical, laundry/ dry-cleaning and hospital industries, and an increase in congenital abnormalities (especially anencephaly and spina bifida) in those working in the glass and pottery industries. This last effect was limited to those working with glazes. Tomlin (1979) surveyed anaesthetists and their families in a region of the United Kingdom, comparing those exposed to anaesthetic gases during their pregnancy with those not exposed (for instance if they had completed their families before becoming anaesthetists). He found that the overall miscarriage rate was higher among those exposed to anaesthetic gases, and the mean birthweight was reduced by 10%. The increase in risk extended to women, not themselves exposed to anaesthetic gases, whose husbands were exposed. Vessey and Nunn (1980), in a later review of the same subject, concluded that there was convincing evidence of a 40% increase in the incidence of miscarriage in exposed women. However, they did not confirm the other findings, finding no firm evidence of risk to the wives of exposed men or of an increased incidence of congenital malformations. The evidence suggested that the effect was mediated by a high concentration of nitrous oxide. Vessey and Nunn (1980) advised that female theatre nurses, anaesthetists and other hospital workers who become pregnant or wish to become pregnant should avoid working in contaminated environments. It was impossible then, and would be difficult in the future with any confidence, to conclude whether scavenging systems would be effective enough to remove the hazard. Kallen et al (1982) examined a cohort of physiotherapists in Sweden giving birth during the years 1973 to 1978, and found the perinatal mortality rate, the proportion of women delivering before 38 weeks' gestation and the proportion of babies with birthweights less than 2.5 kg all statistically no different to expected values. A small increase in perinatal death and malformation was associated with exposure to short-wave diathermy. More recently there has been some concern about the possible risks of working with video display terminals (VDTs). Blackwell and Chang (1988) pointed out that the levels of radiation from VDT screens are very low; for instance, the level of X-rays is less than natural background radiation and the level of ultraviolet radiation is the same from working at a VDT for half an hour as from two minutes' exposure to bright sunlight. The authors concluded that there was no evidence for a link between pregnancy failure and working at VDTs. Miscarriage clusters on the scale reported in some studies arise as a result of random variation.

Exercise

The effects of exercise can be seen to be a minor aspect of the effects of physical work. Evidence exists from animal experiments that vigorous exercise diverts blood away from the uterine bed. Raising the body temperature (such as might occur in a sauna) could theoretically cause a rise in blood lactate levels in the mother, which could in turn increase lactate levels in the fetus (Hytten, 1984). However, no empirical evidence exists in humans to support such concerns. Pommerance et al (1974) found the fitness of women between 35 and 37 weeks' gestation, measured on a bicycle ergometer, to have no effect on length of gestation, pregnancy complications, birthweight or head circumference. Fitness varied inversely with length of labour for multiparous patients. Hauth et al (1982) did electronic fetal monitoring before and after exercise on seven women who went jogging regularly. There was no fetal bradycardia and all traces were reactive. Fetal heart rate rose after jogging and took 22 minutes to return to the level recording before jogging. Similarly Collings et al (1983) recruited 20 women without medical problems and randomized them to a control group or an intervention group. Those in the intervention group were intended to increase their fitness by means of an individualized programme. In this study the obstetric outcomes were all unaffected, although the women did improve their aerobic capacity. There was a rise in mean fetal heart rate from 144 to 148 beats/min during exercise.

As with the effects of work on pregnancy, the conflict between the theoretical and empirical evidence can be resolved by examining the reality of 'exercise'. Animal experiments depend on comparing the effects of hard work on one group with another, already presumably exercising to a certain level. In humans the comparison is between some who lead a more or less completely sedentary existence with others who exercise, probably to a less than maximum capacity, for a limited part of some days in the week. With this in mind there can be no reason for advising against exercising in pregnancy; it may be sensible to advise against anaerobic exercise, certain sports such as scuba diving and water-skiing, and the use of saunas.

Practicalities of pre- and early pregnancy advice

The above is a review of the evidence that could provide a basis for giving advice both before and shortly after conception. Women at the time of conception and afterwards should not smoke (and neither should their partners), should limit their alcohol intake to less than two units of alcohol a day, and should avoid all unnecessary therapeutic drugs. They may continue to work and perhaps should be advised to continue working well into the pregnancy, unless they work in specified occupations that are associated with known risk to the fetus. They may continue taking whatever exercise and eating the diet they are used to. Such a programme is compatible with the simple, at times evangelical, messages which have characterized much of the health promotion practices in the United Kingdom.

Apart from immediate benefits, pregnancy is a time when women and their partners may be particularly receptive to advice about life-style, and may be especially motivated to alter their habits. It has already been pointed out that many pregnant women manage to stop smoking or cut down (MacArthur and Knox, 1988; Madeley et al, 1989). In a survey of 48 primigravid women, Eiser and Eiser (1985) found that 77% had changed their diet since becoming pregnant. The long-term effects of advice given opportunistically in pregnancy could be as important as the immediate benefits to the pregnancy itself.

However, there may be considerable disadvantages in applying such advice to all individuals indiscriminately. First the real risks of smoking and drinking alcohol are, for most women, small. For instance, the average decrease in birthweight as a result of smoking persistently, compared with those who stopped in the first few weeks of pregnancy, was 171 g (MacArthur and Knox, 1988). While this is a significant figure when applied to large populations, the significance to the individual is probably minimal. Second, the evangelical approach denies any advantage that the supposedly unhealthy behaviour may be conferring. In a study of 50 pregnant women, Graham (1976) explored the women's perspectives. Non-smoking mothers identified with the medical view and tended to see smoking as a moral issue. Those who continued to smoke either accepted the medical view and finished up feeling inadequate about their inability to give up, or rejected the scientific evidence. Most important, smoking was found to serve a useful personal function, in helping women cope with other family responsibilities and as a method of breaking up the daily routine and delineating a time for relaxation. It is not stretching credulity too far to imagine that, for some of the most vulnerable women, cigarette smoking may be having a positive effect on the pregnancy by reducing stress.

Finally there is the risk that doctors and other health professionals may become so preoccupied with their own agenda that they may fail to pay attention to the patients' concerns. Stott and Pill (1990) conducted a study of the views of 130 lower social class women in Wales. The women were in favour of their doctors counselling them on specific topics, but many qualified that opinion by stating that, for instance, matters should be raised only if the advice was relevant to the problem they presented or if the patients themselves raised them, and by asserting their right to accept or reject the advice offered. As pregnancy progresses, insistent attention to a habit that women know to be unhealthy but which they have found impossible to give up may merely induce guilt. In the first account of a prepregnancy clinic, Chamberlain (1980) reported that most women referred wanted to discuss fetal and maternal problems from a previous pregnancy, or current gynaecological and medical problems. His findings emphasize the importance of addressing the patients' agenda.

The other major question in addressing the provision of prepregnancy advice is how and whether it can and should be made available without needlessly medicalizing a normal event. As discussed below, a substantial number of pregnancies are unplanned at present and for them a prepregnancy service would not be helpful. It is not clear how many of the remainder would welcome the opportunity to discuss pregnancy before they have conceived. Nor, in the current climate, would it be easy to argue for its importance given the likely costs involved.

It is unarguable that men and women should know that they may have the opportunity to discuss future pregnancy if they wish to do so, provided it can be incorporated into already existing patterns of care. If patients present themselves there is of course an opportunity to review the rubella immune status. This does seem achievable, given that many women consult their general practitioners for contraceptive advice prior to conception and bringing up the subject of future pregnancy at a consultation for contraception need not be obtrusive. The suitability of general practitioners for this role is confirmed from the finding, from a survey of 48 primigravidae, that general practitioners are seen as the most important source of information among health professionals (Eiser and Eiser, 1985).

As doctors are coming increasingly to recognize, there is much more value in a selective approach. Those at most risk, both in terms of background risk and in terms of unhealthy behaviours, are women who are younger, single and from social classes IV and V. They may be the group most in need of advice (and most difficult to reach), although good provision of health education in general and contraceptive services in particular may be the most positive approach for them. The other most important single group are those with insulin-dependent diabetes, where rigorous attention to blood sugar control at the time of conception may have a marked effect on outcome (Rowe et al, 1987). In this case they will be known to their general practitioners and there can be no excuse for not counselling them prior to conception and reviewing their diabetic control. The same argument applies to smaller groups, such as women with phenylketonuria, where high levels of phenylalanine in the mother may damage the developing brain of the fetus.

For the most part, however, giving advice both before and after conception should not become a blanket activity. It should retain a proper sense of proportion about the risks involved and should not take priority over paying attention to the patient's personal concerns.

SCREENING FOR INFECTION

For many years debates on screening have been informed by reference to Wilson's criteria, and it will be helpful to repeat some of them here. Those of particular importance are that the problem to be screened should have a recognized latent or early symptomatic stage, that the natural history of the condition should be adequately understood, that there should be acceptable treatment for the disease and that the cost of case-finding should be economically balanced in relation to civil expenditure on medical care as a whole. In addition, where infectious illness is concerned, the arguments for introducing a screening programme will be influenced by the possibility of immunization. Indeed, when immunization is available the nature of the screening programme is altered; with rubella the condition being screened for is susceptibility to infection, whereas with syphilis the condition is active infection.

Bacteriuria and urinary tract infection

Traditionally pregnant women used to be screened for covert bacteriuria. Between 2 and 7% of pregnant women were found, on screening, to have asymptomatic bacteriuria. If untreated 30% of them would develop acute pyelonephritis; eradication of silent infection was thought to prevent clinical infection (Cunningham, 1987). Recent studies have found flaws in different points of the traditional argument. Campbell-Brown et al (1987) first showed that dipslide screening alone had poor predictive value for bacteriuria verified by suprapubic or catheter specimens. Second, initial treatment of confirmed bacteriuria was successful in only 69 out of 80 cases. Most important, Campbell-Brown et al (1987) confirmed earlier findings by Chng and Hall (1982) that screening failed to prevent all cases of subsequent overt infection since many (in Chng and Hall's study a majority) clinical infections occurred in women who had not had bacteriuria on screening. Finally, only 12.7% of those with bacteriuria on screening but who were not treated subsequently developed overt infection. Foley et al (1987) reported an even lower figure of 6.7%, and concluded that 'Regrettably, this cheap and simple test, which met many of the criteria for the ideal screening test, was based on an initial false premise or the natural history of the disease has altered dramatically.' There can now be no argument in favour of comprehensive screening for bacteriuria in pregnancy. Women with a history of previous clinical infection are at increased risk of further infection in subsequent pregnancy. Screening this group may be justifiable because of their risk status but will not prevent the majority of clinical infections (Chng and Hall, 1982).

Rubella

The consequences of maternal rubella infection in pregnancy are well known. The risks to the fetus are high in the first trimester, with 80% affected when the mother is infected during the first 12 weeks of gestation, falling to 25% at the end of the second trimester, then rising towards 100% in the last month of pregnancy (Miller et al, 1982). Most women are immune at the time of pregnancy as a result of previous infection or immunization policy; in one multicentre study in 1986 overall susceptibility to rubella early in pregnancy was 2.7% in nulliparous women and 1.1% in parous women (Miller et al, 1987). However, this study felt that total immunization was not achievable. Thirty-two women with serologically confirmed rubella infections had previously been immunized or reported immune, and seven infants born to these women had features of congenital rubella infection, so it was concluded that the mother concerned had had primary rubella infection. Under these circumstances, prevention of congenital rubella will depend not on further efforts to achieve 100% immunity in the adult population, but on herd immunity and reduction of epidemics in the population as a whole by high uptake of the measles, mumps and rubella immunization in childhood. However, since the attack rate rises with increasing parity, so that two thirds of women affected by rubella in pregnancy are multiparous (Miller et al, 1982), and since it seems to be possible to reduce susceptibility of the population between the first and subsequent pregnancies, the policy of screening for immunity for rubella with immunization postpartum for the non-immune, at least in the first pregnancy, is sound. It is also self-evident that serological testing before conception is worthwhile if the opportunity arises.

Syphilis

Infection of the fetus is believed not to occur before 20 weeks' gestation, and treatment of infected mothers prevents fetal infection (Sequeira and Tobin, 1984). The natural history therefore provides a latent stage in which effective prevention is possible. However, the overall incidence of congenital syphilis is now very low and there is discussion as to whether the screening programme should be stopped. Mascola et al (1984) showed that congenital syphilis does still occur, and most of the mothers in that survey had received no antenatal care. Stray-Pedersen (1983) has attempted a cost benefit analysis of screening. The calculation was based on a comparison of the cost of screening tests, confirmatory tests and treatment with an estimate of the lifetime costs incurred by the birth of infected children. These comprised direct costs of institutional care and special education, less the cost of normal education that would otherwise have been incurred, and indirect costs of lost income due to disability or death. Assuming an incidence of maternal syphilis of 0.02%, that 60% of their fetuses would be infected, and that of those 20% would end in abortion or intrauterine death, 40% would be normal and 40% would be handicapped, the benefit/cost ratio was 3.8. A further test or tests later in pregnancy, in order to identify those contracting syphilis during the course of pregnancy, would confer fewer benefits and the ratio would be much less. As Clay (1989) has argued, the very low incidence of congenital syphilis can be seen as the result of an effective prevention programme, and therefore an argument for its continuation, rather than an argument for its discontinuation.

Toxoplasmosis

Toxoplasma is a parasite acquired from eating undercooked meat. Fetal infection can occur in the first and second trimesters. It is frequently subclinical in the fetus, but 11–13% of offspring of an affected pregnancy will develop the features of choroidoretinitis, cerebral calcification, hydrocephalus and mental subnormality (Desmonts and Couvreur, 1974). The incidence in the United Kingdom is low, with seven out of 3187 women developing toxoplasmosis during pregnancy in one study (Ruoss and Bourne, 1972). Screening for maternal toxoplasmosis, which exists in France, depends on identifying women without antibody early in pregnancy and repeating serological testing on them later in pregnancy to discover whether they have acquired the infection in the interim (Sequeira and Tobin, 1984). Treatment is unfortunately not wholly effective at eradicating the disease; Desmonts and Couvreur (1974) reported that 50% of infants of untreated mothers were uninfected compared with 76% of infants of treated mothers. In other words, treatment of infected mothers halved the number of affected infants. With this information the arguments for screening pregnant mothers are finely balanced; it could become stronger if the incidence of the disease were to increase or a more effective treatment were developed. There is the possibility that the length of the latent stage is, in this case, a disincentive to the introduction of a screening test, since the effects of the disease are so far removed in time from antenatal care.

Acquired immunodeficiency syndrome

Human immunodeficiency virus (HIV) can be transmitted from mother to infant, although it is not clear whether transmission is intrauterine, intrapartum or by breast milk (Italian Multicentre Study, 1988). About one third of infants born to infected mothers are infected (Bradbeer, 1989). In this case the incomplete knowledge of the disease's natural history together with the absence of effective treatment, quite apart from the ethical problems and acceptability of the screening test itself, rule out a screening programme at present. The issue of testing in high-risk groups is discussed in Chapter 9.

Other infections

With other causes of congenital infection there are apparently insuperable problems when trying to devise a screening programme.

  Cytomegalovirus (CMV) can cause microcephaly and other neurological problems as well as hepatosplenomegaly and thrombocytopenia. Unfortunately there is no treatment for the disease and the only action that can be offered is termination. Since infection can occur late in pregnancy or postnatally, and since only approximately 15% of maternal infections result in disease in infants, termination is not a serious possibility (Hanshaw et al, 1985). This view would be changed by the existence of a safe and effective vaccine.

Listeria monocytogenes can cause second trimester abortion, or pneumonia and meningitis if contracted late in pregnancy. It is believed to affect one in 20 000 births (Spencer, 1987). The problem is that the features of the maternal illness are non-specific, including influenza-like illness, sore throat, diarrhoea and abdominal pain, and the length of time between the maternal illness and miscarriage is short, often as short as one or two days (Fleming et al, 1985; Khong et al, 1986).

Herpes simplex virus is transmitted during parturition from lesions on the cervix and can cause changes similar to CMV as well as encephalitis (Hanshaw et al, 1985). The consensus is that neonatal disease can be prevented if the birth is by caesarean section when the cervical lesions are active. Boehm et al (1981) has described a logical system of culturing suspected lesions for virus particles: if they are present then delivery will be by caesarean section, and if not present then delivery will be vaginally. Sequeira and Tobin (1984) have suggested that the most effective screening test would therefore be a visual examination of the cervix at the beginning of labour.

SCREENING FOR CERVICAL CANCER

Screening for cervical cancer has been practised for many years on the principle that pregnant women are a captive population of sexually active women from whom it is a simple matter to take cytological samples. The argument has been supported by reports of the rising incidence of abnormal smears in the younger age cohorts (Wolfendale et al, 1983), and by published series of pregnant women with abnormal smears (Lee et al, 1981; McDonnell et al, 1981; Hellberg et al, 1987).

However, this argument rests on a fundamental misunderstanding about the purpose of the cervical screening programme. The purpose is not to identify women with cytological abnormalities but to prevent death from invasive cervical cancer. In the United Kingdom the Department of Health has recommended examination of cervical smears every five years for women between the ages of 20 and 64. There would be an argument for taking cervical smears from pregnant women if pregnancy put them at particular risk of invasive cancer, but there is little evidence of any specific effect of pregnancy on cervical abnormalities. The death rates for cervical cancer in younger age groups, as opposed to the numbers of abnormal smears identified, have been rising since 1971, but they remain low, much lower than those in the older age groups (Peto, 1986). The widely held belief of a rapidly progressive form of invasive cervical cancer affecting younger women is probably unfounded (Silcocks and Moss, 1988), and the overall prognosis of cervical cancer for women aged 35 and under is the same as for women aged 36 and over (Smales et al, 1987).

Cervical smears during pregnancy may show cytolysis and therefore be more difficult to interpret (Coleman and Evans, 1988). Abnormal cervical smears have been shown in non-pregnant women to have an adverse psychosexual effect, although this followed the ensuing colposcopy rather than the smear itself (Campion et al, 1988). Such effects in pregnancy are likely to be at least as damaging to the woman and may deflect attention from management of the pregnancy. This problem is further exacerbated by the knowledge that, as with any screening test, when the incidence of the disease to be prevented is low (as with cervical cancer in younger women), then the incidence of false-positive results rises. Kinlen and Cuckle (1984) estimated that screening women between the ages of 20 and 24 would result in a true-positive rate of 0.18 per 1000, and a false-positive rate of 2.4 per 1000. (For this calculation the true-positive rate was defined as the rate of detection of women likely to develop invasive cancer in the following ten years.)

In conclusion, there is no evidence to support a policy of cervical screening in pregnant women. If resources were unlimited, and if policy-makers were confident that it would not divert attention from the more pressing problem of ensuring a comprehensive screening programme in older women, such a policy could be justified (Kinlen and Cuckle, 1984). However, neither of these conditions can be met now, nor are they likely to be met in the future. For women over the age of 25 it is prudent to check that they have had a cervical smear in the last five years. General practitioners should take responsibility not only for implementing the policy but also for informing their specialist obstetrician colleagues so that further wasteful examinations can be avoided. Those women over the age of 25 who have not had a smear in the last five years should be advised to have one. For reasons discussed above there is an argument for deferring it until some time after their delivery; the risks of a major adverse effect on prognosis are small and the benefits in terms of the overall management of pregnancy may be considerable. However, for some women convenience may outweigh such arguments and the decision should be left to them to make.

MANAGEMENT OF UNPLANNED OR UNWANTED PREGNANCY

Despite freely and widely available contraceptive advice, unwanted pregnancy remains a problem in the United Kingdom. In 1988, 183 800 pregnancies were terminated legally. This figure does not encompass all unwanted pregnancies. Cartwright (1976), in a study of 1736 women, found that 71% of first pregnancies were intended, with a lower figure in women under the age of 20. At the time of becoming pregnant, 63% were pleased, while 13% were 'sorry it had happened at all' throughout the pregnancy. Cartwright's figures may be misleadingly high in 1989 if more unwanted pregnancies are prevented or terminated. However, making allowances for this, and for the small numbers of legal terminations done for foreign residents or for fetal abnormality, the burden of unwanted pregnancy must still be substantial.

It is unreasonable to expect that this burden will disappear through better sex education. Luker (1975) interviewed 500 women seeking abortion in California in an attempt to identify the reasons for apparent contraceptive failure. Lack of knowledge was a factor, but in many women there was evidence of some intrapsychic conflict. Contraception carried certain costs. Its use was seen by some as unnatural, deviant behaviour. The notion of planning for intercourse was seen as cold-blooded, as attracting censure, and required women to define themselves in advance as sexually active. In contrast, pregnancy had some benefits connoting fertility and conferring independence and adult status. Such benefits were short-term and vanished as soon as the pregnancy was confirmed.

Many women will therefore set out with mixed or even hostile feelings towards their pregnancies. Doctors, particularly those of first contact, should therefore guard against assuming all pregnancies to be wanted from the outset, even if the women have already decided not to request termination. At the point when pregnancy is first discussed, it is a simple precaution to ask whether the news is welcome or not.

The legal position is determined in the United Kingdom by the Abortion Act, 1967, which came into effect in April 1968. The Act allows termination if '. . . the continuance of the pregnancy would involve risk to the life of the pregnant woman, or of injury to the physical or mental health of the pregnant woman . . . greater than if the pregnancy were terminated . . .'. It also states that '. . . in determining whether the continuance of a pregnancy would involve such risk of injury . . . account may be taken of the pregnant woman's actual or reasonably foreseeable environment.' In practice the first clause quoted above has been widely interpreted to allow abortion on request, at least in the early stages of pregnancy. It has been stated that this was not the intention of Parliament at the time, but Hindell and Simms (1971) have stated that the implications of this wording were recognized at the time the Act was passed. The moral aspects of abortion will not be discussed here, not least because of the argument that it is not a matter for specific medical expertise.

Doctors should, however, profess specific expertise concerning the consequences of abortion. Reviewing 5851 first trimester abortions in Denmark in the years 1981 to 1985, Heisterberg and Kringelbach (1987) reported a complication rate of 6.1%. Complications were haemorrhage, fever or infections requiring antibiotics. The complication rate was higher in women aged less than 25 years and in those with no previous pregnancy. The operative complication rate (e.g. perforated uterus) was very low indeed. The Joint study of the Royal College of General Practitioners and the Royal College of Obstetricians and Gynaecologists (1985) followed up 6105 women who had had abortions. Ten per cent reported some morbidity that was thought to be related to the abortion within three weeks of the operation; 2.1% had major complications (death, uterine perforation, haemorrhage and salpingitis), but this figure fell to 0.8% if women with haemorrhage not requiring transfusion were excluded. In order to determine long-term complications, a later study examined pregnancies which followed abortions in the same group, and compared them with pregnancies in controls which followed completed, but unplanned, pregnancies (Frank et al, 1985, 1987). When compared with all pregnancies, post-abortion pregnancies carried no increase in the rates of stillbirths, preterm deliveries or low birthweight. However, as might be expected, there were higher rates of complications if the group with a previous abortion were compared with the group with a previous completed pregnancy; abortion does not predict for a subsequent normal pregnancy in the way that a completed normal pregnancy does.

The Joint study of the Royal College of General Practitioners and the Royal College of Obstetricians and Gynaecologists (1985) reported psychiatric morbidity, mostly depression, in 2.4%. Ashton (1981) found that half of his sample of 64 patients had experienced regrets since the operation, but in only six were the feelings persistent. Those having abortions for fetal abnormalities detected by prenatal diagnosis may be more at risk from such problems (Donnai et al, 1981).

The evidence suggests that abortion is a safe procedure with acceptably low morbidity, particularly when carried out early on in the first trimester. The duties of doctors consulted by women with unwanted pregnancy are to provide counselling to help the women work through their confusion and ambivalence, and to reduce as far as possible the subsequent feelings of guilt and depression, both by counselling beforehand and, where appropriate, by suitable aftercare (Cheetham, 1977; Ashton, 1981). Advice concerning future contraception is, of course, part of the aftercare. Ideally it should also try to address the difficult area of whatever conflicts contributed to the unwanted pregnancy; the experience of pregnancy and abortion may in itself make women feel less ambivalent towards effective contraception.

There is a licence application currently being made for an oral preparation that will achieve a high rate of successful termination if administered early in pregnancy (Rodger and Baird, 1987). Such a development may reduce still further the physical, and possibly the psychological, consequences of abortion without incurring any drug-induced complications, and it would therefore be welcomed. The only obvious risk is that such a convenient method could put a premium on early decisions in favour of having an abortion. This would be a disadvantage for those who find it difficult to come to an early decision, particularly when others are encouraging them to have an abortion. Such a situation can occur when pressure is applied to young single women by their own families. The requirement for careful non-judgemental counselling could become even more important.

SUMMARY

There is ample evidence to support the familiar message offered to women early in pregnancy that they should stop smoking, limit their alcohol intake to less than two units daily, avoid all unnecessary drugs and eat a normal well-balanced diet. They may continue to take exercise and work (in almost all occupations) without any risk to the fetus. For doctors the challenge is to balance their wish to pass on the scientific evidence with the obligation to address the concerns and needs of their individual patients. Routine screening in early pregnancy should be continued for syphilis and rubella, but the benefits do not justify it for other infectious illness, including urinary tract infection. The arguments for screening for toxoplasmosis in pregnancy are finely balanced; if more effective treatment were available then screening might become worthwhile. Provided a full screening programme for cervical cancer is achieving reasonable coverage for the adult female population, there is no need for additional screening in pregnancy.

Unplanned and unwanted pregnancy is a substantial problem in the United Kingdom and will continue to be so. For those that request it, termination is a safe procedure with low morbidity, especially when carried out early on. Women with unplanned pregnancies are entitled to advice from their doctors in order to help them decide whether they want a termination or not.

REFERENCES

Ajzen I & Fishbein M (1980) *Understanding Attitudes and Predicting Social Behaviour*. Englewood Cliffs: Prentice-Hall.

Ashton JR (1981) The after-care of abortion patients. *Journal of the Royal College of General Practitioners* **31:** 217–222.

Baric L & MacArthur C (1977) Health norms in pregnancy. *British Journal of Preventive and Social Medicine* **31:** 30–38.

Blackwell R & Chang A (1988) Video display terminals and pregnancy. A review. *British Journal of Obstetrics and Gynaecology* **95:** 446–453.

Boehm FH, Estes W, Wright PF & Growdon JF (1981) Management of genital herpes simplex virus infections occurring during pregnancy. *American Journal of Obstetrics and Gynecology* **141:** 735–740.

Bongaarts J (1980) Does malnutrition affect fecundity? A summary of evidence. *Science* **208:** 564–569.

Bradbeer CS (1989) Mothers with HIV. Risks to baby need to be balanced against benefits of breast feeding. *British Medical Journal* **299:** 806–807.

Butler NR & Goldstein H (1973) Smoking in pregnancy and subsequent child development. *British Medical Journal* **iv:** 573–575.

Butler NR, Goldstein H & Ross EM (1972) Cigarette smoking in pregnancy: its influence on birthweight and perinatal mortality. *British Medical Journal* **ii:** 127–130.

Campbell-Brown M, McFadyen IR, Seal DV & Stephenson ML (1987) Is screening for bacteriuria worth while? *British Medical Journal* **294:** 1579–1582.

Campion MJ, Brown JR, McCance DJ et al (1988) Psychosexual trauma of an abnormal cervical smear. *British Journal of Obstetrics and Gynaecology* **95:** 175–181.

Cartwright A (1976) *How many Children?* London: Routledge & Kegan Paul.

Chamberlain G (1980) The prepregnancy clinic. *British Medical Journal* **281:** 29–30.

Cheetham J (1977) *Unwanted Pregnancy and Counselling*. London: Routledge & Kegan Paul.

Chng PK & Hall MH (1982) Antenatal prediction of urinary tract infection in pregnancy. *British Journal of Obstetrics and Gynaecology* **89:** 8–11.

Clay JC (1989) Antenatal screening for syphilis: must continue. *British Medical Journal* **299:** 409–410.

Coleman DV & Evans DMD (1988) *Biopsy, Pathology and Cytology of the Cervix*. London: Chapman & Hall.

Collings CA, Curet LB & Mullin JP (1983) Maternal and fetal responses to a maternal aerobic exercise program. *American Journal of Obstetrics and Gynecology* **145:** 702–707.

Cunningham FG (1987) Urinary tract infections complicating pregnancy. *Baillière's Clinical Obstetrics and Gynaecology* **1:** 891–908.

David TJ (1985) Drugs and environmental agents in the pathogenesis of congenital malformations. In Eskes TKAB & Finster M (eds) *Drug Therapy during Pregnancy*, pp 32–53. London: Butterworths.

Desmonts G & Couvreur J (1974) Toxoplasmosis in pregnancy and its transmission to the fetus. *Bulletin of the New York Academy of Medicine* **50:** 146–159.

Donnai P, Charles N & Harris R (1981) Attitudes of patients after 'genetic' termination of pregnancy. *British Medical Journal* **282:** 621–622.

Eiser C & Eiser JR (1985) Health education needs of primigravidae. *Child: Care, Health and Development* **11:** 53–60.

Eskes TKAB, Nijdam WS, Buys MJRM & van Rossum JM (1985) Prospective study of the use of medication during pregnancy in the Netherlands. In Eskes TKAB & Finster M (eds) *Drug Therapy during Pregnancy*, pp 1–8. London: Butterworths.

Evans HJ, Fletcher J, Torrance M & Hargreave TB (1981) Sperm abnormalities and cigarette smoking. *Lancet* **i:** 627–629.

Fedrick J & Anderson ABM (1976) Factors associated with spontaneous preterm birth. *British Journal of Obstetrics and Gynaecology* **83:** 342–350.

Fleming DW, Cochi SL, MacDonald KL et al (1985) Pasteurized milk as a vehicle of infection in an outbreak of listeriosis. *New England Journal of Medicine* **312:** 404–407.

Foley ME, Farquharson R & Stronge JM (1987) Is screening for bacteriuria worth while? *British Medical Journal* **295:** 270.

Frank PI, Kay CR, Lewis TLT & Parish S (1985) Outcome of pregnancy following induced abortion. Report from the Joint study of the Royal College of General Practitioners and the Royal College of Obstetricians and Gynaecologists. *British Journal of Obstetrics and Gynaecology* **92:** 308–316.

Frank PI, Kay CR, Scott LM, Hannaford PC & Haran D (1987) Pregnancy following induced abortion: maternal morbidity, congenital abnormalities and neonatal death. *British Journal of Obstetrics and Gynaecology* **94:** 836–842.

Frisch RE & McArthur JW (1974) Menstrual cycles: fatness as a determinant of minimum weight for height necessary for their maintenance or onset. *Science* **185:** 949–951.

Garcia J & Elbourne D (1984) Future research on work in pregnancy. In Chamberlain G (ed.) *Pregnant Women at Work*, pp 273–287. London: Royal Society of Medicine.

Golding J & Butler NR (1983) Maternal smoking and anencephaly. *British Medical Journal* **287:** 553–554.

Graham H (1976) Smoking in pregnancy: the attitudes of expectant mothers. *Social Science and Medicine* **10:** 399–405.

Hanshaw JB, Dudgeon JA & Marshall WC (1985) *Viral Diseases of the Fetus and Newborn*. Philadelphia: WB Saunders.

Harlap S & Shiono PH (1980) Alcohol, smoking, and incidence of spontaneous abortions in the first and second trimester. *Lancet* **ii:** 173–176.

Hauth JC, Gilstrap LC & Widmer K (1982) Fetal heart rate reactivity before and after maternal jogging during the third trimester. *American Journal of Obstetrics and Gynecology* **142:** 545–547.

Heisterberg L & Kringelbach M (1987) Early complications after induced first-trimester abortion. *Acta Obstetrica Gynecologica Scandinavica* **66:** 201–204.

Hellberg D, Axelsson O, Gad A & Nilsson S (1987) Conservative management of the abnormal smear during pregnancy. *Acta Obstetrica Gynecologica Scandinavica* **67:** 195–199.

Hemminki K, Mutanen P & Saloniemi I (1983) Smoking and the occurrence of congenital malformations and spontaneous abortions: multivariate analysis. *American Journal of Obstetrics and Gynecology* **145:** 61–66.

Herbst AL, Ulfelder H & Poskanzer D (1971) Adenocarcinoma of the vagina. Association of maternal stilboestrol therapy with tumour appearance in young women. *New England Journal of Medicine* **284:** 878–881.

Herrera MG, Mora JO, De Paredes B & Wagner M (1980) Maternal weight/height and the effect of food supplementation during pregnancy and lactation. In Aebi H & Whitehead R (eds) *Maternal Nutrition during Pregnancy and Lactation*, pp 252–263. Bern: Hans Huber.

Hindell K & Simms M (1971) *Abortion Law Reformed*. London: Peter Owen.

Hytten FE (1980) Nutritional aspects of human pregnancy. In Aebi H & Whitehead R (eds) *Maternal Nutrition during Pregnancy and Lactation*, pp 27–38. Bern: Hans Huber.

Hytten FE (1984) The effect of work on placental function and fetal growth. In Chamberlain G (ed.) *Pregnant Women at Work*, pp 15–25. London: Royal Society of Medicine.

Italian Multicentre Study (1988) Epidemiology, clinical features and prognostic factors of paediatric HIV infectioin. *Lancet* **ii**: 1043–1045.

Jick H, Holmes LB, Hunter JR, Madsen S & Stergachis A (1981) First trimester drug use and congenital disorders. *Journal of the American Medical Association* **246**: 343–346.

Joint study of the Royal College of General Practitioners and the Royal College of Obstetricians and Gynaecologists (1985) Induced abortion operations and their early sequelae. *Journal of the Royal College of General Practitioners* **35**: 175–180.

Jones KL & Smith DW (1973) Recognition of the fetal alcoholic syndrome in early infancy. *Lancet* **ii**: 999–1001.

Jones KL, Smith DW, Ulleland CN & Streissguth AP (1973) Pattern of malformation in offspring of chronic alcoholic mothers. *Lancet* **i**: 1267–1271.

Jones KL, Smith DW, Streissguth AP & Myrianthopoulos NC (1974) Outcome in offspring of chronic alcoholic women. *Lancet* **i**: 1076–1078.

Källen B, Malmquist G & Moritz U (1982) Delivery outcome among physiotherapists in Sweden: is non-ionizing radiation a fetal hazard? *Archives of Environmental Health* **37**: 81–85.

Kalter H & Warkany J (1983) Congenital malformations. *New England Journal of Medicine* **308**: 491–497.

Kardjati S, Kusin JA & De With C (1988) Energy supplementation in the last trimester of pregnancy in East Java: I Effect on birthweight. *British Journal of Obstetrics and Gynaecology* **95**: 783–794.

Khong TY, Frappell JM, Steel HM, Stewart CM & Burke M (1986) Perinatal listeriosis. A report of six cases. *British Journal of Obstetrics and Gynaecology* **93**: 1083–1087.

Kinlen LJ & Cuckle HS (1984) Cancer of the cervix. In Wald NJ (ed.) *Antenatal and Neonatal Screening*, pp 411–419. Oxford: Oxford University Press.

Kline J, Shrout P, Stein Z, Susser M & Warburton D (1980) Drinking during pregnancy and spontaneous abortion. *Lancet* **ii**: 176–180.

Kwok P, Correy JF, Newman NM & Curran JT (1983) Smoking and alcohol consumption during pregnancy: an epidemiological study in Tasmania. *Medical Journal of Australia* **1**: 220–223.

Laurence KM, James N, Miller M & Campbell H (1980) Increased risk of recurrence of pregnancies complicated by neural tube defects in mothers receiving poor diets and possible benefit of dietary counselling. *British Medical Journal* **281**: 1592–1594.

Lee RB, Neglia W & Park RC (1981) Cervical carcinoma in pregnancy. *Obstetrics and Gynecology* **58**: 584–589.

Lenz W & Knapp K (1962) Thalidomide embryopathy. *Archives of Environmental Health* **5**: 100–105.

Luker K (1975) *Taking Chances: Abortion and the Decision not to Contracept*. Berkeley: University of California Press.

Lumley J, Correy JF, Newman NM & Curran JT (1985) Cigarette smoking, alcohol consumption and fetal outcome in Tasmania 1981–2. *Australian and New Zealand Journal of Obstetrics and Gynaecology* **25**: 33–38.

MacArthur C & Knox EG (1988) Smoking in pregnancy: effects of stopping at different stages. *British Journal of Obstetrics and Gynaecology* **95**: 551–555.

Madeley RJ, Gillies PA, Power FL & Symonds EM (1989) Nottingham mothers stop smoking project—baseline survey of smoking in pregnancy. *Community Medicine* **11**: 124–130.

Mascola L, Pelosi R, Blount JH, Binkin NJ, Alexander CE & Cates W (1984) Congenital syphilis. Why is it still occurring? *Journal of the American Medical Association* **252**: 1719–1722.

McDonnell JM, Mylotte MJ, Gustafson RC & Jordan JA (1981) Colposcopy in pregnancy. A twelve year review. *British Journal of Obstetrics and Gynaecology* **88**: 414–421.

McKnight A & Merrett JD (1986) Smoking in pregnancy—a health education problem. *Journal of the Royal College of General Practitioners* **36**: 161–164.

Meyer MB, Jonas BS & Tonascia JA (1976) Perinatal events associated with maternal smoking during pregnancy. *American Journal of Epidemiology* **103**: 466–476.

Miller CL, Miller E & Waight PA (1987) Rubella susceptibility and the continuing risk of infection in pregnancy. *British Medical Journal* **294**: 1277–1278.

Miller E, Cradock-Watson JE & Pollock TM (1982) Consequences of confirmed maternal rubella at successive stages of pregnancy. *Lancet* ii: 781–784.

Mills JL & Graubard BI (1987) Is moderate drinking associated with an increased risk for malformation? *Pediatrics* 80: 309–314.

Mills JL, Rhoads GG, Simpson JL et al (1989) The absence of a relation between the periconceptual use of vitamins and neural-tube defects. *New England Journal of Medicine* 321: 430–435.

Milunsky A, Jick H, Jick SS et al (1989) Multivitamin/folic acid supplementatio₊ in early pregnancy reduces the prevalence of neural tube defects. *Journal of the American Medical Association* 262: 2847–2852.

Murphy JF, Dauncey M, Newcombe R, Garcia J & Elbourne D (1984) Employment in pregnancy: prevalence, maternal characteristics, perinatal outcome. *Lancet* i: 1163–1166.

Naeye RL (1978) Relationship of cigarette smoking to congenital anomalies and perinatal growth. *American Journal of Pathology* 90: 289–294.

Newman NM & Correy JF (1980) Effects of alcohol in pregnancy. *Medical Journal of Australia* 2: 5–10.

Olegård R, Sabel K-G, Aronsson M et al (1979) Effects on the child of alcohol during pregnancy. *Acta Paediatrica Scandinavica Supplement* 275: 112–121.

Peters TJ, Adelstein P, Golding J & Butler NR (1984) The effects of work in pregnancy: short- and long-term associations. In Chamberlain G (ed.) *Pregnant Women at Work*, pp 87–104. London: Royal Society of Medicine.

Peto R (1986) Geographic patterns and trends. In Peto R & Zur Hausen H (eds) *Viral Etiology of Cervical Cancer*, pp 3–16. New York: Cold Spring Harbor Laboratory.

Pommerance JJ, Gluck L & Lynch VA (1974) Physical fitness in pregnancy: its effect on pregnancy outcome. *American Journal of Obstetrics and Gynecology* 119: 867–876.

Rodger MW & Baird DT (1987) Induction of therapeutic abortion in early pregnancy with mifeprostone in combination with prostaglandin pessary. *Lancet* ii: 1415–1418.

Rowe BR, Rowbotham CJF & Barnett AH (1987) Pre-conception counselling, birth weight, and congenital abnormalities in established and gestational diabetic pregnancy. *Diabetes Research* 6: 33–35.

Rubin PC, Craig GF, Gavin K & Sumner D (1986) Prospective survey of use of therapeutic drugs, alcohol and cigarettes during pregnancy. *British Medical Journal* 292: 81–83.

Ruoss CF & Bourne L (1972) Toxoplasmosis in pregnancy. *Journal of Obstetrics and Gynaecology of the British Commonwealth* 79: 1115–1118.

Rush D, Stein Z & Susser M (1980) A randomized trial of prenatal nutritional supplementation in New York City. *Pediatrics* 65: 683–697.

Saurel MJ & Kaminski M (1983) Pregnant women at work. *Lancet* i: 475.

Sequeira PJL & Tobin JO'H (1984) Intrauterine infections: syphilis, viral diseases, toxo- plasmosis, and chlamydial infections. In Wald NJ (ed.) *Antenatal and Neonatal Screening*, pp 358–381. Oxford: Oxford University Press.

Sexton M & Hebel JR (1984) A clinical trial of change of maternal smoking and its effect on birth weight. *Journal of the American Medical Association* 251: 911–915.

Shaarawy M & Mahmoud KZ (1982) Endocrine profile and semen characteristics in male smokers. *Fertility and Sterility* 38: 255–257.

Silcocks PBS & Moss SM (1988) Rapidly progressive cervical cancer: is it a real problem? *British Journal of Obstetrics and Gynaecology* 95: 1111–1116.

Simpson WJ (1957) A preliminary report on cigarette smoking and the incidence of pre- maturity. *American Journal of Obstetrics and Gynecology* 73: 808–815.

Smales E, Perry CM, Ashby MA & Baker JW (1987) The influence of age on prognosis in carcinoma of the cervix. *British Journal of Obstetrics and Gynaecology* 94: 784–787.

Smithells RW, Sheppard S, Schorah CJ et al (1980) Possible prevention of neural-tube defects by periconceptual vitamin supplementation. *Lancet* i: 339–340.

Smithells RW, Nevin NC, Seller MJ et al (1983) Further evidence of vitamin supplementation for prevention of neural tube defect recurrences. *Lancet* i: 1027–1031.

Spencer JAD (1987) Perinatal listeriosis. *British Medical Journal* 295: 349.

Stott NCH & Pill RM (1990) 'Advise yes, dictate no'. Patients' views on health promotion in the consultation. *Family Practice* (in press).

Stray-Pedersen B (1983) Economic evaluation of maternal screening to prevent congenital syphilis. *Sexually Transmitted Diseases* 10: 167–172.

Tafari N, Naeye RL & Gobezie A (1980) Effects of maternal undernutrition and heavy physical work during pregnancy on birth weight. *British Journal of Obstetrics and Gynaecology* **87**: 222–226.

Tomlin PJ (1979) Health problems of anaesthetists and their families in the West Midlands. *British Medical Journal* **i**: 779–784.

Vessey MP & Nunn JF (1980) Occupational hazards of anaesthesia. *British Medical Journal* **281**: 696–698.

Vessey MP, Wright NH, McPherson K & Wiggins P (1978) Fertility after stopping various different methods of contraception. *British Medical Journal* **i**: 265–267.

Wolfendale MR, King S & Usherwood MMcD (1983) Abnormal cervical smears: are we in for an epidemic? *British Medical Journal* **287**: 526–528.

2

Routine testing and prophylaxis

PETER B. TERRY

The antenatal care of women during pregnancy is designed to detect conditions of relevance to both the mother and her fetus. It provides an excellent opportunity to screen for conditions that may cause problems later in pregnancy, to provide prophylaxis, and to discuss aspects of health education. The routine tests are usually undertaken early in pregnancy, but not exclusively so (Table 1), and prophylaxis is undertaken during the antenatal period or during the early postnatal period. Some tests may be used to screen the whole population while others are offered to clearly identifiable groups on the basis of epidemiological studies. Some investigations, if found positive, will inevitably lead to other non-routine tests and in some cases treatment of the mother, her fetus or the neonate. It is

Table 1. Antenatal investigations.

Routine first visit tests
  Blood group
  Rhesus typing
  Antibody screen
  Full blood count
  Urinalysis
  Hepatitis B antigen
  Mid-stream urine
  Blood pressure
  Rubella antibody screen
  Serology for syphilis
  Ultrasound scan
  Cervical smear

Routine later visit tests
  Haemoglobin at 30 weeks
  Antibody screen at 28 and 34 weeks for rhesus negative
  Antibody screen at 34 weeks for rhesus positive
  Urinalysis at each visit
  Blood pressure at each visit
  Serum α-fetoprotein at 16 weeks for neural tube defects
  Serum α-fetoprotein (+ oestriol, HCG) for Down's syndrome in those aged 32 to 40
  Ultrasound scan at 18 weeks for fetal abnormality

Selective testing
  Haemoglobin electrophoresis in many ethnic groups
  Calcium and alkaline phosphatase in many ethnic groups
  Chest X-ray in some ethnic groups

Baillière's Clinical Obstetrics and Gynaecology—
Vol. 4, No. 1, March 1990
ISBN 0–7020–1476–1

important therefore that every attempt is made to counsel the mother before undertaking any investigation so that she is fully aware of the implications of either a positive result or of refusing to undergo any given investigation.

Routine testing in a population will depend largely on the prevalence of the condition in question. This is particularly so in the fields of infectious disease and haemoglobinopathies. A further consideration, which is related to the prevalence of the condition, is the amount of resource available to the medical practitioners. It may seem extremely wasteful to test routinely for a condition with a low prevalence. Nevertheless, from both a moral and often an economic point of view, the routine testing for serious and potentially life-threatening conditions is cost-effective.

Finally, with the expansion of antenatal diagnosis in all its forms together with changing patterns of fertility and an increase in medical litigation in certain parts of the world, it is important to consider a number of conditions for which routine testing or screening has been advocated but is not generally available. The aspiration to a pregnancy which is not only planned but also perfect has been widespread in Western societies for many years. Maternal health is desirable and avoidable neonatal wastage unacceptable. The trend towards smaller families in developing communities must be supported by the appropriate high standards of obstetric care together with testing for relevant pathologies.

HAEMATOLOGICAL INVESTIGATIONS

Haemoglobin estimation

Anaemia as measured by the haemoglobin concentration is extremely common in pregnancy, with a prevalence of between 40 and 60% (Levin and Algazy, 1975; Letzky and Weatherall, 1984). However, the normal physiological changes that occur during pregnancy result in an increase in the plasma volume of approximately 40% and an increase in the red cell volume of approximately 28% (Chesley, 1972). Therefore these physiological changes will usually lead to a reduction in the haemoglobin concentration and an increase in the incidence of anaemia, if measured by the haemoglobin concentration. Logically, and because of these changes, the concept and possibly the definition of anaemia during pregnancy should be different (Lind, 1983). As a consequence of the haemodilution effect the normal haemoglobin concentration may fall to a mean of 10.4 g/dl and the haematocrit to 30% at about 32–33 weeks of pregnancy (Levin and Algazy, 1975). If lower values are found, anaemia, as defined as a haemoglobin deficiency, may be present.

In a number of pathological conditions during pregnancy higher haemoglobin levels may be found and anaemia masked because of a decrease in haemodilution (MacGillivray, 1983a). Reduced haemodilution can occur in association with fetal growth retardation (Koller et al, 1979). A haemoglobin concentration as a routine test in an uncomplicated pregnancy usually undertaken at booking and again early in the third trimester of pregnancy is of value in screening for anaemia assuming that the haemodilution effect of pregnancy is taken into account. In complicated pregnancies where the haemodilution effect may not have occurred or where the haemoglobin concentration is below 10.5 g/dl further tests will be required as part of the investigation of anaemia.

In iron-deficiency anaemia a decreased mean cell volume (MCV) will be one of the earliest detectable effects (Taylor and Lind, 1976; Letzky and Weatherall, 1984). The serum ferritin level is useful as a test of the body iron stores (Blake et al, 1981; Letzky and Weatherall, 1984; Okuyama et al, 1985). However, Taylor et al (1982) have shown that the serum ferritin level decreases during the first and second trimester of pregnancy.

In summary, it appears that haemoglobin concentration early in the first trimester is a useful screening test for anaemia, in particular iron-deficiency anaemia, and will detect women with pre-existing anaemia due to parasitic infestation with organisms such as hookworm or those who have depleted iron stores through excessive loss at menstruation. Haemoglobin estimation later in pregnancy in the early third trimester is useful in uncomplicated pregnancies as a method of picking up women whose iron status may have been low pre-pregnancy and who have developed iron-deficiency anaemia during the pregnancy. Interpretation of haemoglobin concentrations in pregnancy and in particular in those with complicated pregnancies presents problems but can be helped by examining the MCV, ferritin levels or red cell morphology.

Routine iron supplementation during pregnancy

Much debate has surrounded the routine supplementation of women with iron during pregnancy. The rationale for routine supplementation has been presumably the physiological reduction in the haemoglobin concentration that occurs. Alternatively it may have been assumed that women are either iron deficient at the start of pregnancy or unable to absorb enough iron to provide for themselves and their fetus. Hytten and Leitch (1971) attempted to add up the iron costs of a pregnancy in terms of the fetus, the placenta, blood loss and lactation and the iron savings during pregnancy as a result of amenorrhoea and found that the net cost was between 0 and 750 mg of iron. In addition, Heinrich et al (1968) have estimated the absorption of iron during pregnancy and found an increase of approximately 90% towards term. It appears that the additional iron costs of pregnancy can be adequately met by the increased absorption of iron. Therefore it would appear that there is no requirement for iron supplementation.

On the other hand, and in addition to the physiological decrease in the haemoglobin concentration, there is also a reduction in the plasma iron levels of about 35% and, as has already been mentioned, a decrease in the ferritin levels during the first two trimesters of pregnancy. Iron supplementation will reverse the reduction in the haemoglobin concentration and reduce the fall in the ferritin levels. However, while women not given iron supplementation will usually maintain their MCV at a normal non-pregnant mean of 85 fl, those given iron supplementation increased their MCV to 89 fl and in some cases showed marked macrocytosis. On the basis of this evidence there would seem to be little indication to provide routine iron supplementation for pregnant women as long as one is prepared to accept that the reduction in the haemoglobin concentration and ferritin levels is physiological. Indeed, supplementation would appear to be non-physiological and suggest a failure of women to adapt to the pregnant state. Following the general principle that all drugs should be avoided in pregnancy unless specifically indicated, supplementation may, by causing macrocytosis in some cases, be disadvantageous. A reasonable policy would be to supplement if the haemoglobin concentrations fall below 10 g/dl associated with a reduced MCV (82 fl or less). It should be borne in mind that the life span of the red cell is 120 days and that the MCV may well lag behind changes in the haemoglobin concentration.

Haemoglobinopathy

Women heterozygous for the sickle cell trait, α-thalassaemia or β-thalassaemia can be identified by undertaking haemoglobin electrophoresis at booking. The importance of identifying such an abnormality, which may give rise to a mild microcytic anaemia during pregnancy, is to attempt to identify those cases in which screening of the partner and prenatal diagnosis, if appropriate, can be offered. It is important to screen the mothers as early in the first trimester as possible so that chorionic villus sampling can be offered. Women who are heterozygous for the sickle cell trait have pregnancies that may be complicated by urinary tract infection and low birthweight (Terry, 1986). Finally, identification of these women at an early stage will prevent inappropriate treatment with iron of cases that develop mild anaemia.

The screening policy of a unit will depend entirely upon the population served. The sickle cell status of all Afro-Caribbeans should always be established at the first possible opportunity, if only because at some stage these women may require an anaesthetic and therefore risk a sickle cell crisis if appropriate steps are not taken. In some areas of Europe (e.g. Greece, Italy) the prevalence of thalassaemia is high and the screening of all women is to be recommended. In addition, a similar policy would be appropriate for low-risk geographical areas dealing with a high-risk migrant population. As a result of migration from Southeast Asia to Europe an increasing number of units will appreciate the need to undertake haemoglobin electrophoresis as a routine screening procedure on all pregnant women (Weatherall and Letzky, 1984).

Important principles are involved in the management of patients who are heterozygous for haemoglobinopathy. They should be treated as high-risk pregnancies and careful maternal and fetal monitoring undertaken. In addition, these women, although often anaemic, are very rarely iron deficient and iron supplementation should be avoided. However, they do often have a folic acid deficiency, which can be confirmed by undertaking a red cell folate estimation and treated with folic acid supplementation. It is important to characterize the haemoglobinopathy since the clinical features of the heterozygous state may vary.

Other haematological disorders

Megaloblastic anaemia due to folic acid deficiency can occur in pregnancy, usually in association with multiple pregnancy, rapidly successive pregnancies or malnutrition. Usually an adequate diet will provide sufficient folic acid for the normal pregnancy but if a deficiency is present it will usually respond to supplementation.

Of the other genetic haematological disorders, the only one which occurs commonly in some populations is the red cell enzyme defect glucose-6-phosphate dehydrogenase (G6PD) deficiency. This is the most common X-linked disorder, with a frequency of greater than 10% of males in some populations, especially in blacks from central Africa, some areas of the Mediterranean (lowland Sardinia), and some populations from Southeast Asia. The incidence in Northwest Europe is probably less than 1% of males (WHO Technical Report, 1972). There are a large number of variants which can produce different clinical pictures. Since it is sex linked, the incidence of homozygous females is low (Grech and Vicatou, 1973). The clinical importance is that in about a third of heterozygous females of the more severe variety the proportion of abnormal cells is high enough to predispose to clinically significant haemolysis. The other important clinical problem is neonatal hyperbilirubinaemia which can be severe if the neonate is exposed to infection, certain drugs or the inhalation of fava bean pollen.

Screening for G6PD deficiency is relatively simple. In general terms the condition is too mild to consider antenatal diagnosis and selective abortion, and testing of the pregnant woman or the neonate should only be undertaken if clinically indicated.

There are a number of other rare genetic haematological disorders, including haemophilia, Christmas disease, von Willebrand's disease, factor XI deficiency and platelet abnormalities. Whilst diagnosis of a family trait is important so that antenatal diagnosis can be offered, these conditions are too rare to make widespread screening a practical proposition.

Blood group typing

Haemorrhage is still one of the main causes of maternal death. Blood group typing of a woman early in pregnancy is useful if only to reduce time-consuming blood group matching if an emergency cross-match is required. However, it is important from the point of view of the neonate and the future reproductive career of the woman to assess the rhesus status together with any blood group antibodies that may be present.

Rhesus disease

Before the advent of screening and treatment of rhesus disease, approximately 9% of children born to rhesus-negative mothers were affected and about 15% of the affected neonates died. As a result of screening and treatment (prevention), rhesus haemolytic disease occurs in less than 2 in 1000 neonates and the mortality among the affected neonates is less than 2%

(Bowman, 1984). Of the three antigens (C, D and E), D is by far the most important. A rhesus-negative woman exposed to the D rhesus antigen will develop antibodies which can cross the placenta and cause haemolysis of the red cells of a rhesus-positive fetus. Prevention is achieved by avoiding exposure to the rhesus-positive antigen or, if this has occurred during pregnancy, the woman should be given an injection of anti-D to prevent sensitization. Despite a variation in the prevalence of rhesus negativity (15% of Caucasians, 7% of American blacks, 0.1% of Chinese and Japanese), the need to screen for and act where necessary on the basis of the rhesus status of a pregnant woman is undisputed. It is probable that rhesus negativity has occurred in black and Asian populations as a result of genetic mixing with Caucasians. With increased mobility it is likely that the prevalence of rhesus negativity will rise in those populations with a low current prevalence.

Screening not only enables prevention during pregnancy and after delivery by an injection of anti-D, but also demonstrates those women at risk of developing rhesus disease during the current pregnancy by identifying those rhesus-negative women with low levels of rhesus antibody. These women can subsequently be monitored during the pregnancy and action taken if it appears that the fetus is developing haemolytic anaemia.

Antenatal rhesus prophylaxis. The value of giving anti-D immunoglobulin prophylactically after the delivery of a rhesus-positive neonate to a rhesus-negative mother, or after induced or spontaneous abortion in rhesus-negative mothers, is well-established. Thornton et al (1989) have suggested giving anti-D immunoglobulin antenatally at 28 and at 34 weeks in order to decrease the number of new sensitizations which occur as a result of the undiagnosed feto-maternal transfusion. However, as pointed out by Hussey (1989), this trial compared routine antenatal prophylaxis with no prophylaxis. The problem with such a policy is that some of the rhesus-negative women will have rhesus-negative fetuses (approximately 30%) and are therefore being unnecessarily injected. It can be difficult to differentiate between passively administered antibodies and those resulting from new sensitizations in the antenatal period. This will undoubtedly lead to unnecessary alarm and maternal and fetal monitoring. In addition, antenatal prophylaxis with anti-D immunoglobulin is generally given to high-risk pregnancies (after amniocentesis, antepartum haemorrhage or external cephalic version) and the basis for the original comparison by Thornton et al (1989) is possibly invalid. Until further evidence in favour of antenatal prophylaxis for all rhesus-negative women becomes available, a more satisfactory policy is to administer anti-D immunoglobulin after events that may lead to a transfer of fetal blood into the maternal circulation.

Irregular blood group antibodies

Other blood group antibodies may arise during pregnancy, giving rise to haemolytic disease of the newborn in rhesus-positive mothers due to antigenic disparity involving one of the other rhesus blood groups or antigens of other blood groups. This alloimmunization most commonly occurs as a result of the mother having previously received a blood transfusion or as a result of a previous pregnancy. It would be possible to prevent sensitization occurring by administering an appropriate immunoglobulin in the same way as is done for rhesus-negative women, but it would be extremely costly and time-consuming to undertake such investigation and treatment in all pregnant women, as well as costly to produce the appropriate immunoglobulin. Some antibodies are incapable of causing haemolytic disease of the newborn (Lewis and P1 antibodies), while the other rhesus and non-rhesus antigens most commonly result in a mild form of haemolytic disease in the newborn. Routinely screening for these other antibodies in the antenatal period, usually at booking and at approximately 36 weeks in those women who have had previous blood transfusions, not only alerts the obstetrician to women with high levels of antibodies which may give rise to severe types of haemolytic disease but also provides identification of a population who are at an increased risk if blood transfusion is required. In addition, compatible blood can be selected in advance for the treatment of the neonate if required. The Kell blood group is a good example of another system which occasionally causes severe problems (Farr and Gray, 1988) and anti-K antibodies are found in patients who have had multiple transfusions.

One study (Solola et al, 1983) of 6000 women in Tennessee found irregular antibodies in 100 women. Of these only six were judged to be potentially haemolytic. In no case would the clinical management have been jeopardized by omitting antenatal testing and relying on the antibody testing performed during routine transfusion testing alone. On the basis of this evidence these workers suggested that the routine screening of all rhesus-positive women could not be justified on cost benefit grounds. This is an opinion that is not commonly accepted by obstetricians; Bowell et al (1986) in a large study of 70 000 serum samples in Oxford proposed that serum should be screened at booking and the traditional tests for unsensitized rhesus-negative mothers and those who have been previously transfused should be undertaken at 28 weeks and 34–36 weeks. The remaining rhesus-positive women should be tested at 34–36 weeks.

In summary, all mothers should have their blood group established early in pregnancy together with serological evaluation. Rhesus-negative women should be screened at 28 and 34 weeks, unless antibodies have been detected at the first screening when more careful surveillance would be required. In addition, women at increased risk of developing irregular blood group antibodies should be screened again during the third trimester.

BIOCHEMICAL TESTS

Urinalysis

The urine of pregnant women should be tested at each antenatal visit for the presence of protein and glucose. This is usually undertaken as a screening procedure by the semiquantitative dipstick method which, although it has a high sensitivity, has a specificity of only 70% and is complicated by intra- and inter-observer error (Shaw et al, 1983).

Urine samples that are positive for protein should be investigated by undertaking a quantitative test. MacGillivray (1983b) suggested that if on quantitative testing the excretion of protein is less than 250 mg/l, the result should not be regarded as pathological. Proteinuria may indicate a urinary tract infection or renal disease, but undoubtedly the overwhelming need for its detection in pregnancy is because of its association with pregnancy-induced hypertension and the accompanying risk to both the mother and fetus (Naeye and Friedman, 1979; MacGillivray and Campbell, 1980). Since pregnancy-induced hypertension is a disease that predominately occurs in the late second trimester and in the third trimester, it seems reasonable to increase the frequency of urinalysis as pregnancy advances, such that at the end of pregnancy the urine is tested every two weeks. Interpretation of the severity and the need to intervene in pregnancy-induced hypertension is made on the basis of both the urinalysis for proteinuria and the patient's blood pressure. While these two clinical features usually go hand-in-hand, it is important to appreciate that, especially in multiracial populations, the rise in blood pressure may be more significant than the absolute value. Also, in some fulminating cases of pregnancy-induced hypertension, proteinuria may appear before a significant blood pressure rise.

Finally, an elevation in the serum uric acid above 0.36 mmol/l before 32 weeks' gestation in patients with hypertension in pregnancy has been shown to be associated with a high perinatal mortality (Redman et al, 1976). Although possibly useful in the management of individual cases, the serum uric acid has not found widespread support as a screening test.

Gestational diabetes

The presence of glucose in the urine as detected by a semiquantitative dipstick method is common, especially in women with a lowered renal threshold and in the postprandial period. For this reason the use of such a test as a screen for gestational diabetes is best undertaken on second fasting specimens, even though this may be positive in women with a lowered renal threshold for glucose. Nevertheless, the value of undertaking urinalysis to detect the presence of glucose is to allow further investigations in an attempt to diagnose those women with impaired glucose tolerance associated with pregnancy ('gestational diabetes'). Once impaired glucose tolerance during pregnancy has been diagnosed, the management is fairly straightforward and involves rigorous carbohydrate control, with diet and often insulin, together with careful monitoring of the control and of the fetus. There is some disagreement about the need to treat mild glucose intolerance in pregnancy, but the analysis of the previous pregnancies of women who subsequently were found to have abnormal carbohydrate tolerance showed an increase in the perinatal mortality rate (Gabbe et al, 1977; Gyves et al, 1977).

Controversy in this area relates to two debates: firstly, the definition of abnormal glucose tolerance as judged by the results of the various glucose tolerance tests, and secondly, whether screening by urinalysis is sufficient to pick up those women with abnormal glucose tolerance.

Much of the debate relating to the definition of impaired glucose tolerance during pregnancy relates to the fact that the condition is more common than pre-existing diabetes during pregnancy and also to differences in the responses to the oral and the intravenous glucose challenges. These have different results which are dependent on the different methods of glucose challenge. Glucose tolerance in pregnancy in normal women is usually impaired and the cut-off point at which such an impairment is regarded as pathological is largely arbitrary. Certainly to challenge a pregnant woman with a substantial oral or intravenous glucose load is unphysiological. In addition, Fraser (1983) has documented differences in carbohydrate handling in women who eat high-fibre diets compared with those who eat low-fibre diets.

Screening for gestational diabetes. The absence of a gold standard for the glucose tolerance test has arisen because of the different doses and modes of administering the glucose load. The differences in the criteria for abnormality compound the problems associated with screening for gestational diabetes. The condition, however diagnosed, is associated with fetal and neonatal morbidity in terms of macrosomia, traumatic and operative delivery, and neonatal metabolic derangements such as hypoglycaemia. These are similar to those found in patients with pre-existing diabetes (Coustan and Carpenter, 1985). However, because of the different diagnostic criteria and the problems associated with intervention in patients with both pre-existing diabetes and gestational diabetes, the association between perinatal morbidity, mortality and gestational diabetes must be questioned.

Screening on the basis of glycosuria in pregnancy, although widespread, has a low sensitivity in the region of 60% (Lind, 1984), since not all diabetics have glycosuria all the time. Considerable observer bias occurs in the interpretation of the semiquantitative dipsticks and the specificity of the test is not high because all pregnant women may have some glucose in the urine at some stage. Similarly, the presence of glycosuria after a standard glucose load has not been shown to be a reliable test.

Sutherland et al (1979) reported on the use of the maternal and past obstetric history as a method of screening. The factors in the history included fasting glycosuria, a family history of diabetes, obesity, congenital abnormality, polyhydramnios, previous large babies, previous small babies and previous fetal and neonatal loss. They were able to show convincingly an association between an abnormal intravenous glucose tolerance test and a higher perinatal mortality rate in women in whom the intravenous tolerance test had been performed because of the presence of one or more of the aforementioned risk factors. Although such evidence would support the importance of identifying those women with abnormal glucose tolerance tests, it was difficult to quantify the increased risk associated with the abnormal glucose tolerance test over and above that which already existed because of other high-risk factors. Lind (1984) and Coustan and Carpenter

(1985) established the reliability of screening on history alone and found a sensitivity of approximately 63% and a specificity of 56%. A further factor which is often overlooked by those who would advocate screening on the basis of history is that the most significant factor that would indicate glucose tolerance testing relates to a woman's performance in a previous pregnancy and the outcome of that pregnancy; such risk factors are clearly not available to women in their first pregnancy.

The most reliable screening test has been shown to be the blood sugar level. A number of methods have been advocated including a random sample, a postprandial sample after a known interval or a postprandial sample after a standard meal (Lind, 1984; Marquette et al, 1985). These tests should be performed in the second or early third trimester and both the sensitivity and specificity have been reported to be as high as 80–90%. This is not surprising, however, since the screening method is simply a modified version of the gold standard, i.e. the glucose tolerance test. Such a screening procedure is clearly costly both in terms of finances and the organization required.

In summary, screening for gestational diabetes by urinalysis or by the estimation of the blood sugar level on a random or non-random basis is advocated by many. Others (Jarrett, 1984) would regard there to be no reason to introduce widespread screening on the basis of there being little evidence that there is any benefit associated with establishing the diagnosis.

Steroids and placental proteins

Pregnancy-specific steroids and placental proteins have been under investigation as methods of, in the first instance, diagnosing pregnancy and, thereafter, determining the well-being of the pregnancy. Although used extensively, and almost routinely, in the past as placental function tests, all have been found to lack both the sensitivity and specificity required.

Human chorionic gonadotrophin

Human chorionic gonadotrophin (HCG) is possibly the only pregnancy-related hormone that is routinely used. Its function is mainly in the diagnosis of pregnancy and for this the use of a urinary sample tested by a monoclonal antibody enzyme immunoassay technique for the qualitative determination of HCG is probably all that is required. Test kits are available which can detect HCG in the urine in concentrations as low as 50 mIU/ml and such estimations have probably replaced other, less sensitive, kit methods. A quantitative estimation of HCG may be required in some conditions (molar pregnancy, ectopic pregnancy) but is not routinely used. Although the level of HCG in the circulation is related to the length of gestation, the variability is too great for it to be of any value in establishing the duration of the pregnancy. However, a quantitative estimation of HCG has been advocated, together with the maternal age, serum α-fetoprotein and unconjugated oestriol estimation, to detect Down's syndrome early in pregnancy (Wald et al, 1988).

α-fetoprotein

In addition to a low serum α-fetoprotein being associated with Down's syndrome and a high value with an open neural tube defect, there is evidence that a high value in the absence of a neural tube defect is associated with low birthweight (Smith, 1980; Brock et al, 1982; Buckland et al, 1984). Although not diagnostic, with a low sensitivity and specificity, the test is performed routinely in many areas and a high serum α-fetoprotein should be regarded as a risk factor.

Schwangerschaftsprotein 1

Schwangerschaftsprotein 1 (SP1) has been advocated as a suitable placental protein to be measured early in pregnancy in order to establish the length of gestation as there is a fairly close relationship between the level of SP1 and the gestation (Ahmed and Klopper, 1986). However, apart from being unable to diagnose twin pregnancy and the debate concerning what is and is not an appropriate gestation gold standard (Hall, 1986), further evidence would suggest that the relationship between SP1 and the gestation is not as close as originally thought (Thomson et al, 1988).

Other placental proteins

A large number of other placental proteins have been identified, including pregnancy-associated plasma protein A (PAPP-A), pregnancy-associated plasma protein B (PAPP-B), placental protein 5 (PP5) and placental protein 10 (PP10). While interesting, there is little evidence to suggest that these placental proteins will find a routine application in the management of pregnant women in the near future.

Oestriol

For many years oestriol was used as a placental function test in the third trimester of pregnancy. The rationale for this is the involvement of the fetal liver, fetal adrenal and placenta in the synthesis of oestriol from pregnenolone. Oestriol therefore found a use in the monitoring of high-risk pregnancies and those in which a problem such as intrauterine growth retardation had been identified. It has been suggested as a screening investigation to identify otherwise undiagnosed intrauterine growth retardation (Beischer et al, 1968; Dickey et al, 1972). Any screening tests for intrauterine growth retardation must have a reasonably high sensitivity and specificity similar to any other diagnostic test. In addition, it is important that such a screening test will identify pathological pregnancies which would remain undiagnosed by other simpler means. Finally, it is necessary that those cases diagnosed only by the placental function test and not by other simpler means have clinically significant pathology. In relation to the last point, and while birthweight for gestational age is often taken as the gold standard for fetal growth, it is important to realize that there is an enormous variation in birthweight and that no account can be taken of the potential for growth in an individual fetus. A fetus with the potential to grow to an above average weight may be growth retarded and yet well within the normal range of birthweight for gestational age.

On the basis of the above requirements of a diagnostic test, the use of oestriol to screen for fetal growth retardation has not found widespread support.

Human placental lactogen

Human placental lactogen (HPL) was identified by Josimovich and MacLaren (1962) in the blood of pregnant women as a protein with lacto-genic properties and which was immunologically related to pituitary growth hormone. Spellacy et al (1975) claimed that an assay of HPL would be a useful placental function test and reduce perinatal mortality. The relation-ship between fetal growth and HPL is uncertain and indeed fetal growth has been recorded in the absence of HPL (Nielsen et al, 1979). It is probable that the level of HPL is related more to the size of the placenta than to the fetal weight. HPL is measured in either the serum or the plasma by a simple radio-immunoassay and advocates of this test as a screening test routinely performed in pregnancy suggest that it should be undertaken at approxi-mately 36 weeks, although performing it at any other time during the third trimester is probably just as effective. Letchworth and Chard (1972) in 333 unselected patients found that those with levels below 4 µg/ml after 36 weeks had a 30% risk of fetal distress and neonatal asphyxia, while Grudzinskas et al (1981) found that in 2609 unselected subjects the sensitivity was 22% and the predictive value for intrauterine growth retardation, neonatal asphyxia and perinatal death if the HPL level was below the tenth centile was 18%. England et al (1974) also found an increased risk (31.6%) of fetal distress, neonatal asphyxia and intrauterine growth retardation in 547 normal subjects with HPL levels of less than 3.5 µg/ml.

The problems with using HPL as a screening test to predict growth retardation or fetal distress are exactly the same as those that apply to oestriol estimation. It has not been shown that HPL will identify clinically significant cases that could not be identified more readily by other means. Also there is an enormous overlap in the range of HPL in relation to the birthweight, thus leading to many false-negative and false-positive results.

In addition to HPL and oestriol, other substances, including alkaline phosphatase and progesterone as well as the newer placental proteins, have been suggested as possible placental function tests. While many practitioners will find oestriol and HPL useful in the monitoring of high-risk pregnancies or those in which growth retardation has already been identified, most obstetricians have abandoned the use of such tests, relying mainly on more dynamic tests such as cardiotocography and ultrasound techniques as well as the usual clinical measurements of weight gain, blood pressure, fundal height and estimates of fetal movements.

There is even less justification for the use of placental function tests as a screening technique in an unselected population. While there is undoubtedly an association between abnormal placental function tests and abnormal pregnancies, there is no evidence that placental function tests add to the current methods of identifying those pregnancies which are at increased risk and they may even be positively disadvantageous because of the false-positive results that are obtained.

NUTRITIONAL SUPPLEMENTATION

Good nutrition studies in pregnancy are rare because of the energy input/ output calculation difficulties and the need to assess diets in terms of not only protein, fat and carbohydrates, but also trace elements and vitamins.

Carbohydrate and protein supplementation

Two studies in humans that monitored the effects of famine were those of Antonov (1947) and Smith (1947). Antonov studied the results of the siege of Leningrad and Smith the Dutch famine of 1944–1945. Both, not surprisingly, noted a reduction in birthweight as a result of famine. There was an increase in perinatal mortality during the siege of Leningrad but no increase following the Dutch famine. Campbell and MacGillivray (1975) showed that a 1200 Calorie diet in the last trimester reduced birthweight. The effect of a restricted as opposed to a severely restricted diet is less certain, but Lechtig et al (1975a,b) in a study of calorie versus protein and calorie supplementation in the situation of moderate malnutrition in Guatemala showed a reduction in the incidence of low birthweight with both regimens. Viegas et al (1982) in a selected group of 'nutritionally at-risk' Asian mothers demonstrated enhanced intrauterine growth with protein/energy supplementation in the third trimester, but an almost equal reduction in birthweight if the same supplementation was given to those not 'nutritionally at-risk'. The criteria by which mothers in this study were deemed to be at-risk must be questioned. It is probable that in moderately well nourished mothers dietary supplementation has little or no effect; Stein and Susser (1975) showed the effects on birthweight of famine over a level of 1500 Calories were negligible. Nevertheless, Ademowore et al (1972) concluded that adequate nutrition during pregnancy was a better indicator of larger infant size than total weight gain, and Rush et al (1972) suggested that nutrition during pregnancy is a determinant of birthweight.

Vitamin requirements

The use of vitamin supplementation before or around the time of conception to prevent neural tube defects is considered in Chapter 1. Hurley (1980) has shown that the administration of a diet deficient in vitamins in experimental animals produces spontaneous abortions and congenital abnormalities. The vitamin requirements of non-pregnant women have been determined either as a result of experimental studies or as a result of estimates. Such requirements are often published by nationally administered advisory bodies and are subject to variation. There is a common assumption, however, that pregnant women need to consume larger quantities of vitamins in order to support the increased metabolic rate and fetal growth. The increased vitamin intake advised for pregnant women is largely arbitrary and takes no account of maternal adaptation to pregnancy resulting in an increased level of absorption or utilization. While non-pregnant women will absorb adequate vitamin levels from a normal diet, there is no reason to suspect that a similar diet will not also provide sufficient for pregnant women and this represents a more reasonable philosophy than the one which assumes that pregnant women are likely to become deficient of vitamins as a result of a physiological process.

Vitamin supplementation

Vitamin intake during pregnancy should be sufficient to prevent any clinical signs or symptoms of vitamin deficiency. The outcome of the pregnancy should be good or, at least, if the outcome is adverse, it should not have been associated with any vitamin deficiency. There should be at the end of the pregnancy normal chemical tests of vitamin status in both the mother and the neonate. While studies on the signs and symptoms of deficiency and on pregnancy outcome are fairly straightforward, there are very few studies that determine the vitamin status of the mother at the end of pregnancy. This is mainly because the vitamin status during pregnancy has yet to be assessed. There are, however, some studies for some vitamins.

Willoughby and Jewell (1968) showed that blood levels of folic acid in the folate supplemented group were twice as high as the unsupplemented group six weeks postpartum. In this study the supplemented group received 330 μg per day. Despite this, King (1983) has estimated that the requirements during pregnancy are very similar to the recommended intake for non-pregnant women of 800 μg per day.

Vitamin D deficiency during pregnancy can result in significant neonatal problems, particularly with calcium homeostasis, dental enamel dysplasia and on rare occasions frank neonatal rickets. Vitamin D deficiency is uncommon in the white population and is much more likely to occur among immigrant populations, particularly Asians. This is probably due to a combination of cultural and dietary factors (Brooke et al, 1981a).

Brooke et al (1980) studied Asian women in pregnancy. The unsupplemented group received a placebo, while the supplemented group received 1000 units of vitamin D daily from 28 weeks. The unsupplemented group had very low levels of 25-hydroxy-vitamin D (25-OHD) associated with elevated bone alkaline phosphatase activity, suggesting some clinical osteomalacia. The unsupplemented women also gained less weight during pregnancy. In the neonates there were no cases of symptomatic hypocalcaemia in the supplemented group, but five cases in the unsupplemented group; there were no differences in the birthweight. In addition there was a suggestion that the infants of mothers who were supplemented grew better in the first year of life than the infants of unsupplemented mothers (Brooke et al, 1981b).

As a result of these studies, vitamin D deficiency in Asian immigrant populations would appear to be a significant problem sufficient enough to cause clinically recognizable symptoms in the neonate and, on occasions, in the mother. It is therefore appropriate to supplement Asian women living in countries with less sunshine with vitamin D. The recommended dose in pregnancy is 400 units per day throughout pregnancy or 1000 units per day in the last trimester.

Metz et al (1965) has shown that serum vitamin B_{12} levels, although they fall during pregnancy, usually return to normal by six weeks postpartum irrespective of whether a vitamin B_{12} supplement is given. The fall of serum vitamin B_{12} levels during pregnancy occurs even if high levels of supplementation are given. It has been suggested that an impairment of vitamin B_{12} absorption could account for this, but Brown et al (1977) showed that, in mice, vitamin B_{12} absorption is increased during pregnancy. The conclusion must be that the lowering of the serum vitamin B_{12} levels in late pregnancy does not seem to be related to any inadequacy of the vitamin and has not been shown to be associated with any pathology. There is no reason to recommend vitamin B_{12} supplements for pregnant women. The amount provided by the average diet (3–5 µg daily) is close enough to the recommended intake of 4 µg for this to be sufficient to meet the needs of pregnancy.

Vir et al (1980) have looked at the thiamine status of women in pregnancy. There does not seem to be any decline in the thiamine status during pregnancy and the recommended intake of 0.6 mg per 1000 Calories is adequately provided for in a normal diet.

In summary, there appears to be a lack of information concerning vitamin requirements during pregnancy and, in particular, there is no evidence to suggest that vitamin supplementation is required with a normal diet, apart from vitamin D supplementation in some populations.

Trace elements

There is very little information on trace element requirements during pregnancy. Buamah et al (1984) compared the maternal serum zinc concentrations in 244 normal pregnancies and 15 abnormal pregnancies and found that they were lower in those with anencephalic pregnancies but normal in those whose pregnancies that ended with spontaneous abortion. Soltan and Jenkins (1982) showed that the plasma zinc concentrations were significantly lower in 54 women giving birth to congenitally abnormal babies. Subclinical deficiency in zinc has been suggested by Aggett and Harries (1979) to be commoner than previously thought. The role of many trace elements in non-pregnant subjects is unclear and the role and the requirements for such elements in pregnancy even more uncertain. Flynn et al (1981) showed an association between alcoholism, low zinc status and congenital malformation. From this evidence there would appear to be an association between low zinc levels and congenital abnormality, but it must be stressed that at the current time this is simply an association and no causal link has been found. However, in a double-blind randomized controlled trial of zinc supplementation during pregnancy, Mahomed et al (1989) showed no benefit to the mother or her fetus.

SUMMARY

Routine testing and prophylaxis is considered in terms of haematological disorders, biochemical testing, hormonal testing, screening for gestational diabetes and nutritional deficiencies. Within these headings the place of routine supplementation of pregnant women with iron, vitamins, trace elements and an increased protein/calorie intake is discussed. Screening for haemoglobinopathies, irregular blood group antibodies and gestational diabetes is dealt with in detail. The place for routine prophylaxis with anti-D is considered. Biochemical and hormonal testing is covered with particular reference to the use of biochemical and hormonal assays as placental function tests and their use in assessing fetal well-being. In this respect the use of biochemical and hormonal tests to screen a pregnant population for intrauterine growth retardation is also discussed.

REFERENCES

Ademowore AS, Courey NG & Kime JS (1972) Relationship of maternal nutrition and weight gain to newborn birthweight. *Obstetrics and Gynecology* **39:** 460–464.
Aggett PJ & Harries JT (1979) Current status of zinc in health and disease states. *Archives of Disease in Childhood* **54:** 909–917.
Ahmed AG & Klopper A (1986) Estimation of gestational age by last menstrual period, by ultrasound and by SP1 concentration: comparison with date of delivery. *British Journal of Obstetrics and Gynaecology* **93:** 122–127.
Antonov AN (1947) Children born during the siege of Leningrad in 1942. *Journal of Pediatrics* **30:** 250–259.
Beischer NA, Bhargava VL, Brown JB & Smith MA (1968) The incidence and significance of low oestriol excretion in an obstetric population. *Journal of Obstetrics and Gynaecology of the British Commonwealth* **75:** 1024–1033.
Blake DR, Waterworth RF & Bacon PA (1981) Assessment of iron stores in inflammation by assay of serum ferritin concentrations. *British Medical Journal* **283:** 1147–1148.
Bowell PJ, Allen DL & Entwistle CC (1986) Blood group antibody screening tests during pregnancy. *British Journal of Obstetrics and Gynaecology* **93:** 1038–1043.
Bowman JN (1984) Rhesus haemolytic disease. In Wald NJ (ed.) *Antenatal and Neonatal Screening*, pp 314–344. Oxford: Oxford University Press.
Brock DJH, Barron L, Watt M, Scrimgeour JB & Keay AJ (1982) Maternal plasma alpha fetoprotein levels and low birthweight: a prospective study throughout pregnancy. *British Journal of Obstetrics and Gynaecology* **89:** 348–351.
Brooke OG, Brown IRF, Bone CDM et al (1980) Vitamin D supplements in pregnant Asian women: effects on calcium status and fetal growth. *British Medical Journal* **280:** 751–754.
Brooke OG, Brown IRF, Cleave HJW & Sood A (1981a) Observations on the vitamin D state of pregnant Asian women in London. *British Journal of Obstetrics and Gynaecology* **88:** 18–26.
Brooke OG, Butters F & Wood C (1981b) Intrauterine vitamin D nutrition and postnatal growth in Asian infants. *British Medical Journal* **283:** 1024.
Brown J, Robertson J & Gallagher N (1977) Humoral regulation of vitamin B_{12} absorption by pregnant mouse small intestine. *Gastroenterology* **72:** 881–885.
Buamah PK, Russell M, Bates G, Milford Ward A & Skillen AW (1984) Maternal zinc status: a

determination of central nervous system malformation. *British Journal of Obstetrics and Gynaecology* **91**: 788–790.

Buckland CM, Thom H & Campbell AGM (1984) Maternal serum alpha fetoprotein levels in low birthweight singleton pregnancies. *Journal of Perinatal Medicine* **12**: 127–132.

Campbell DM & MacGillivray I (1975) The effect of a low calorie diet or a thiazide diuretic on the incidence of pre-eclampsia and on birthweight. *British Journal of Obstetrics and Gynaecology* **82**: 572–577.

Chesley LC (1972) Plasma and red cell volumes during pregnancy. *American Journal of Obstetrics and Gynecology* **112**: 440–450.

Coustan DR & Carpenter MW (1985) Detection and treatment of gestational diabetes. *Clinical Obstetrics and Gynecology* **28**: 507–515.

Dickey RF, Grannis GF, Hanson FW, Schumacher A & Ma S (1972) Use of the estrogen/creatinine ratio and the 'estrogen index' for screening of normal and 'high risk' pregnancies. *American Journal of Obstetrics and Gynecology* **113**: 880–886.

England P, Lorrimer D, Fergusson JC, Moffatt AM & Kelly AM (1974) Human placental lactogen: the watchdog of fetal distress. *Lancet* **i**: 5–6.

Farr V & Gray E (1988) Pregnancy outcome in mothers who develop Kell antibodies. *Scottish Medical Journal* **4**: 300–303.

Flynn A, Miller SI, Marthier SS et al (1981) Zinc status of pregnant alcoholic women: a determinant of fetal outcome. *Lancet* **i**: 572–574.

Fraser RB (1983) High fibre diets in pregnancy. In Campbell DM & Gillmer MGD (eds) *Nutrition in Pregnancy*, pp 269–277. London: Royal College of Obstetricians and Gynaecologists.

Gabbe SG, Mestman JH, Freeman RK, Anderson GV & Lowensohn RI (1977) Management and outcome of Class A diabetes mellitus. *American Journal of Obstetrics and Gynecology* **127**: 465–469.

Grech JL & Vicatou M (1973) Glucose-6-phosphate dehydrogenase deficiency in Maltese newborn infants. *British Journal of Haematology* **25**: 261–269.

Grudzinskas JG, Gordon YB, Wadsworth J, Menabawcy M & Chard T (1981) Is placental function testing worthwhile? An update on placental lactogen. *Australian and New Zealand Journal of Obstetrics and Gynaecology* **21**: 103–105.

Gyves MT, Rodman HM, Little AB, Fanaroff AA & Merkatz IR (1977) A modern approach to management of pregnant diabetics: a two year analysis of perinatal outcomes. *American Journal of Obstetrics and Gynecology* **128**: 606–616.

Hall MH (1986) Estimation of gestational age by last menstrual period, by ultrasound and by SP1 concentration: comparison with date of delivery. *British Journal of Obstetrics and Gynaecology* **93**: 649–650.

Heinrich HC, Bartels H, Heinisch E et al (1968) Intestinale ^{59}Fe resorption und pralatenter eisenmangel wahrend der graviditat der menschen. *Klinische Wochenschrift* **46**: 199–202.

Hurley LS (1980) *Developmental Nutrition*. Englewood Cliffs, New Jersey: Prentice-Hall Inc.

Hussey R (1989) Antenatal prophylaxis with anti-D immunoglobulin. *British Medical Journal* **299**: 568.

Hytten FE & Leitch I (1971) *The Physiology of Human Pregnancy*, pp 1–43. Oxford: Blackwell.

Jarrett RJ (1984) Diabetes mellitus and gestational diabetes. In Wald NJ (ed.) *Antenatal and Neonatal Screening*, pp 382–395. Oxford: Oxford University Press.

Josimovich JB & MacLaren JA (1962) Presence in the human placenta and term serum of a highly lactogenic substance immunologically related to pituitary growth hormone. *Endocrinology* **71**: 209–220.

King JC (1983) Vitamin requirements during pregnancy. In Campbell DM & Gillmer MDG (eds) *Nutrition in Pregnancy*, pp 33–44. London: Royal College of Obstetricians and Gynaecologists.

Koller O, Sagen N, Ulstein M & Vaula D (1979) Fetal growth retardation associated with inadequate haemodilution in otherwise uncomplicated pregnancy. *Acta Obstetrica et Gynaecologica Scandinavica* **58**: 9–13.

Lechtig A, Delgado H, Lasky R et al (1975a) Maternal nutrition and fetal growth in developing countries. *American Journal of Diseases of Children* **129**: 553–556.

Lechtig A, Habicht JP, Delgado H et al (1975b) Effect of food supplementation during pregnancy on birthweight. *Pediatrics* **56**: 508–520.

Letchworth AT & Chard T (1972) Placental lactogen levels as a screening test for fetal distress and neonatal asphyxia. *Lancet* **i:** 704–706.

Letzky EA & Weatherall DJ (1984) Acquired haematological diseases. In Wald NJ (ed.) *Antenatal and Neonatal Screening*, pp 283–297. Oxford: Oxford University Press.

Levin J & Algazy KM (1975) Haematologic disorders. In Burrow GN & Ferris TF (eds) *Medical Complications during Pregnancy*, pp 689–737. Philadelphia: WB Saunders.

Lind T (1983) Iron supplementation during pregnancy. In Campbell DM & Gillmer MDG (eds) *Nutrition in Pregnancy*, pp 181–191. London: Royal College of Obstetricians and Gynaecologists.

Lind T (1984) Antenatal screening for diabetes mellitus. *British Journal of Obstetrics and Gynaecology* **91:** 833–834.

MacGillivray I (1983a) *Pre-eclampsia, the Hypertensive Disease in Pregnancy*, pp 83–84. London: WB Saunders.

MacGillivray I (1983b) *Pre-eclampsia, the Hypertensive Disease in Pregnancy*, pp 128–131. London: WB Saunders.

MacGillivray I & Campbell DM (1980) The effects of hypertension and oedema on birthweight. In Bonnar J, MacGillivray I & Symonds EM (eds) *Pregnancy Hypertension*, pp 307–311. Lancaster: MTP Press.

Mahomed K, James DK, Golding J & McCabe R (1989) Zinc supplementation during pregnancy: a double blind randomised controlled trial. *British Medical Journal* **299:** 826–830.

Marquette GP, Klein VR, Repke JT & Niebyl JR (1985) Cost-effective criteria for glucose screening. *Obstetrics and Gynecology* **66:** 181–184.

Metz J, Festenstein H & Welch P (1965) Effect of folic acid and vitamin B_{12} supplementation on tests of folate and vitamin B_{12} nutrition in pregnancy. *American Journal of Clinical Nutrition* **16:** 472–479.

Naeye RL & Friedman EA (1979) Causes of perinatal death associated with gestational hypertension and proteinuria. *American Journal of Obstetrics and Gynecology* **133:** 8–10.

Nielsen PV, Pedersen H & Kampmann EM (1979) Absence of human placental lactogen in an otherwise uneventful pregnancy. *American Journal of Obstetrics and Gynecology* **135:** 322–326.

Okuyama T, Tawada T, Furuya H & Villee CA (1985) The role of transferrin and ferritin in the fetal–maternal–placental unit. *American Journal of Obstetrics and Gynecology* **152:** 344–350.

Redman CWG, Beilin LJ, Bonnar J & Wilkinson RH (1976) Plasma urate measurements in predicting fetal death in hypertensive pregnancy. *Lancet* **i:** 1370–1373.

Rush D, Davis H & Susser M (1972) Antecedents of low birthweight in Harlem, New York City. *International Journal of Epidemiology* **1:** 375–387.

Shaw AB, Risdon P & Lewis Jackson JD (1983) Protein creatinine index and Albustix in assessment of proteinuria. *British Medical Journal* **287:** 929–932.

Smith CA (1947) Effects of maternal undernutrition upon the newborn infant in Holland (1944–1945). *Journal of Pediatrics* **31:** 229–243.

Smith ML (1980) Raised maternal serum alpha fetoprotein levels and low birthweight babies. *British Journal of Obstetrics and Gynaecology* **87:** 1099–1102.

Solola A, Sibai B & Mason JM (1983) Irregular antibodies: an assessment of routine prenatal screening. *Obstetrics and Gynecology* **61:** 25–30.

Soltan MH & Jenkins DM (1982) Maternal and fetal plasma zinc concentration and fetal abnormality. *British Journal of Obstetrics and Gynaecology* **89:** 56–58.

Spellacy WN, Buhi WC & Birk SA (1975) Effectiveness of human placental lactogen as an adjunct in decreasing perinatal deaths. *American Journal of Obstetrics and Gynecology* **121:** 835–844.

Stein Z & Susser M (1975) The Dutch famine. Parts I and II. *Pediatric Research* **9:** 70–83.

Sutherland HW, Stowers JM & Fisher PM (1979) Detection of chemical gestational diabetes. In Sutherland HW & Stowers JM (eds) *Carbohydrate Metabolism in Pregnancy and the Newborn*, pp 436–461. Berlin: Springer.

Taylor DJ & Lind T (1976) Haematological changes during normal pregnancy: iron induced macrocytosis. *British Journal of Obstetrics and Gynaecology* **83:** 760–767.

Taylor DJ, Mallen C, McDougall N & Lind T (1982) Effect of iron supplementation on serum ferritin levels during and after pregnancy. *British Journal of Obstetrics and Gynaecology* **89:** 1011–1017.

Terry PB (1986) *Perinatal mortality and birthweight in a multiracial population.* MD thesis, University of Edinburgh.

Thomson MA, Duncan RO & Cunningham P (1988) The value of serum placental lactogen and Schwangerschaftsprotein 1 to determine gestation in an antenatal population. *Human Reproduction* **3**: 463–465.

Thornton JG, Page C, Foote G et al (1989) Efficacy and long term effects of antenatal prophylaxis with anti-D immunoglobulin. *British Medical Journal* **298**: 1671–1673.

Viegas OAC, Scott PH, Cole TJ et al (1982) Dietary protein energy supplementation of pregnant Asian mothers at Sorrento, Birmingham. II. Selective during third trimester only. *British Medical Journal* **285**: 592–595.

Vir SC, Love AGH & Thompson W (1980) Vitamin B_6 status during pregnancy. *International Journal for Vitamin and Nutrition Research* **50**: 403–411.

Wald NJ, Cuckle HS, Densem JW et al (1988) Maternal serum screening for Down's syndrome in early pregnancy. *British Medical Journal* **297**: 883–887.

Weatherall DJ & Letzky EA (1984) Genetic and haematological disorders. In Wald NJ (ed.) *Antenatal and Neonatal Screening*, pp 155–191. Oxford: Oxford University Press.

WHO Technical Report Series (1972) No. 509.

Willoughby MLN & Jewell FG (1968) Folate status throughout pregnancy and in the post-partum period. *British Medical Journal* **4**: 356–360.

3

Routine or selective ultrasound scanning

GÉRARD BREART
VIRGINIE RINGA

Since its introduction in obstetrics, ultrasound examination has become an indispensable tool for antenatal care. However, one may wonder if the actual use (Blondel et al, 1989) corresponds to the scientific evidence. The main unresolved issue is its routine use in low-risk populations (Pearce, 1987). Therefore this chapter will review the scientific evidence on the value of routine scanning as opposed to scanning on specific indications.

METHODOLOGICAL CONSIDERATIONS

The evaluation of a screening procedure should have three components: diagnostic efficacy, effect on medical practice and overall effect (medical, psychosocial and economic consequences) (Cadman et al, 1984).

The estimation of the *diagnostic efficacy* is generally based on the comparison of the results of the evaluated procedure with a 'gold standard' (e.g. comparison of the diagnoses of malformations made during the pregnancy to the diagnoses made at birth) (Sackett et al, 1985). The diagnostic performance is generally expressed by four indices:

Sensitivity (S_e)—The probability that a patient with the disease will be detected

$$= \frac{\text{True positives}}{\text{Patients with the disease}}$$

Specificity (S_p)—The probability that a patient without the disease will not be detected

$$= \frac{\text{True negatives}}{\text{Patients without the disease}}$$

Positive predictive value (PPV)— The probability that a positive subject will have the disease

$$= \frac{\text{True positives}}{\text{True positives} + \text{false positives}}$$

Baillière's Clinical Obstetrics and Gynaecology—
Vol. 4, No. 1, March 1990
ISBN 0–7020–1476–1

Negative predictive value (NPV)—The probability that a negative subject will not have the disease

$$= \frac{\text{True negatives}}{\text{True negatives} + \text{false negatives}}$$

Whereas the first two indices express the intrinsic diagnostic value, the last

Table 1. Predictive values of a screening procedure ($S_e = 70\%$, $S_p = 90\%$) in two populations with different prevalences.

(a) Population A: SGA prevalence of 0.20.

		SGA		
		Yes	No	Total
IUGR	Yes	1400	800	2200
	No	600	7200	7800
	Total	2000	8000	10000

PPV = 1400/2200 = 0.64
NPV = 7200/7800 = 0.92

(b) Population B: SGA prevalence of 0.05.

		SGA		
		Yes	No	Total
IUGR	Yes	350	950	1300
	No	150	8550	8700
	Total	500	9500	10000

PPV = 350/1300 = 0.27
NPV = 8550/8700 = 0.98

SGA = small for gestational age; IUGR = intrauterine growth retardation; S_e = sensitivity; S_p = specificity; PPV = positive predictive value; NPV = negative predictive value.

Table 2. Methodology of the six randomized controlled trials.

	Wladimiroff and Laar (1980)		Bennett et al (1982)		Neilson et al (1984)	
Population	General, hospital based		General, hospital based		Low risk, hospital based	
Fetal measurements	Single measurement of chest area		Biparietal diameter		Product of crown to rump length and trunk area	
Diagnosis	Small and large for dates		Gestational age		Small for dates	
Regimens	Scan between 32 and 36 weeks	Scanning on indication	Scan at 16 weeks Results known	Results withheld	Scan between 34 and 36 weeks Results known	Results withheld
Sample size	341	364	531	531	433	444

IUGR = intrauterine growth retardation.

two are more interesting for the clinician because decisions are based on predictive values. Predictive values which depend on the intrinsic diagnostic value of the screening procedure also vary with the level of risk in the population to which the procedure is applied.

Table 1 shows the results of the same screening procedure for detection of intrauterine growth retardation (IUGR) ($S_e = 70\%$, $S_p = 90\%$) applied to two populations, with different prevalences of smallness for gestational age (20% and 5%). In the first population the positive predictive value is 0.64 and the negative predictive value is 0.92, whereas in the second population the corresponding figures are 0.27 and 0.98. This example shows the influence of the prevalence on the predictive value.

The relationship between PPV, NPV and S_e, S_p and prevalence (P) is given by the following formulas:

$$PPV = \frac{S_e P}{S_e P + (1 - S_p)(1 - P)}$$

$$NPV = \frac{S_p (1 - P)}{S_p (1 - P) + P (1 - S_e)}$$

According to these formulas, a decrease in prevalence leads to a decrease in PPV and an increase in NPV. In the example, two thirds of the positive subjects are true positive in the first population, whereas only one quarter is true positive in the second.

The influence of the prevalence on the predictive value is of particular importance when evaluating a screening procedure. Since screening generally means that the procedure is applied to low-risk groups, a low PPV must be expected. Because of the low predictive value, iatrogenic consequences of false positive diagnoses might exceed the beneficial effect of the consequences of an early diagnosis.

Evaluation of the *effect on medical practice* and of the *overall effect* should be based on comparisons of the results observed among a group exposed to

Eik-Nes et al (1984)		Bakketeig et al (1984)		Secher et al (1986)		Waldenström et al (1988)	
General, hospital based		Single fetus, hospital based		General, hospital based		General, hospital based	
Biparietal and abdominal diameters, etc.		Biparietal and abdominal diameters, etc.		Biparietal and abdominal diameters		Biparietal diameter	
Gestational age, location of placenta, number of fetuses, IUGR and malformations		Gestational age, date of delivery, location of placenta, number of fetuses, IUGR and fetal position		Small for dates		Gestational age, expected day of delivery	
Two scans at 18 and 32 weeks	Scanning on indication	Two scans at 19 and 32 weeks	Scanning on indication	Two scans at 32 and 37 weeks	Scanning on indication	One scan between 13 and 19 weeks	No scan before 19 weeks
809	819	510	499	1570	1741	2389	2412

the screening procedure with a group not exposed to the screening procedure. The most rigorous way of constituting the comparison groups is a randomized controlled trial. Therefore, to evaluate the consequences of one or several routine ultrasound examinations during pregnancy, this chapter will mainly be based on analysis of the published randomized trials (Wladimiroff and Laar, 1980; Bennett et al, 1982; Bakketeig et al, 1984; Eik-Nes et al, 1984; Neilson et al, 1984; Secher et al, 1986; Waldenström et al, 1988) whose methodology is detailed in Table 2.

All the published studies compare one or two systematic scans with scanning on indication and they concern low-risk populations. This chapter will, therefore, try to analyse the advantages and disadvantages of routine scanning as opposed to scanning on indication. It will look in turn at the diagnostic efficacy, the effects on medical practice and the overall effect.

REVIEW OF THE EVALUATIVE STUDIES

One aim of antenatal care is for the mother to give birth to a healthy neonate. This objective can be reached mainly by preventing or treating preterm birth, intrauterine growth retardation and congenital anomalies, which are the most important causes of perinatal morbidity and long-term handicaps.

Preterm birth

Policies have been proposed to prevent preterm birth (Papiernik et al, 1986; Sureau et al, 1986). They are based on early determination of risk factors (social characteristics, past medical history, clinical signs) leading to preventive measures such as social support, modification of working conditions, cerclage and betamimetics. Ultrasound examination does not have a major role in the determination of these risk factors, except for multiple pregnancy (which is discussed in Chapter 7).

Intrauterine growth retardation

No preventive policy has been proven, on a wide scale, to be effective in reducing the incidence of intrauterine growth retardation (IUGR), nor has any treatment been proven to be effective in improving the growth of a growth-retarded fetus (Chalmers et al, 1989). Therefore, current care regarding IUGR aims at early diagnosis leading to intensive care (including repeated ultrasound examinations, electronic fetal monitoring and antenatal admission). The objective of this care is to look for superimposed signs of fetal distress which might indicate elective delivery to avoid irreversible neurological damage and long-term handicap. It is generally believed that the earlier the diagnosis, the better the care will be.

Ultrasound examinations have a key role since numerous studies have shown that they increase the diagnostic performance of the clinical examination alone. This is observed in the four randomized controlled trials

(RCTs) which compare systematic scanning during the eighth month of the pregnancy with scanning on indication (Table 3). The results observed in these RCTs are in agreement with the results observed in other studies (Bouyer and Ringa, 1987) (Table 4). Table 4 shows that, even for well-trained ultrasonographers, the rates of false positives and false negatives are high. This is not surprising and is probably due to the imprecise definition of IUGR as well as to the poor performance of ultrasound examinations. However, whatever the reason, it turns out that half of the fetuses who are considered growth retarded during pregnancy will be delivered with a

Table 3. Sensitivity of the diagnostic procedure for intrauterine growth retardation in four randomized controlled trials.

Reference	Sensitivity of scanning (%)	
	Systematic	On indication
Wladimiroff and Laar (1980)	86	42
Neilson et al (1984)	94	31
Eik-Nes et al (1984)	'Severe growth retardation was recognized in the ultrasound group'	
Secher et al (1986)	62	45

Table 4. Sensitivity, specificity and predictive value for the diagnosis of intrauterine growth retardation by ultrasound examination as reported in different studies. From Bouyer and Ringa (1987).

Parameter	Reference	S_e	S_p	PPV	NPV	P
BPD	Ferrazzi et al (1986)	72–89	71–78	41–61	92–95	18.6
BPD	Warsof et al (1986)	25	93	39	87	10
BPD	Benson et al (1986)	28–88	62–94	21–44	92–98	10
BPD	Whetham et al (1976)	70	94	70	94	16
BPD	Campbell and Dewhurst (1971)	73	98	28	68	26
BPD	Lee and Chard (1983)	24.2	92.5	18.2	94.6	6.5
AC	Pearce and Campbell (1987)	83	79	39	87	14.3
AC	Ferrazzi et al (1986)	72–89	78–84	51–71	87–96	18.6
AC	Warsof et al (1986)	35	91	49	86	10
TA	Wladimiroff and Laar (1980)	82	96	70	94	16
HC	Warsof et al (1986)	48	93	61	89	10
HG	Hughey (1984)	65	—	6	—	1.7
CRL + TA	Neilson et al (1980)	94	98	39	99	8
CRL + TA	Neilson et al (1984)	94	90	28	99.7	3.8
BPD + AD	Secher et al (1986)	38.2	97	59.8	93.3	10
BPD + AD	Secher et al (1987)	31	96	45	93	6.6
BPD + AD	Persson and Kullander (1983)	60	99	65	98	4
BPD + AD	Eik-Nes (1983)	77	78	16	98	5
FL/AC	Ott (1985)	67	52	26	86	19.9
FL/AC	Benson et al (1986)	34–49	78–83	18–20	92–93	10
HC/AC	Benson et al (1986)	82	94	62	98	10

S_e = sensitivity; S_p = specificity; PPV = positive predictive value; NPV = negative predictive value; P = prevalence; BPD = biparietal diameter; AC = abdominal circumference; TA = trunk area; HC = head circumference; HG = head growth; CRL = crown–rump length; AD = abdominal diameter; FL = femoral length.

Table 5. Obstetric management in the randomized controlled trials where ultrasound examinations were done for the diagnosis of intrauterine growth retardation (IUGR).

	Neilson et al (1984)		Eik-Nes et al (1984)		Bakketeig et al (1984)		Secher et al (1986)	
	Systematic	On indication	Systematic	On indication	Systematic	On indication	Systematic	On indication
SGA babies								
Number	17	16						
Antepartum admission:								
Number (%)	4 (24)	4 (25)						
Mean days (SD)	3.1 (1.7)	1.8 (0.8)						
Number admitted for IUGR	2	3	'Severe growth retardation recognition led to more active obstetric intervention of the fetuses at risk causing more postnatal days of hospital care for dysmaturity'					
Induction number (%)	4 (24)	7 (44)						
Overall								
Number	433	444	809	819	496	478	1570	1741
Antepartum admission:								
Number (%)	43 (10)	46 (10)	184 (23) ($P<0.01$)	269 (33)	104 (21) ($P<0.005$)	58 (12)	?	?
Mean days (SD)	1.0 (0.2)	0.9 (0.2)	1.0	1.0	1.7	0.72		
Number admitted for IUGR	3	5			10	4		
Induction:								
Total number (%)	129 (31)	129 (29)			32 (6.5)	38 (7.9)	174 (11.1)	202 (11.6)
Number for IUGR (%)	12 (3)	9 (2)			—	—	—	—
Caesarean section:								
Elective number (%)	17 (4)	24 (5)			8 (1.6)	5 (1.0)		
Emergency number (%)	37 (9)	32 (7)			21 (4.2)	12 (2.5)		

SGA = small for gestational age.

birthweight adequate for gestational age (AGA). Because of this high rate of error, it is particularly important to study the consequences of the diagnosis to see if there are more disadvantages than advantages in routinely scanning pregnant women for IUGR.

To lead to improvement in the health of a growth-retarded baby, improvement in diagnostic performance should lead to modification in obstetrical behaviour, reflected in changes in antenatal intensive care, hospitalization, induction of labour, caesarean section and preterm elective delivery.

Table 5 gives the obstetric results seen in the RCTs where the results of the ultrasound examinations were revealed to the obstetricians responsible for the care of the mother and the newborn. To evaluate the impact of ultrasound scanning on medical practice, Eik-Nes et al (1984) and Bakketeig et al (1984) measured both the number and duration of antenatal hospitalizations. The former observed a significant decrease in admissions in the routinely scanned group (184 versus 269, $P<0.01$), whereas the latter made the opposite observation (104 versus 58, $P<0.005$). In the Eik-Nes et al (1984) trial, the number of hospital days was the same in both groups, while in the Bakketeig et al (1984) trial it was higher in the routinely scanned group (819 versus 145, $P<0.005$). With the same criteria, Neilson et al (1984) and Secher et al (1987) observed no difference. Thus the RCTs do not show constant patterns of modification in obstetric practices as a result of routine ultrasound. However, modifications in surveillance are noted by Hughey (1984), who showed an increase in the use of non-stress tests and ultrasound examinations among a routinely scanned group compared with a selectively scanned group. Cochlin (1984) in a non-randomized controlled study did not observe a significant difference in prenatal admissions, but did observe a significant decrease in the use of X-rays and a slight increase in the number of premature neonates in the scan group due to the small but significant number of early inductions for IUGR. According to these studies the clearest effect of routine scanning is on antenatal care (antenatal admission and the use of electronic fetal monitoring). An effect on the mode of delivery is seen in only one study (Hughey, 1984). This might be related to the number of cases studied, since to have 0.95 chance of observing a doubling of the rate of preterm elective delivery each group (routine scan or not) should include at least 7000 women.

Besides the influence of routine scanning on the content of antenatal care, the main question is the effect of the routine scan on the health of the baby. To specifically evaluate the potential benefit of an antenatal diagnosis for small for gestational age (SGA) babies, we have looked in the published studies comparing routine and selective scanning at the outcome of SGA babies. In the clinical trials, Neilson et al (1984) did not observe any significant difference in Apgar scores; however, there were only 33 SGA babies (17 in the routine group, 16 in the selective group). Eik-Nes et al (1984) reported that 'severe growth retardation was recognized in the ultrasound group . . ., and this resulted in fewer deaths due to growth retardation in the ultrasound screened group. Among the controls, four (out of eight) of the lost fetuses presented undetected growth retardation with sudden

Table 6. Comparison of perinatal outcome in 167 small for gestational age (SGA) infants from 1687 routinely scanned and 8350 selectively scanned private patients. From Hughey (1984).

	Routinely scanned	Selectively scanned
Number of SGA infants	28	139
Stillborn	2/28 (7%)	8/139 (6%)
Neonatal deaths	2/28 (7%)	5/139 (4%)
Perinatal deaths	4/28 (14%)	13/139 (9%)
Apgar score <7 at 1 min	10/26 (38%)	32/131 (24%)
Apgar score <7 at 5 min	3/26 (12%)	28/131 (6%)

intrauterine death'. Hughey (1984) in a non-randomized controlled study (Table 6) did not observe any significant difference in the outcomes of SGA babies belonging to either the routinely scanned group or to the selectively scanned group.

The published studies which evaluate the effect of routine scan on the outcome of SGA babies failed to demonstrate any beneficial effect, but because of the number of patients involved in these studies they have not ruled out such an effect. However, none of the studies show any favourable trend.

Besides the weaknesses in the methodology of the published reports (Ringa et al, 1989), the lack of significant difference between routinely or selectively scanned groups might be due to limits in effectiveness in the management of IUGR. 'Active management' leading to preterm elective delivery can only be beneficial for a small proportion of SGA babies—the most severe—which are more likely to be diagnosed in a selectively scanned group. Therefore the increase in diagnostic efficacy with routine ultrasound examination might lead mainly to an increase in the number of diagnoses of moderate IUGR, for whom the benefit of 'intensive antenatal care' can only be small, if any, and very difficult to prove.

Therefore, it seems reasonable to consider that, because of the rate of false negatives, because of the diagnostic gain concentrated on moderate cases, and because the ability to effectively manage SGA fetuses is not very good, the benefit of a routine scan for detecting IUGR is likely to be minimal. Because of the likely small benefit, it is important to take into consideration the disadvantages of ultrasound, particularly the consequences of a false-positive diagnosis, which might lead to anxiety, excessive hospitalization, excessive intervention and even to iatrogenic preterm birth which could be more harmful for the neonate than no diagnosis of IUGR. Further research is needed to improve the quality of the diagnosis of IUGR to select the fetuses who are really at risk in utero and who are more likely to benefit from early delivery. Further research is also needed on the consequences of false-positive diagnoses.

On the basis of the results presented here, a systematic ultrasound examination around 32 or 34 weeks of gestation for the detection of IUGR among pregnant women without specific pathology can only be of small benefit (if any). Because of the small benefit expected, the ratio of advantages to disadvantages might be in favour of a routine scan only if the quality of the examination is very high, but even this remains to be proven and no survey has looked at the consequences of a false-positive diagnosis.

Congenital anomalies

For congenital anomalies, there is no possibility of prevention. The proposed policies in this field aim at an antenatal diagnosis which might lead to termination of pregnancy, to early intervention for surgical correction or, more rarely, to in utero intervention. Here again the diagnosis is mainly based on ultrasonography.

Several studies reviewed by Boog and Bandaly (1987) have systematically evaluated the diagnostic efficacy of ultrasound applied to low-risk, hospital-based populations. Table 7 shows that the sensitivity varies from 33% for chromosomal anomalies to 100% for anencephaly. These figures are comparable with those published more recently by Rosendahl and Kivinen (1989) (Table 8) and Macquart-Moulin et al (1989), and are in agreement with the first results published by Campbell and Pearce (1983) on the diagnostic possibilities of ultrasound examination, but there might be an overestimation of the diagnostic efficacy of systematic ultrasound when applied to the general population. Lys et al (1989), in Belgium, showed that systematic ultrasound led to the diagnosis of malformation for 27 fetuses out of 8313 pregnancies (3‰) and Kullendof et al (1984) in Lund showed that a two-scan regimen led

Table 7. Sensitivity (S_e) of ultrasound examination for the diagnosis of the most common anomalies as reported for hospital-based populations by Boog and Bandaly (1987). The number given is the number of true positives, with the number of false positives given in parentheses.

	Schmidt et al (1985) ($n = 209$)	Hansmann and Gembruch (1984) ($n = 304$)	Hill et al (1985) ($n = 83$)	Boog and Bandaly (1987) ($n = 275$)	S_e (%)
Anencephaly	31 (0)	48 (0)	4 (0)	19 (0)	100
Spina bifida	5 (7)	23 (7)		9 (1)	79
Encephalocele			1 (0)	3 (0)	100
Hydrocephaly	12 (0)	27 (0)	2 (0)	12 (0)	100
Microcephaly	6 (1)	11 (0)	0 (1)	1 (0)	90
Holoprosencephaly	2 (1)		1 (0)	4 (0)	88
Polycystic kidneys		12 (2)	1 (1)	5 (0)	86
Renal agenesis	16 (1)	24 (6)	3 (0)	5 (1)	86
Hydronephrosis		15 (0)	2 (0)	40 (0)	100
Urethral obstruction			2 (0)	4 (0)	100
Oesophageal atresia	0 (1)		0 (2)	4 (5)	33
Intestinal atresia		5 (2)		12 (0)	89
Diaphragmatic hernia	1 (2)		1 (0)	5 (0)	78
Exomphalos		20 (2)	0 (2)	9 (0)	90
Gastroschisis		4 (0)	1 (0)	1 (1)	86
Cardiac malformations	1 (11)		3 (15)	17 (13)	42
Limb malformations	3 (0)	11 (2)	4 (6)	15 (2)	77
Chromosomal aberrations			1 (8)	8 (10)	33

Table 8. Sensitivity of ultrasound examinations. From Rosendahl and Kivinen (1989).

Anomaly	n	Antenatal diagnosis	Abnormal ultrasound
Central nervous system	17	12 (71%)	15
Gastrointestinal tract and abdominal wall	25	12 (48%)	19
Cardiovascular system	22	8 (36%)	17
Chromosomal aberrations	17	4 (23%)	12
Skeletal malformations	5	2 (40%)	3
Genitourinary tract	34	24 (71%)	25

to the diagnosis of malformation for 23 fetuses out of 6090 pregnancies (4‰). These figures are higher in hospital-based studies: 6‰ for Rosendahl and Kivinen (1989), 12‰ for Hill et al (1985) and 36‰ for Boog and Bandaly (1987). These observed differences in detection rates might reflect differences in the populations studied as well as in the type and quality of the ultrasound examinations. Besides sensitivity, evaluation of the diagnostic efficacy should also include evaluation of the specificity. Data on this are scarce. The data from Rosendahl and Kivinen (1989) and Boog and Bandaly (1987) showed a very good specificity (Table 9), whereas Lys et al (1989) in their population-based study report a 98% specificity (three false positives out of 144 non-malformed births). As for IUGR, the published data show the diagnostic power of ultrasound examination, but they also show that the diagnostic efficacy depends on the type of examination (Campbell and Pearce, 1983; Sabbagha et al, 1985; Sollie et al, 1988). The high level of sensitivity and specificity reported corresponds to stage II ultrasound examinations performed or supervised by specialists, which might not be feasible for every pregnant woman. Sollie et al (1988) have studied the diagnostic efficacy of a selective policy for ultrasound examination for the diagnosis of congenital

Table 9. Diagnostic efficacy of ultrasound examination.

(a) Results of Rosendahl and Kivinen (1989).

		Malformation		
		Yes	No	Total
Diagnosed in utero	Yes	54	5	59
	No	39	8914	8953
	Total	93	8919	9012

$S_e = 54/93 = 58\%$; $S_p = 8914/8919 = 99.9\%$.
$PPV = 91\%$; $NPV = 99.6\%$.

(b) Results of Boog and Bandaly (1987).

		Malformation		
		Yes	No	Total
Abnormal scan	Yes	229	11	240
	No	46	6359	6405
	Total	275	6370	6645

$S_e = 229/275 = 83\%$; $S_p = 6359/6370 = 99.8\%$.
$PPV = 95\%$; $NPV = 99.3\%$.
S_e = sensitivity; S_p = specificity; PPV = positive predictive value; NPV = negative predictive value.

Table 10. Diagnostic value of the selection criteria for stage II ultrasound examination (Sollie et al, 1988).

	Malformation		
	Yes	No	Total
Qualifying for stage II examination	36	145	181
Not qualifying for stage II examination	24	1854	1878
Total	60	1999	2059

$S_c = 36/40 = 60\%$; $S_p = 1854/1999 = 93\%$.
$PPV = 20\%$; $NPV = 99\%$.

Abbreviations as for Table 9.

anomalies. In their population (hospital-based), they proposed a stage II ultrasound examination only for high-risk women (IUGR, polyhydramnios, immature premature contractions, history of congenital malformations). Table 10 gives the results of their policy. The selection criteria led to the scanning of 9% of the population and this group included 60% of the malformations (36/60). The authors do not give the number of diagnoses actually made antenatally among the 36, but they report a sensitivity of 83% for stage II ultrasound examinations. Therefore their policy probably led to the antenatal diagnosis of about 50% of the malformed fetuses present in their population. This figure is lower than those reported by groups using systematic ultrasound. However, these numbers are difficult to compare because of the difference in the populations and in the settings. We did not find any paper comparing, in the same population, systematic stage II ultrasound versus ultrasound on indication for the diagnosis of malformation. Therefore it is difficult to estimate the gain due to systematic stage II ultrasound scanning. It seems reasonable to think that it will increase the sensitivity from 50 to 80%; Sollie et al (1988) mentioned that the 24 infants excluded from the procedure had markedly fewer severe congenital anomalies than the 36 who did qualify for stage II ultrasound scanning, and 11 of the 24 had minor anomalies most likely not detectable by ultrasound examination. It is not certain that the increase in diagnostic efficacy is worth the generalization of stage II ultrasound examination, as the generalization of this procedure is likely to be accompanied by a decrease in specificity and might not be feasible because of lack of personnel. Another point to be considered is the time of diagnosis in regard to positive action. In their paper Macquart-Moulin et al (1989), in a population where 80% of the population had two ultrasound examinations or more, observe that 28% of the major fetal anomalies detected in utero were diagnosed before 23 weeks of gestation but that 14% were not diagnosed by 32 weeks of gestation. These data are close to those published by Boog and Bandaly (1987) and consistent with developmental physiology.

The second stage of evaluation is the evaluation of the consequences of the diagnosis on the decisions made. Kullendorf et al (1984) reported that nine of the 23 diagnoses led to early terminations of pregnancy. Lys et al (1989) in their paper noted that, among the 27 diagnosed malformations, 14 led to termination of pregnancy (two during the first trimester, five during the second and seven during the third), three had induction and one a caesarean section because of the malformation, one ended by a spontaneous abortion, and eight had a spontaneous onset of labour. Five neonates had surgery during the neonatal period which had been scheduled antenatally. Of the 54 malformations included in Rosendahl and Kivinen's paper (1989), 23 (42.6%) survived, one of whom was severely handicapped. Spontaneous abortion occurred in the second trimester in two cases, one fetus died in utero, 11 infants died during the first week, and three died during the first month of life. In 14 cases the parents decided to terminate the pregnancy because of the obviously poor fetal prognosis. Caesarean section was performed in 20 of 35 pregnancies with mature fetuses (57%). No intrauterine interventions were performed. Eighteen infants underwent postnatal surgery, 14 of whom recovered with good results. These data clearly show that an antenatal diagnosis has an impact on antenatal care. Goujard (1989) showed in Paris that the modification in antenatal diagnosis led to a decrease in the incidence of severe congenital malformations at birth.

To estimate the overall impact of a routine scan for the diagnosis of congenital anomalies, comparative studies are necessary. Among the published RCTs, screening for fetal anomalies was only considered by Eik-Nes et al (1984), and they observed a lower number of days in special care nursery for infants with malformations born to routinely scanned mothers. However, this seemed to be mainly due to one malformed infant.

The results presented here show the diagnostic power of ultrasound examinations for congenital anomalies. Most studies involved stage II ultrasound performed by specialists and therefore probably represent an overestimation of the diagnostic efficacy of the procedure if applied to the general population. Evaluative studies comparing the overall impact of the two strategies (systematic search for congenital anomalies or scanning on indication) are needed. Taking into account the difficulty of performing an examination for the diagnosis of malformation and the lack of evaluative studies assessing the real impact of the procedure, it could be wise to have ultrasound examination for the diagnosis of malformations performed only by specialists, whatever is the mode of selection of the patients coming to see them.

Determination of gestational age

In the presence of any pathology during pregnancy, the main prognostic factor when considering elective delivery is gestational age. Therefore precise determination of gestational age is a prerequisite for any decision. In addition, in the absence of any pathology, it is of interest per se to determine if the pregnancy is overdue and if induction is indicated. Evaluating the value of the ultrasound examination in determining the gestational age is difficult since there is no obvious 'gold standard'. Therefore the evaluation has to be indirect, and two types of studies have been done.

Some studies have looked at the statistical correlation between ultrasound parameters and gestational age estimated from the date of last menstrual period (LMP). These studies generally show a good correlation (correlation coefficient = 0.9) but they cannot prove that estimation based upon ultrasound examination is better than estimation based upon LMP since there is no external reference which can say what is the truth. However, these studies show that ultrasound parameters are good predictors of duration of pregnancy. These studies have also looked at the variability of these parameters and showed that it increases with the duration of pregnancy.

Another type of study gives a good estimate of the precision of the ultrasound parameters. In these studies authors have selected a group of women whose date of the beginning of the pregnancy was precisely known (LMP known, regular cycles) and have made serial measurements of ultrasound parameters throughout pregnancy.

All these studies have been reviewed by Bouyer and Ringa (1987), who produced a table (Table 11) giving the precision of the estimation of gestational age based upon ultrasound echography. These results show that a good estimate of the gestational age can be obtained through ultrasound examination, but they also show that such an estimate might be less precise than the estimation based upon the LMP when the date of the beginning of the pregnancy is known by other means (induction of ovulation, body temperature).

Table 11. Precision of the estimation of gestational age by gestational age and ultrasound parameters. From Bouyer and Ringa (1987).

Gestational period (weeks)	Ultrasound parameter	Precision (days)
5–6	Gestational sac	± 3
7–12	Crown–rump length	± 4
13–17	Biparietal diameter (BPD)	± 9
14–22	Femoral length (FL)	± 7
18–24	Biparietal diameter (BPD) + abdominal circumference (AC)	± 8
25–41	BPD + AC + FL	± 20

To evaluate the impact of the estimation of gestational age by ultrasound, the first step is to look at the changes made as a result of using ultrasound. Several studies (Bennett et al, 1982; Persson and Kullander, 1983; Belfrage et al, 1987; Rudigoz et al, 1987) have shown that correction of the expected date of delivery according to ultrasound occurred in about one fifth of the pregnancies. To evaluate the direct impact of such adjustments it is important to know the direction of the change (postponement or advancement of the date of delivery). Table 12 shows that Belfrage et al (1987) and Bennett et al (1982) observed conflicting results. If the correction leads more often to postponement one should expect a decrease in induction for 'overdue pregnancy', whereas if it leads more often to an advancement the reverse should be observed. Table 13 shows the results observed for the rate of induction in the RCTs where determination of gestational age by ultrasound examination was part of the evaluation. Determination of gestational age was the major indication in the trials conducted by Bennett et al (1982) and by Waldenström et al (1988). The former found that the number of inductions of labour for post-term pregnancy was the same in both groups,

Table 12. Correction of date of delivery according to an early ultrasound examination.

Date of delivery (weeks)	Belfrage et al (1987)	Bennett et al (1982)
Postponed by		
1–2	10%	—
2–3	3%	—
>3	3%	—
Total	16%	3%
Advanced by		
1–2	3%	—
2–3	0.5%	—
>3	0.5%	—
Total	4%	13%

Table 13. Rates of induction observed in randomized controlled trials in which estimation of gestational age was an indication for ultrasound examination.

	Routine scanning			Scanning on indication	
Reference	n	(%)		n	(%)
Bennett et al (1982)	104	(19.6)	NS	107	(20.2)
Eik-Nes et al (1984)[*]	—	(1.9)	P<0.01	—	(7.8)
Bakketeig et al (1984)	32	(6.3)	NS	38	(7.6)
Waldenström et al (1988)	—	(5.9)	P<0.001	—	(9.1)

NS = not significant.
[*] Treatment for overdue pregnancy.

Table 14. Low Apgar scores and perinatal deaths observed in randomized controlled trials.

	Low 1 min Apgar score		Perinatal deaths	
Reference	Routine scanning (n)	Scanning on indication (n)	Routine scanning (n)	Scanning on indication (n)
Bennett et al (1982) (<4)	37	35	5	3
Neilson et al (1984) (<7)	37	40	0	1
Eik-Nes et al (1984) (<7)	41	35	3	8
Bakketeig et al (1984) (<7)	34	23	5	3
Secher et al (1986) (<7)	212	271	8	7
Waldenström et al (1988)	—	—	12	12

Table 15. Seven guidelines for deciding whether a screening programme does more good than harm (Sackett et al, 1985).

1. Has the programme's effectiveness been demonstrated in a randomized trial?

If an effectiveness trial with a positive result has not been carried out:

2. Are there efficacious treatments for the primary disorder and/or efficacious preventive manoeuvres for its sequelae?
3. Does the current burden of suffering warrant screening?
4. Is there a good screening test?
5. Does the programme reach those who could benefit from it?
6. Can the health system cope with the screening programme?
7. Will positive screenees comply with subsequent advice or interventions?

whereas the latter observed a reduction in induced labours performed for suspected post-term pregnancies in the screened group (1.7% versus 3.7%, $P<0.0001$). In the study of Eik-Nes et al (1984) the determination of gestational age was only one of the indications mentioned, and they reported a significant decrease in the frequency of 'treatment for overdue pregnancy' in the routinely scanned group (1.9% versus 7.8%, $P<0.01$).

The trend to a decrease in induction for overdue pregnancy when correction of expected date of delivery occurred has also been reported by Belfrage et al (1987) and by Cochlin (1984). To know if the reduction in induction is good for the infants, data are necessary on pregnancies not induced because of the correction in the scanned group and on the induced pregnancies in the control group. One of the criteria could be a reduction in iatrogenic preterm births. Only Eik-Nes et al (1984) addressed this question and found that four of the control infants delivered following induction for post-term pregnancy were judged premature by paediatricians, and infants spent fewer days in the special care nursery for hyperbilirubinaemia in the experimental group.

Again, the published data on estimation of gestational age by ultrasound show clearly the diagnostic value of this procedure and its direct impact on the management of the pregnancy. But the impact on the health of the neonates as well as on the quality of decision made during pregnancy is more difficult to evaluate.

Overall impact of systematic screening

In the previous sections the effects of ultrasound examination has been studied indication by indication. However, the RCTs have also studied the overall impact of systematic screening (Table 14).

To assess the consequences of ultrasound scanning on the infants' health, all the studies chose Apgar scores and perinatal deaths as indicators, and all but Eik-Nes et al (1984) studied birthweight. No difference was found in Apgar score. Only Eik-Nes et al (1984) reported a decrease in the number of perinatal deaths in the routinely scanned group (three versus eight, $P=0.1$). An increase in the mean birthweight of the babies born to screened mothers compared with those born to non-screened mothers (singletons: 3521 g versus 3479 g, $P=0.008$) was observed by Waldenström et al (1988).

CONCLUSIONS

According to the data presented here, what conclusions can be reached on the value of systematic scanning? To answer this question one can be helped by the seven guidelines proposed by Sackett et al (1985) to decide whether a screening programme does more good than harm (Table 15).

1. Has the programme's effectiveness been demonstrated in a randomized trial?
This review as well as other reviews and meta-analyses of the RCTs

(Thacker, 1985; Grant, 1986; Ringa et al, 1989) concluded that the published RCTs do not give strong evidence of the usefulness of a programme of routine scanning compared with scanning on indication. However, because of some methodological problems (number of patients included in the trials, judgement criteria), the observed results do not exclude a beneficial effect of such a programme, but this benefit cannot be very high. Because the benefit is likely to be small, the decision to implement a programme should be done only after a complete discussion of the six other guidelines considered below.

2. Are there efficacious treatments for the condition(s) screened?

It is likely that a severely growth retarded fetus will benefit from elective preterm delivery but it is not certain that it will be beneficial in the case of moderate growth retardation. For congenital anomalies we do not know exactly what the benefits of several proposed interventions are (Vintzileos et al, 1987). This guideline implies that the implementation of a screening programme should be accompanied by guidance on what to do in cases of anomaly.

3. Does the current burden of suffering warrant screening?

It is certainly important to diagnose severe anomalies during pregnancy, but the answer is not obvious for minor anomalies.

4. Is there a good screening test?

This point is particularly important because the value of the programme depends on it. This review showed that the diagnostic value of echography cannot be questioned. However, the published papers come from well-trained teams. Therefore the implementation of a routine scan programme should be preceded by specific training. This training should outline the variation in predictive values when screening in low-risk populations and the difficulties and risk of error in the diagnosis of IUGR. This training should also stress that echography is a diagnostic tool among others and when there are conflicting results between ultrasound examination and, say, date of LMP for the estimation of gestational age, ultrasound might be less precise.

The implementation of routine programmes should be accompanied by evaluative studies looking in particular at the level and the consequences of false diagnoses. Another point should be stressed concerning the timing of the scan. The diagnostic value of echography depends on the gestation when the examination is done. Therefore, in places where all pregnant women already have ultrasound examinations it is certainly better to have them done at a fixed time rather than at any time.

5. Does the programme reach those who could benefit from it?

In France, Poisson-Salomon et al (1987) have shown that the diffusion of the use of ultrasound was not based on the level of risk.

6. Can the health system cope with the screening programme?

This should be examined in two ways. Is the health system ready to accept the extra cost generated by the procedure (examination, resulting surveillance and admission, etc.)? Are there enough competent people to take charge of the examinations and their consequences?

7. Will positive screenees comply with subsequent advice or interventions?

This question can be broadened to the psychological consequences of the scanning.

The answers to the previous questions are not unequivocal and may vary from one place to another. Therefore one can expect to have different decisions in different places. This might partly explain the difference in conference consensus statements and in professional recommendations (Royal College of Obstetricians and Gynaecologists, 1984; Tournaire et al, 1987).

Because of the conflicting results published (good diagnostic value without any proof of the beneficial effect on health), no change in policy of scanning should be implemented without built-in evaluation to look at the medical, psychological and socio-economical effects of this change and particularly at the consequences of false-positive diagnoses.

Based upon the scientific evidence, according to the classification proposed by Battista and Fletcher (1988), we could say that there is poor evidence to support the recommendation of routine ultrasound examination, but recommendations may be proposed on other grounds.

REFERENCES

Bakketeig LS, Eik-Nes SH, Jacobsen G et al (1984) Randomized controlled trial of ultrasonographic screening in pregnancy. *Lancet* **ii**: 207–211.

Battista RN & Fletcher SW (1988) Making recommendations on preventive practices: methodological issues. *Journal of Preventive Medicine* **4(supplement)**: 53–67.

Belfrage P, Fernström I & Hallenberg G (1987) Routine or selective ultrasound examinations in early pregnancy. *Obstetrics and Gynecology* **69**: 747–750.

Bennett MJ, Little G, Dewhurst J & Chamberlain G (1982) Predictive value of ultrasound measurement in early pregnancy: a randomized controlled trial. *British Journal of Obstetrics and Gynaecology* **89**: 338–341.

Benson CB, Doubilet PM & Saltzman DH (1986) Intra-uterine growth retardation: predictive value of US criteria for antenatal diagnosis. *Radiology* **160**: 415–417.

Blondel B, Ringa V & Bréart G (1989) The use of ultrasound examinations, intrapartum fetal heart rate monitoring and betamimetic drugs in France. *British Journal of Obstetrics and Gynaecology* **96**: 44–51.

Boog G & Bandaly F (1987) Le diagnostic échographique des malformations foetales. In Tournaire M, Bréart G, Papiernik E & Delecour M (eds) *Apport de l'Échographie en Obstétrique*, pp 253–273. Paris: Vigot.

Bouyer J & Ringa V (1987) Age gestationnel et retard de croissance. In Tournaire M, Bréart G, Papiernik E & Delecour M (eds) *Apport de l'Échographie en Obstétrique*, pp 197–209. Paris: Vigot.

Cadman O, Chambers L, Feldman WR & Sackett DL (1984) Assessing the effectiveness of community screening programs. *Journal of the American Medical Association* **251**: 1580–1585.

Campbell S & Dewhurst CJ (1971) Diagnosis of small-for-dates fetus by serial ultrasonic cephalometry. *Lancet* **ii**: 1002–1006.

Campbell S & Pearce JM (1983) The prenatal diagnosis of fetal structural anomalies by ultrasound. *Clinics in Obstetrics and Gynaecology* **10**: 475–506.

Chalmers I, Enkin M & Keirse M (eds) (1989) *Effective Care in Pregnancy and Childbirth.* Oxford: Oxford University Press.

Cochlin DL (1984) Effects of two ultrasound scanning regimens on the management of pregnancy. *British Journal of Obstetrics and Gynaecology* **91**: 885–890.

Eik-Nes SH (1983) Prediction of fetal growth deviation by ultrasonic biometry. II. Clinical application. *Acta Obstetrica et Gynecologica Scandinavica* **62**: 117–123.

Eik-Nes SH, Okland O, Aure JC & Ulstein M (1984) Ultrasound screening in pregnancy: a randomized controlled trial. *Lancet* **i:** 1347.

Ferrazzi E, Nicoloni U, Kustermann A & Pardi G (1986) Routine obstetrics ultrasound: effectiveness of cross-sectional screening for fetal growth retardation. *Journal of Clinical Ultrasound* **14:** 17–22.

Goujard J (1989) Approche épidémiologique des malformations congénitales. In Gillet M et al (eds) *Diagnostic Anténatal des Malformations Foetales par l'Échographie.* Paris: Vigot (in press).

Grant A (1986) Controlled trials of routine ultrasound in pregnancy. *Birth* **13:** 22–28.

Hansmann M & Gembruch U (1984) Gezielte sonographische Ausschlussdiagnostik Fetaler Fehlbildungen in Risikogruppen. *Gynäkologe* **17:** 19–32.

Hill LM, Breckle R & Gehrking WC (1985) Prenatal detection of congenital malformations by ultrasonography. Mayo Clinic experience. *American Journal of Obstetrics and Gynecology* **151:** 44–50.

Hughey MJ (1984) Routine ultrasound for detection and management of the small-for-gestational-age fetus. *Obstetrics and Gynecology* **64:** 101–107.

Kullendorf CM, Larsson LT & Jörgensen C (1984) The advantage of antenatal diagnosis of intestinal and urinary tract malformations. *British Journal of Obstetrics and Gynaecology* **91:** 144–147.

Lee JN & Chard T (1983) Determination of biparietal diameter in the second trimester as a predictor of intra-uterine growth retardation. *International Journal of Gynaecology and Obstetrics* **21:** 213–215.

Lys F, De Wals P, Borlée-Grimée I et al (1989) Evaluation of routine ultrasound examination for the prenatal diagnosis of malformation. *European Journal of Obstetrics, Gynecology and Reproductive Biology* **30:** 101–109.

Macquart-Moulin G, Julian V, Chapel F & Ayme S (1989) Sensibilité de l'échographie obstétricale dans le diagnostic anténatal des anomalies foetales majeures. *Revue d'Epidémiologie et de Santé Publique* **37:** 197–205.

National Institutes of Health Development Conference Consensus Statement (1984) *Diagnostic Ultrasound Imaging in Pregnancy.* Washington: US Department of Health and Human Services.

Neilson JP, Whitfield CR & Aitchison TC (1980) Screening for the small-for-dates fetus: a two-stage ultrasound examination schedule. *British Medical Journal* **280:** 1203–1206.

Neilson JP, Munjanja SP & Whitfield CR (1984) Screening for small for dates fetuses: a controlled trial. *British Medical Journal* **289:** 1179–1182.

Ott WJ (1985) Femur length, neonatal crown-heel length and screening for intra-uterine growth retardation. *Obstetrics and Gynecology* **65:** 460–464.

Papiernik E, Bréart G & Spira N (eds) (1986) *Prevention of Preterm Birth,* 442pp. Paris: INSERM.

Pearce JM (1987) Making waves: current controversies in obstetric ultrasound. *Midwifery* **3:** 25–28.

Pearce JM & Campbell S (1987) A comparison of symphysis–fundal height and ultrasound as screening tests for light-for-gestational age infants. *British Journal of Obstetrics and Gynaecology* **94:** 100–104.

Persson PH & Kullander S (1983) Long-term experience of general ultrasound screening in pregnancy. *American Journal of Obstetrics and Gynecology* **146:** 942–947.

Poisson-Salomon AS, Bréart G & Maillard F (1987) Diffusion of obstetrical echography in France between 1976 and 1981. *International Journal of Epidemiology* **16:** 234–238.

Ringa V, Blondel B & Bréart G (1989) Ultrasound in obstetrics: do the published evaluative studies justify its routine use? *International Journal of Epidemiology* **18:** 489–497.

Rosendahl H & Kivinen S (1989) Antenatal detection of congenital malformations by routine ultrasonography. *Obstetrics and Gynecology* **73:** 947–951.

Royal College of Obstetricians and Gynaecologists (1984) Report of Working Party on routine ultrasound examination in pregnancy. London: Royal College of Obstetricians and Gynaecologists.

Rudigoz RC, Gaucherand P & Le Maout G (1987) Age gestationnel et biométrie foetale (I). In Tournaire M, Bréart G, Papiernik E & Delecour M (eds) *Apport de l'Échographie en Obstétrique,* pp 173–196. Paris: Vigot.

Sabbagha RE, Sheikh Z, Tamura RK et al (1985) Predictive value, sensitivity and specificity of ultrasonic targeted imaging for fetal anomalies in gravid women at high risk for birth defects. *American Journal of Obstetrics and Gynecology* **152:** 822–827.

Sackett DL, Haynes RB & Tugwell P (1985) *Clinical Epidemiology*, 370pp. Boston: Little, Brown and Company.

Schmidt W, Leucht W, Boos R et al (1985) Sonographische Diagnostik schwerer fetaler Fehlbidungen. *Geburtshilfe und Frauenheilkunde* **45:** 511–524.

Secher NJ, Hansen PK, Lenstrup C & Eriksen PS (1986) Controlled trial of ultrasound for light for gestational age (LGA) infants in late pregnancy. *European Journal of Obstetrics, Gynecology and Reproductive Biology* **23:** 307–313.

Secher NJ, Hansen PK, Lenstrup C, Eriksen PS & Morsing G (1987) A randomized study of fetal abdominal diameter and fetal weight estimation for detection of light-for-gestation infants in low-risk pregnancies. *British Journal of Obstetrics and Gynaecology* **94:** 105–109.

Sollie JE, Van Geijn H & Arts N (1988) Validity of a selective policy for ultrasound examination of fetal congenital anomalies. *European Journal of Obstetrics, Gynecology and Reproductive Biology* **27:** 125–132.

Sureau C, Blot Ph, Cabrol C, Cavaillé F & Germain G (1986) *Control and Management of Parturition*, 272pp. Paris: John Libbey INSERM.

Thacker SB (1985) Quality of controlled clinical trials. The case of imaging in ultrasounds in obstetrics: a review. *British Journal of Obstetrics and Gynaecology* **92:** 437–444.

Tournaire M, Bréart G, Papiernik E & Delecour M (eds) (1987) *Apport de l'Échographie en Obstetrique*. Paris: Vigot.

Vintzileos AM, Campbell WA, Nochimson DJ & Weinbraum PJ (1987) Antenatal evaluation and management of ultrasonically detected fetal anomalies. *Obstetrics and Gynecology* **69:** 640–660.

Waldenström U, Axelsson O, Nilsson S et al (1988) Effects of routine one stage ultrasound screening in pregnancy: a randomized controlled trial. *Lancet* **ii:** 585–588.

Warsof SL, Cooper DJ, Little D & Campbell S (1986) Routine ultrasound screening for antenatal detection of intra-uterine growth retardation. *Obstetrics and Gynecology* **67:** 33–39.

Whetham JC, Muggah H & Davidson S (1976) Assessment of intra-uterine growth retardation by diagnostic ultrasound. *American Journal of Obstetrics and Gynecology* **125:** 577–580.

Wladimiroff JW & Laar J (1980) Ultrasonic measurement of fetal body size: a randomized controlled trial. *Acta Obstetrica et Gynecologica Scandinavica* **59:** 177–179.

4

Identification of high risk and low risk

MARION H. HALL

Antenatal care could theoretically be disaggregated into a number of specific goals, with each element of screening or intervention subject to evaluation of its efficacy, acceptability and cost-effectiveness. However, what is usually practised is a global standard package which is recommended for all and accepted by all but a few women, at least in the United Kingdom, where there are no charges for care. Would it be better to differentiate between high-risk women requiring extra tests and specialist attention, and low-risk women with different needs? This chapter will discuss some of the reasons for advocating this, and the extent to which it is possible.

Identification of high risk may be practised at the booking visit early in pregnancy (a) to select those women who should be recommended for confinement in a specialist obstetric unit, and (b) to select women who should be offered additional screening, surveillance, therapy or reassurance during the antenatal period, such measures being usually under specialist control. By whom should this identification be made? It seems reasonable that specialists should see and examine the women for whom they will be partly or wholly responsible, but there is debate as to whether all women should be seen by specialists at least once (as suggested by the Working Party of the Royal College of Obstetricians and Gynaecologists) (Working Party on Antenatal and Intrapartum Care, 1982) or whether specialists should simply agree with other health professionals upon protocols as to which women should be referred (as in Holland) or whether, as autonomous primary care providers, midwives or general practitioners (GP) should decide on referral of each individual woman. Booking for confinement is to some extent an academic question in settings where virtually all women are booked for delivery in specialist hospitals. Where integrated or isolated general practitioner units or schemes for team midwifery care in specialist hospitals or at home exist, then agreed protocols, with or without a routine specialist visit, are usual as facilities are less sophisticated (Melhuish, 1985; Chamberlain, 1987); since transfer from a distance will be more hazardous and disruptive for the mother, protocols will usually be more stringent for isolated general practitioner units and home confinements.

It is obvious that risk status may change from low to high during the pregnancy, for example by the development of hypertension, but since this may happen at any time, protocols covering the eventuality of newly occurring risk factors are likely to be more useful than a routine specialist visit in late pregnancy. It is also obvious that for most risk factors the majority of women at risk will not in fact develop the complication of which they were at risk, and if it is clear that they are no longer at risk, they should be (but often are not) referred back to primary care.

This chapter will discuss the identification of high risk and low risk for the purposes of booking for confinement and planning care for pregnancy. It should be emphasized, however, that the demonstration of a risk factor does not necessarily imply that specialist unit confinement, extra specialist antenatal visits or intervention will actually reduce the likelihood of the complication occurring or reduce the resultant morbidity, and such measures can be justified only if benefit is likely.

For some risk factors, especially social ones, midwife or GP care may actually offer more benefit than specialist care, but the main argument in favour of midwifery or GP care is that pregnancy and parturition are physiological and care is therefore best provided by professionals with an optimistic, holistic approach, oriented towards the normal. Midwives are specialists in the care of normal pregnancy, and GPs have the advantage of being responsible for the care of the woman and her family before and after, as well as during, the pregnancy.

MATERNAL CHARACTERISTICS

Parity

Both in cross-sectional (Baird and Thomson, 1969) and longitudinal analysis (Bakketeig and Hoffman, 1979), perinatal mortality is increased in first births, partly because both maternal adaptation to pregnancy and parturition itself are more successful after a previous event, and also because some complications such as pregnancy-induced hypertension are commoner in the first pregnancy (Campbell et al, 1985). However, primigravidae now constitute almost half of the pregnant population in the United Kingdom and most have no serious complications. Confinement under specialist care need not be mandatory on the grounds of primigravidity alone. The woman pregnant for the first time should, however, have more antenatal checks than the multigravid woman in order to detect pregnancy-induced hypertension. The likelihood of the condition occurring and hence the productivity of visits intended to detect it is greater after 33 weeks' gestation (Hall et al, 1980), but it has been argued (Redman, 1982; Wallenburg, 1989) that extra visits should be made in the second trimester on the grounds that the condition is more morbid for mother and baby if it does develop then. No data has been produced, however, to support the contention that extra visits would reduce this morbidity. Concentrating care on primigravidae in Aberdeen (Hall et al, 1985c) did not result in any reduction in the proportion of cases detected antenatally.

Very high parity is so uncommon in the developed world that it is difficult to be sure to what extent it is now a risk factor independent of the adverse social factors by which it is often accompanied. In the absence of malpresentation, specialist unit confinement may be unnecessary, and may be contraindicated by a history of quick labours if the specialist unit is distant from home. Clearly women of high parity should be assessed in late pregnancy to identify malpresentation.

Age

Very young teenagers are at a higher risk of having low birthweight babies (Leading article, 1989a) but this may be attributable to late booking, unwanted pregnancy (Bury, 1985), poor uptake of and compliance with care, and lack of social support. Perhaps the best arguments for specialist unit confinement are that skeletal growth may not be complete and that epidural analgesia may be required because of inadequate preparation for and support during labour.

Increased maternal age is undoubtedly a risk factor for fetal chromosome anomaly, but the increase is gradual and the age at which chorion villus biopsy or amniocentesis should be offered is arbitrary and the uptake variable. After choosing an appropriate level of risk, the sensitivity and specificity of age as a risk factor can be improved by combining it with an assay of serum α-fetoprotein, and possibly oestriol and chorionic gonado-trophin (Wald et al, 1988).

The risk of dystocia in labour in older primigravidae (Baird, 1969) is an indication for specialist unit confinement, but not for extra antenatal care. Maternal age is a non-specific risk factor for maternal and perinatal mortality, but the age used as a cut-off point in primigravidae varies between 30 in Britain (Ministry of Health, 1959) and 35 in Holland (van Alten, 1986). Similarly, multigravidae are categorized at 35 and 45 years, respectively. An increasing proportion of first-time mothers are over 30 years (Holloway and Brook, 1988) and a cut-off point of 30 years may not be justified as this becomes the norm, but where a problem such as hypertension occurs in an older mother, referral for specialist treatment should be prompt.

Height

Short stature may be used as a risk factor, especially in primigravidae, mainly on the basis that those women who are short because they have not reached their genetic potential, perhaps because of nutritional problems in childhood, are more likely to have a higher perinatal mortality (Baird and Thomson, 1969) and also a contracted pelvis.

It would be customary to book short women for specialist unit confine-ment on the grounds that operative or instrumental delivery is more likely to be required (Chng et al, 1980). The appropriate cut-off point will vary according to the height distribution in the population. A height of 152 cm is often used, but the data of Bull (1983) suggest that 160 cm may be more reasonable.

Women of short stature are more likely to have a baby which is small for gestational age using tables uncorrected for maternal size. It is not clear whether this is physiological or pathological (Carr-Hill and Pritchard, 1985).

Growth should certainly be monitored in short women, since the delivery of an unduly large or small baby may cause problems in labour.

Weight

Women who are underweight for height are at risk of having a growth retarded baby (van der Spuy et al, 1988) and fundal height checking, perhaps with serial ultrasound, is indicated, together with monitoring of maternal weight gain.

Obesity (overweight for height) is a risk factor for fetal macrosomy and pre-eclampsia (Treharne et al, 1979; Harrison et al, 1980). Extra visits for blood pressure checks, using an obese cuff, are indicated. In addition, both during pregnancy and in labour, it may be difficult to identify the lie and presentation, and obese women should be seen by a specialist with a scan available in late pregnancy and booked for confinement under specialist care. Anaesthesia can also be dangerous (Report on Confidential Enquiries into Maternal Deaths, 1989) and should if possible be avoided in flying squad circumstances.

Growth should be carefully monitored in view of the risk of macrosomy leading to shoulder dystocia.

Smoking

Maternal smoking of more than ten cigarettes per day increases the risk of perinatal mortality and intrauterine growth retardation, and reduces the risk of pre-eclampsia (Leading article, 1989b), but would not normally influence plans for booking or antenatal care. Advice about smoking is discussed in Chapter 1 and smoking habit should be taken into account when planning monitoring of fetal growth.

Socio-economic factors

That lack of social and economic support has adverse effects upon pregnancy outcome is indisputable (Chalmers, 1985). Occupational data on the woman and her partner may be of value, not only to assess the likelihood of socio-economic disadvantage, but also to identify any specific occupational hazards, as discussed in Chapter 1. Other characteristics which may be associated with disadvantage are race (Committee to Study the Prevention of Low Birth Weight, 1985), age at completion of full-time education and uncertainty of gestation (Hall and Carr-Hill, 1985; Hall et al, 1985a).

The value of social interventions in pregnancy is discussed in Chapter 5 and care for women with social problems in Chapter 9.

Pelvic examination findings

Vaginal examination is often routinely done at booking, but has been carefully scrutinized by O'Donovan et al (1988), who concluded that the likelihood of finding a remediable problem was remote.

PREVIOUS MEDICAL HISTORY

The management of women with active medical disorders is discussed in Chapter 8.

Inactive medical problems of relevance would include a previous history of surgery to the female genital tract, which would indicate specialist unit confinement and discussion of the mode of delivery.

A prior history of infertility or ectopic pregnancy is usually regarded as requiring specialist unit confinement and extra surveillance. The actual risk is not well documented, being confounded by other factors such as age, but the fear that there may be few or no subsequent pregnancies tends to raise anxiety in all concerned and influence patterns of care.

PREVIOUS OBSTETRIC HISTORY

Some pregnancy problems tend to recur and others predispose to different adverse outcomes in future pregnancies. The ascertainment of risk arising from the previous obstetric history requires the use of an appropriate control group, but this is not always easy and may require very large data sets, such as the Norwegian Birth Registry (Bakketeig et al, 1979), to consider uncommon outcomes or those with a low recurrence risk. Some of the problems are: (a) data should if possible be recorded prospectively to avoid ascertainment bias; (b) cases must be excluded who could not experience the adverse outcome being considered whether in the previous pregnancy or the index one; (c) pregnancy sequences of the same size and type should be compared (though it is now rarely possible to look at sequences of more than three pregnancies); (d) if possible, early pregnancy outcomes should be included in the analysis; and (e) cases with missing data may have to be excluded or considered separately, but this may introduce bias if the groups being compared do not have the same proportion of missing data (Hall et al, 1985a).

Previous early pregnancy failure

This outcome is difficult to study as very early pregnancy may not be recognized, and a variable proportion of recognized miscarriages are admitted to hospital and the diagnosis confirmed histologically. Another problem is that retrospective records analysis often provides inadequate detail as to whether events occurred in the first or second trimester.

There is a recurrence risk, but no evidence that any antenatal treatment influences the prognosis (Speert, 1954; Vlaanderen and Treffers, 1987). The recurrence risk of ectopic pregnancy is around 15%. The main relevance of a history of early pregnancy failure is that a scan at seven weeks' gestation will confirm an ongoing intrauterine pregnancy. Maternal anxiety may lead to extra surveillance after this.

Previous second trimester miscarriage may be considered together with preterm labour, especially if the history is suggestive of cervical incompetence.

Previous induced abortion

A history of a prior uncomplicated early induced abortion does not constitute a significant risk factor (World Health Organization, 1979; Hogue et al, 1982). Whether late induced abortion or repeated abortion should be considered a risk factor is not well established, nor is the efficacy of preventive measures.

Previous preterm labour

Longitudinal studies of pregnancy careers show that women with a previous preterm birth have a threefold risk of preterm birth in the second pregnancy compared with those with one previous term birth (Bakketeig and Hoffman, 1981). A similar study was done in Aberdeen (Carr-Hill and Hall, 1985), where reliable data on induction was available and the study could be restricted to women with only spontaneous onset labours in singleton live births; data on early pregnancy outcomes was also available. Some results from this study are summarized in Table 1.

Table 1. Incidence of spontaneous preterm birth after various previous obstetric histories.

First birth	Second birth	% incidence of spontaneous preterm labour in next birth
Term	—	4.7
Preterm	—	15.4
Term	Term	4.0
Preterm	Preterm	32.0
Term	Preterm	23.5
Preterm	Term	12.0

A history of one prior spontaneous or induced abortion did not significantly change the above risks.

In spite of this clearly elevated risk, the proportion of preterm births which can be attributed to or accounted for by a previous preterm delivery is small. In the above study, only 76 out of 337 (22.6%) preterm second births were in the group with a previous history, so that any intervention could have only limited success if applied to only 22% of the cases with an adverse outcome.

Identification of a risk of preterm labour, whether on the basis of previous history or on factors such as maternal age or cervical changes (Bouyer et al, 1986), might lead to extra surveillance, perhaps including serial vaginal examinations, ultrasound scans, cervical cerclage or prolonged bedrest. Few of these measures could properly be applied to the whole pregnant population. Where they have been applied generally, some interventions such as work leave and rest at home seem to have been more successful in low-risk groups than in high-risk ones (Papiernik et al, 1985).

Previous intrauterine growth retardation or macrosomy

That there is a correlation between birthweight in consecutive births to the same mother was noted by Carr-Hill and Samphier (1983). This may also be expressed as a recurrence risk for intrauterine growth retardation (IUGR) or macrosomy of two to three times (Bakketeig et al, 1979). However, the attributable risk is low, and the outcome for growth retarded second babies is actually worse where there is no previous history, which limits the value of previous history as an indication for specific action. Extra surveillance, including serial ultrasound scan, is often offered to women with a previous IUGR baby, but whether any clinical benefit results from IUGR detection is doubtful (Neilson et al, 1984).

Previous third stage complications

A history of previous third stage complications is significant for antenatal care only in respect of the booking for confinement. Women with a previous history of third stage complications on one occasion have around three times the risk in a second pregnancy compared with women without such a history (Hall et al, 1985b). Because of the potential hazard to the mother, anyone with a history of retained placenta or postpartum haemorrhage should be booked for confinement in a specialist unit with facilities for blood transfusion.

Previous perinatal death

This is indeed a risk factor, but the recurrence risk and the appropriate plan for care depends entirely upon the cause of death, gestation birthweight, and other previous medical and obstetric history.

Previous caesarean section

Enkin (1989) has reviewed the literature on mode of delivery after previous caesarean birth, and concluded that the presence of a lower segment scar in the uterus is not in itself an indication for a repeat caesarean section (CS), for which a specific indication should be required.

No special antenatal care is required, except that a specialist review in late pregnancy could check whether any indication for repeat CS has arisen. Because of the risk of uterine rupture in labour, delivery must be in a specialist unit with facilities for prompt operation.

Previous forceps delivery

Only if a previous forceps delivery had resulted in serious fetal or maternal trauma would there be an indication for CS in subsequent deliveries. With a previous uncomplicated forceps delivery, delivery will usually be spontaneous in the next pregnancy (see Table 2) though in a significantly smaller proportion of women than those with a previous spontaneous delivery.

Table 2. Percentage distribution of mode of delivery in second birth by mode of delivery in first birth (Aberdeen 1964–1983).

Mode of delivery in second birth	Mode of delivery in first birth				
	CS ($n = 884$)	Forceps ($n = 3511$)	Breech ($n = 266$)	SVD ($n = 1113$)	All modes ($n = 12\,953$)
CS	64.6	3.4	4.9	1.8	6.6
Forceps	21.6	9.3	8.6	2.8	6.0
Breech	0.5	1.5	6.8	1.6	1.6
SVD	13.3	85.8	79.7	93.7	85.8
Total	100	100	100	100	100

CS = caesarean section; SVD = spontaneous vaginal delivery.

Good practice in antenatal care would entail scrutiny of the notes of the previous forceps delivery at the booking visit to identify any suspicion of cephalopelvic disproportion, and attention to the estimated fetal weight and the station of the head in late pregnancy. In the absence of any such problems, confinement in a general practitioner unit is not contraindicated.

Previous pre-eclampsia

The recurrence risk of pre-eclampsia does not follow the same pattern as with the complications already considered, since it occurs primarily in the first pregnancy. Thus, primiparity itself is the main risk factor (Campbell et al, 1985). This longitudinal study also showed that previous spontaneous or induced abortion did not reduce the risk in the first viable pregnancy, and that a woman in her second pregnancy with a previous history of albuminuric pre-eclampsia would have the same risk as all primigravidae. The practical implications of this for antenatal care are discussed earlier in this chapter.

IDENTIFICATIONS OF LOW RISK

It is clear that many, though not all, women prefer to be delivered as near as possible to their own homes, by staff already known to them and in a homely atmosphere (O'Brien, 1978). This can sometimes be provided even in a large hospital.

When women are asked to compare antenatal care in hospital with that from the general practitioner (Hall et al, 1985c), they prefer the general practitioner, and there is recent evidence that this form of care may be cheaper for them (Meldrum, 1989). Midwifery care is also very acceptable to women who have had the opportunity to experience it (Flint and Poulengeris, 1987).

The argument about whether home, general practitioner unit or hospital confinement is safest for low-risk women cannot be resolved because of the poor quality of the available evidence, which was summarized by Campbell and MacFarlane (1987). Like is rarely compared with like. The relevance of this issue to the provision of antenatal care is that the booking visit is often expected to (a) select those women who need little or no specialist antenatal

Table 3. Percentage of women transferred from GP/midwife to specialist care in the antepartum period and during labour in various studies.

Reference	% transferred antepartum	% transferred in labour*
Chng et al (1980)	30	15
Bull (1980)	24	12
Ris (1986)	10	22
van Alten (1986)	16	8
Young (1987)	19	8
Reynolds et al (1988)	20	15
Prentice and Walton (1989)	31	22
Bull (1989)	16	14
van Alten et al (1989)	17	10
Marsh and Channing (1989)	12	16

* The percentage transferred in labour was calculated from data in the papers using as a denominator the number of women still booked for GP/midwife care at onset of labour.

care; and (b) select those who could be delivered under the care of the midwife or general practitioner. However, many recent studies, summarized in Table 3, have shown that a considerable proportion (up to 30%) of the low-risk women had to be transferred to specialist care during the antenatal period, usually because of hypertension, antepartum haemorrhage, IUGR, malpresentation, etc. Transfer rates were usually higher in primigravidae. Whether all transfers were essential is not usually explored.

The proportion transferred is likely to vary according to the stringency of the original booking criteria and whether they were actually applied (Chng et al, 1980), but the proportion originally booked for GP care is not always explained. Most authors seem to be using similar criteria to determine risk and yet the proportion originally booked for primary care in Holland is always much higher than in Britain. It has been argued that low primary care booking rates and high transfer rates deprive women of the care they want. However, although the antepartum transfer rates may be high, all units report that of those still booked for GP/midwife confinement at the end of the antenatal period, a substantial proportion are transferred in labour. These transfer rates are summarized in Table 3. There is no clear evidence that low antepartum transfer rates are associated with high intrapartum transfer rates, but it could be argued that the antepartum transfer rates were too low since they failed to select out the women who would need transfer in labour. Another relevant consideration here is that the perinatal mortality of those who are transferred to specialist care is high. This is not surprising since they are transferred because of a problem, but might indicate that transfer was too late. These questions cannot be resolved without randomized studies, which are unlikely to occur.

This approach could also be used in the opposite direction. Since many of the women under specialist care because of a risk factor do not in fact have any complication, in at least some cases (e.g. risk of IUGR where growth has been monitored and found to be normal) the women could theoretically be transferred back to the care of the GP or midwife. Perhaps this should be considered more often, provided that it does not result in even more discontinuity in care.

SUMMARY

Identification of high risk is only moderately successful at the booking visit; most risk factors only give a relative risk of around three, so that most of the high-risk group do not experience the adverse outcome, and most adverse outcomes occur in low-risk women. Risk factors are useful in planning for confinement and extra care, but since new problems can arise at any time and most antenatal admissions are for conditions arising in spite of antenatal care (Chng et al, 1980), some care should be offered to all women. Traditional schedules of care, however, have no scientific justification.

Identification of low risk is also fallible and there seems to be an irreducible minimum of unpredictable problems which will arise even in low-risk women. Methods need to be found to reduce the lack of continuity which often results from unscheduled transfers of care.

REFERENCES

Baird D (ed.) (1969) Dystocia. *Combined Textbook of Obstetrics and Gynaecology*, pp 365–412. Edinburgh & London: E & S Livingstone.

Baird D & Thomson AM (1969) General factors underlying perinatal mortality rates. In Butler NR & Alberman ED (eds) *Perinatal Problems*, pp 16–35. Edinburgh & London: E & S Livingstone.

Bakketeig LS & Hoffman JH (1979) Perinatal mortality by birth order within cohorts based on sibling size. *British Medical Journal* iii: 693–696.

Bakketeig LS & Hoffman HJ (1981) Epidemiology of preterm birth: results from a longitudinal study of births in Norway. In Elder MG & Hendricks CH (eds) *Preterm Labour*, pp 17–46. London: Butterworths.

Bakketeig LS, Hoffman HJ & Harley EE (1979) The tendency to repeat gestational age and birthweight in successive births. *American Journal of Obstetrics and Gynecology* **135**: 1086–1103.

Bouyer J, Papiernik E & Dreyfus J (1986) Facteurs de risque de prematurite etablis lors des consultations prenatales. *Colloque INSERM* **138**: 123–138.

Bull MJV (1980) Ten years' experience in a general practice obstetric unit. *Journal of the Royal College of General Practitioners* **30**: 208–215.

Bull MJV (1983) Obstetrics: selection of patients for GP care. *Maternal and Child Health* **8**: 84–90.

Bull MJV (1989) Referral to general practitioner units. *British Medical Journal* **299**: 1402.

Bury JK (1985) Commentary: teenage pregnancy. *British Journal of Obstetrics and Gynaecology* **92**: 1081–1082.

Campbell DM, MacGillivray I & Carr-Hill R (1985) Pre-eclampsia in a second pregnancy. *British Journal of Obstetrics and Gynaecology* **92**: 131–140.

Campbell R & MacFarlane A (1987) *Where to be Born? The Debate and the Evidence*, 72pp. Oxford: National Perinatal Epidemiology Unit, Radcliffe Infirmary.

Carr-Hill R & Hall MH (1985) The repetition of spontaneous preterm labour. *British Journal of Obstetrics and Gynaecology* **92**: 921–928.

Carr-Hill R & Pritchard C (1985) *The Development and Exploitation of Empirical Birthweight Standards*. London: Macmillan Press.

Carr-Hill R & Samphier M (1983) Birthweight and reproductive careers. *Journal of Biosocial Science* **15**: 453–464.

Chalmers I (1985) Short, Black, Baird, Himsworth and social class differences in fetal and neonatal mortality rates. *British Medical Journal* **291**: 231–232.

Chamberlain G (1987) Less than one a day. In Chamberlain G & Gunn P (eds) *Birthplace*, pp 263–276. London: John Wiley & Sons.

Chng PK, Hall MH & MacGillivray I (1980) An audit of antenatal care: the value of the first antenatal visit. *British Medical Journal* 281: 1184–1186.

Committee to Study the Prevention of Low Birth Weight, Division of Health Promotion and Disease Prevention (1985) *Preventing Low Birthweight.* Washington DC: National Academy Press.

Enkin M (1989) Labour and delivery following previous caesarean section. In Chalmers I, Enkin M & Keirse MJNC (eds) *Effective Care in Pregnancy and Childbirth*, pp 1196–1215. Oxford: Oxford University Press.

Flint C & Poulengeris P (1987) *The 'Know Your Midwife' Report.* London: C Flint, 49 Peckerman's Wood.

Hall MH & Carr-Hill R (1985) The significance of uncertain gestation for obstetric outcome. *British Journal of Obstetrics and Gynaecology* 92: 452–460.

Hall MH, Chng PK & MacGillivray I (1980) Is routine antenatal care worthwhile? *Lancet* ii: 78–80.

Hall MH, Carr-Hill R, Fraser C, Campbell DM & Samphier ML (1985a) The extent and antecedents of uncertain gestation. *British Journal of Obstetrics and Gynaecology* 92: 445–451.

Hall MH, Halliwell R & Carr-Hill R (1985b) Concomitant and repeated happenings of complications of the third stage of labour. *British Journal of Obstetrics and Gynaecology* 92: 732–738.

Hall MH, Macintyre S & Porter M (1985c) *Antenatal Care Assessed*, pp 139. Aberdeen: Aberdeen University Press.

Harrison GG, Udall JN & Morrow G (1980) Maternal obesity, weight gain in pregnancy and infant birthweight. *American Journal of Obstetrics and Gynecology* 136: 411–412.

Hogue CJR, Cates W & Tietze C (1982) The effects of induced abortion on subsequent reproduction. *Epidemiologic Reviews* 4: 66–94.

Holloway S & Brook DJH (1988) Changes in maternal age, distribution and their possible impact on demand for prenatal diagnostic services. *British Medical Journal* 296: 978–981.

Leading article (1989a) Adolescent pregnancy. *Lancet* ii: 1308–1309.

Leading article (1989b) Smoke screen round the fetus. *Lancet* ii: 1310–1311.

Marsh GN & Channing DM (1989) Audit of 26 years of obstetrics in general practice. *British Medical Journal* 298: 1077–1080.

Meldrum P (1989) *Costing Antenatal Visits. Health Economics Unit Discussion Paper, 02/89.* Aberdeen: University of Aberdeen.

Melhuish AH (1985) Different settings for intrapartum care: the isolated unit. In Marsh GN (ed.) *Modern Obstetrics in General Practice*, pp 256–264. Oxford: Oxford University Press.

Ministry of Health (1959) *Cranbrook Committee Report. Report of the Maternity Services Committee.* London: HMSO.

Neilson JP, Munjanja SP & Whitfield CR (1984) Screening for small for dates fetuses: a controlled trial. *British Medical Journal* 289: 1179–1182.

O'Brien M (1978) Home and hospital confinement: a comparison of the experience of mothers having home and hospital confinements. *Journal of the Royal College of General Practitioners* 28: 460–466.

O'Donovan P, Gupta JK, Savage J, Thomson JG & Lilford RJ (1988) Is routine antenatal booking vaginal examination necessary for reasons other than cervical cytology if ultra-sound examination is planned? *British Journal of Obstetrics and Gynaecology* 95: 556–559.

Papiernik E, Bouyer J & Dreyfus J (1985) Risk factors for preterm births and results of a prevention policy. The Hagenau Perinatal Study 1971–1982. In Beard RW & Sharp F (eds) *Preterm Labour and its Consequences*, pp 15–20. London: Royal College of Obstetricians and Gynaecologists.

Prentice A & Walton SM (1989) Outcome of pregnancies referred to a general practitioner unit in a district hospital. *British Medical Journal* 299: 1090–1092.

Redman C (1982) Screening for pre-eclampsia. In Enkin M & Chalmers I (eds) *Effectiveness and Satisfaction in Antenatal Care*, pp 182–197. London: Spastics International Medical Publications.

Report on Confidential Enquiries into Maternal Deaths England and Wales 1982–1984 (1989) *Department of Health Report on Health and Social Subjects 34.* London: HMSO.

Reynolds JL, Yudkin PL & Bull MJV (1988) General practitioner obstetrics: does risk prediction work? *Journal of the Royal College of General Practitioners* **38:** 307–310.

Ris M (1986) Obstetrical care in the Netherlands. The place of midwives and specific aspects of their role. In Kaminski M, Breart G, Buekens P, Huisjes HJ, McIlwaine G & Selbmann H (eds) *Perinatal Care Delivery Systems*, pp 167–177. Oxford: Oxford University Press.

Samphier M & Thompson B (1981) The Aberdeen Maternity and Neonatal Databank. In Mednick SA & Baert AE (eds) *Prospective Longitudinal Research*, pp 61–65. Oxford: Oxford University Press.

Speert H (1954) Pregnancy progress following repeated abortion. *American Journal of Obstetrics and Gynecology* **68:** 665–693.

Treharne IAL, Sutherland HW, Stowers JM & Samphier M (1979) Reproduction in obese women. In Sutherland HW & Stowers JM (eds) *Carbohydrate Metabolism in Pregnancy and the Newborn*, pp 479. Berlin: Springer Verlag.

van Alten D (1986) Obstetric care in the Netherlands. Principles and results. In Kaminski M, Breart G, Buekens P, Huisjes HJ, McIlwaine G & Selbmann H (eds) *Perinatal Care Delivery Systems*, pp 178–186. Oxford: Oxford Medical Publications.

van Alten D, Eskes M & Treffers P (1989) Midwifery in the Netherlands. The Wormerveer study: selection, mode of delivery, perinatal mortality and infant morbidity. *British Journal of Obstetrics and Gynaecology* **96:** 656–662.

van der Spuy ZM, Steer PJ, McKuster M, Steele SJ & Jacobs HS (1988) Outcome of pregnancy in underweight women after spontaneous and induced ovulation. *British Medical Journal* **296:** 962–965.

Vlaanderen W & Treffers PE (1987) Progress of subsequent pregnancies after recurrent spontaneous abortion in first trimester. *British Medical Journal* **295:** 92–93.

Wald NJ, Cuckle HS & Densem JW (1988) Maternal serum screening for Down's syndrome in early pregnancy. *British Medical Journal* **297:** 883–887.

Wallenburg HCS (1989) Detecting hypertensive disorders of pregnancy. In Chalmers I, Enkin M & Keirse MJNC (eds) *Effective Care in Pregnancy and Childbirth*, pp 382–402. Oxford: Oxford University Press.

Working Party on Antenatal and Intrapartum Care (1982). London: Royal College of Obstetricians and Gynaecologists.

World Health Organization (1979) Gestation; birthweight and spontaneous abortion in pregnancy after induced abortion. *Lancet* **i:** 142–145.

Young G (1987) Are isolated maternity units run by general practitioners dangerous? *British Medical Journal* **294:** 744–746.

5

Social and midwifery support

ROBERT BRYCE

THE LIMITATIONS OF MEDICAL SUPPORT

Antenatal care in most Western countries is either directly provided by, or supervised by, obstetricians or general practitioner-obstetricians. Cynicism and despondence regarding the value of this 'traditional' antenatal care is widespread, even amongst those providing the care. It is therefore surprising that most retrospective reports by women about this care have indicated general satisfaction with it (Porter and MacIntyre, 1984; Canadian Medical Association, 1986). Several factors may work, however, to bias these results in favour of traditional care. Generally these women had recently undergone a pregnancy in these arrangements and consequently felt some obligation to report that these arrangements were the best possible ones (Porter and MacIntyre, 1984). There is a tendency to respond negatively to new arrangements until they have been experienced, which may also have influenced women to respond unfavourably to an alternative form of care. Also, the responses of women to questions about their care could have been influenced by their perceptions of what the interviewer wanted them to indicate (Lumley, 1985; Oakley, 1985). This latter criticism also applies to those retrospective assessments of women's satisfaction with obstetrical care which have drawn negative conclusions (Oakley, 1979).

The principal criticisms of traditional antenatal care focus on the social aspects of the care in that it is impersonal, and that advice and information are either insufficiently or inappropriately provided (Garcia, 1982). The impersonal nature of traditional antenatal care is a particular problem for women who attend public clinics where they often see several different doctors during their pregnancies. Women's criticisms of the medical aspects of their care have likewise focused on poor communication of the results of screening tests rather than on the screening tests themselves (Reid and Garcia, 1989). These perceived deficiencies in antenatal care could be categorized as deficient social support (the social gratification received through interaction with others). Thoits (1982) has operationalized social support in two ways: expressive support (sympathy, empathy, understanding, affection, acceptance and acting as a confidant) and instrumental support (information, advice and material aid).

Some authors have argued that women expect social support to be a part of their antenatal care (Oakley, 1979; Garcia, 1982), although it is not clear that most women put great importance on it. Interviews in mid-pregnancy of 135 women attending a public hospital antenatal clinic in Australia and of 45 of their care-providers found that the women's responses to 'What should you get from antenatal care?' rated screening and management of physical problems as three times more important than advice or information and as five times more important than reassurance (Bryce et al, 1987). A desire for continuity of medical care was infrequently stated. The providers, on the other hand, rated screening and advice or information equally. Dissatisfaction with antenatal care was more frequent in women of higher education levels.

Notwithstanding the limitations of observational research and the bias of data collection from women already in traditional antenatal care, it is clear that this care provides unsatisfactory social support to many women. However, a significant improvement in the support provided may not be possible within the current medical model of antenatal care. Because of the nature of training for junior doctors, rotation of these staff is necessary and will lead to a lack of continuity of medical care-givers for women over the several months of their care. Furthermore, most hospital clinics do not have sufficient staff to provide prolonged consultations at each antenatal visit. Finally, and most importantly, medical training focuses on the diagnosis and treatment of illness rather than on the ability to communicate and to appropriately reassure a healthy person. Many doctors are uncomfortable with the provision of expressive social support to women and furthermore do not see it as part of their duty. Ethnic and social differences between doctors and the women attending antenatal clinics also contribute to the inability of this relationship to provide adequate support.

The training of medical students in many universities now includes training in behavioural medicine and this approach gives some hope that the doctor of the future will be better equipped to provide the support that women seek. Another possible way to improve the supportive quality of each antenatal visit is to reduce the quantity of visits. This was proposed a decade ago by Hall et al (1980), but generally practice has not changed in this area, with healthy women being seen an average of ten times during their pregnancies.

Alternative sources of social support in pregnancy to medical ones are now being sought by some women. These sources may be found outside of hospital care, with women seeking antenatal care and childbirth in their homes. There is a developing trend in Western society towards this style of care, driven by pregnant women themselves. Home birth and antenatal care by alternative providers are believed by medical practitioners to carry greater risks to the health of the mother and infant than traditional care and hospital birth. If those who hold this belief wish to reverse the trend towards non-medical care, the medical care needs to be made more supportive and consequently more attractive to all pregnant women.

ALTERNATIVE SOURCES OF SUPPORT

While antenatal care provided by medical staff may be the common in Western countries at present, this has not always been the case. Originally, family members provided any care that was necessary and later midwives from the same culture provided the care. Medical involvement in obstetrics really only appeared in the twentieth century, and with this advent, care and childbirth moved from the home to the hospital (DeVries, 1989). This progression in caregivers and in the place of care also describes a pattern of care which moves from a situation most conducive to effective social support to one least conducive to it.

Spencer (1982) argues that (expressive) social support is most effectively provided in a relationship where the receiver of the support perceives herself to be 'at the same level' as the provider, rather than the receiver being in a position of inferiority. Such relationships are difficult to create artificially, as even in a normally-formed social relationship, judgemental behaviour and the provision of gratuitous advice are common. Furthermore, this hypothesis means that the provision of instrumental support would be to the detriment of the provision of expressive support as, by providing instrumental support, the provider becomes an authority.

Family workers have been used as an additional source of nonjudgemental support to medical care in the antenatal period. An example of such providers are the travailleuse familiale of France (Spencer, 1982). These women, without formal qualifications, are chosen mainly on the basis of their characters, and given training in social, health and domestic subjects. They enter families on request and provide emotional support as well as domestic help, and act as advocates for pregnant women. A similar role has been developed for lay workers in Manchester, England (Spencer et al, 1989). Untrained lay women (doulas) have also been used to provide support for women in labour in Guatemala (Klaus et al, 1986).

Antenatal care by a midwife, either as an alternative or as an addition to medical care, has been proposed as being more supportive than medical care. Various categories of midwives can be found performing antenatal care including lay midwives who do not have formal training in midwifery, certified midwives who have trained in midwifery but not in general nursing, and nurse-midwives who are registered both as general nurses and as midwives.

Lay midwives are in a good position to provide effective expressive social support to pregnant women. Their training is often based on personal experience and their view of pregnancy is more spiritual than medical (Gaskin, 1978), although it cannot be assumed that their care is not judgemental or advice orientated. Their practices are normally limited to a relatively small number of low-risk clients with whom they have plenty of time for exploring emotional issues. The setting of the care in the home also provides an environment conducive to free communication.

Certified midwives or nurse-midwives generally work in hospital settings with varying degrees of medical supervision (Robinson, 1989). In general, the more independent the practice, the lower-risk the clientele. This once again provides an opportunity for a greater focus on emotional issues. Traditional midwifery training suffers from the same problems as medical training in that it is illness-orientated without a strong emphasis on communication skills; however, as with medical training, this is improving. Women probably feel more at ease discussing emotional problems with their midwife than with their doctor because the midwife has a perceived lower authority status than the doctors, often appears less busy, and is generally of the same sex. However, the authority status of the midwife and the emphasis in midwifery training on the provision of advice to pregnant women are both barriers to the provision of effective expressive support. Because of this, systems of social support by midwives, supplemental to medical antenatal care, have deliberately avoided gratuitous advice (R. Bryce, unpublished data).

Within medical care itself, it is probable that antenatal care provided by a general practitioner, either independently or in a shared-care arrangement with an obstetrician, is more supportive for women than care from a specialist obstetrician alone (Klein and Zander, 1989). The care is provided in a surgery or office which is familiar to the woman, the doctor and the woman are familiar with one another and there is an existing understanding of the woman's background. All these factors are conducive to improved communication of emotional problems.

THE EFFECTS OF SOCIAL SUPPORT

The effects on physical outcomes

Retrospective and prospective studies of social support in pregnancy have generally found an association between poor social support and adverse pregnancy outcomes (Norbeck and Tilden, 1983; Chalmers, 1984; Boyce et al, 1986). Berkowitz and Kasl (1983) failed to confirm this association and Nuckolls et al (1972), in an often-quoted study, found the association between poor support and adverse physical outcome only to be present in those women experiencing a high level of stress.

It has been assumed that the relationship between good support and good pregnancy outcome is causal. The theory of the action of social support is that it may act as a buffer between a stress and an adverse physical or emotional response by providing the perception in the woman of an ability to cope or by dampening her physiological responses to the stress. Social support may also affect women's health behaviour so as to avoid stressful events (Cohen, 1988). However, a causal relationship between social support and the physical outcome of pregnancy cannot be assumed, as the association is confounded by social class and by stress. For example, several studies have found associations between social class and adverse pregnancy outcomes such as preterm birth, with an increasing proportion of preterm births with decreasing social class (Kaminski et al, 1973; Fedrick and Anderson, 1976; Berkowitz, 1985). Also, stress is most common in women of the lower social classes and is associated with preterm birth (Newton et al,

1979; Newton and Hunt, 1984). Despite these doubts about causation, the hypothesis that the provision of increased social support in pregnancy will improve its outcome has been extensively tested.

The interventions which could be perceived as supportive and which have been investigated in pregnancy may be broadly grouped into antenatal education, enhanced antenatal care, and care by midwives. Antenatal education provides instrumental social support in the form of advice and information. Although it may also provide some expressive support, education regarding adverse health behaviours such as smoking may be perceived negatively by recipients. The randomized controlled trials of antenatal education which have addressed physical outcomes are summarized in Table 1. Two randomized controlled trials of anti-smoking advice

Table 1. Physical effects of antenatal education.

Reference	Sample size	Intervention	Outcome
Donovan, 1977	552	Anti-smoking	No effect
Sexton and Hebel, 1984	783	Anti-smoking	↑ birthweight
MacArthur et al, 1987	982	Anti-smoking	No effect
Zimmermann-Tansella et al, 1979	34	Childbirth preparation	↑ vacuum extraction
Timm, 1979	118	Childbirth preparation	No effect
Nelson et al, 1980	56	Childbirth preparation	↓ length of labour
Beck et al, 1980	72	Childbirth preparation	No effect

found no difference in birthweight for those receiving the advice compared with controls (Donovan, 1977; MacArthur et al, 1987), but one trial with intensive anti-smoking intervention found a 92 g increase in mean birthweight in the babies of women who received the intervention (Sexton and Hebel, 1984). Four small trials of preparation for childbirth have addressed physical outcomes. Zimmerman-Tansella et al (1979) found an increase in vacuum extractions for women receiving education and Nelson et al (1980) found a decreased length of labour for women who studied a Leboyer approach to childbirth. The other two trials failed to identify any physical effects of antenatal education (Timm, 1979; Beck et al, 1980). Kehrer and Wohin (1979) described data on 404 infants from a randomized controlled trial of income subsidy for black Americans. No significant effect was seen on birthweight from the subsidy. Rush et al (1980) provided nutritional supplementation to urban black American women in pregnancy in a randomized trial with 770 women. No significant effects were seen on birthweight or gestation.

Enhanced antenatal care has been advocated for the prevention of preterm birth. An element of this care is increased social support. Seven non-randomized trials using historical or concurrent controls all described reductions in preterm birth associated with the identification of high-risk patients, the introduction of special clinics for high-risk women, the education of patients and providers about the signs of preterm labour, and the liberal use of tocolytic drugs (Sokol et al, 1980; Herron et al, 1982;

Goujon et al, 1984; Papiernik et al, 1985a, b; Hardy et al, 1987; Konte et al, 1988). The antenatal care was generally provided by medical staff. In many cases differences were apparent between the cases and the controls which were not related to the interventions, such as more public patients, (Goujon et al, 1984) or more late booking for antenatal care (Papiernik et al, 1985b) in the control groups. These sources of bias in the non-randomized trials may explain the lack of effect of enhanced antenatal care on physical outcomes in the randomized controlled trials.

Table 2. Physical effects of enhanced antenatal care.

Reference	Sample size	Intervention	Outcome
Scott, 1984	11 000	Behaviour modification	No effect
Main et al, 1985	132	Preterm prevention	No effect
Lovell et al, 1987	235	Hold own case notes	↑ instrumental delivery
Spencer et al, 1989	1288	Family workers	No effect

The randomized controlled trials of the physical effects of enhanced antenatal care are summarized in Table 2. A small trial of a preterm birth prevention programme for black American women similar to the programmes that appeared to be so successful in comparison with non-randomized controls failed to show any difference in the incidence of preterm birth between those allocated to the programme and controls; however this trial only had the statistical power to demonstrate profound effects (Main et al, 1985). A trial of women holding their own case notes (which should provide instrumental support) found an increase in instrumental deliveries in those women who held their own notes (Lovell et al, 1987). A large trial of behaviour modification for socially disadvantaged women in Nova Scotia, Canada, did not demonstrate any overall effects on birthweight (Scott, 1984). A recent important study in this area evaluated the effects of family workers in Manchester, who aimed specifically to provide social support in the homes of women at risk of having low birthweight infants (Spencer et al, 1989). The methodology and statistical power were good, but no differences in birthweight or gestation were observed between the women receiving the visits and the controls.

It is interesting to note that there were so few physical differences seen in these trials between the women who received the enhanced antenatal support and the controls. This contrasts with findings of Klaus et al (1986), who observed significant benefits for women allocated to additional support in labour compared with those having an unsupported labour. They allocated women in labour in Guatemala to receive support from a doula or to have a traditional labour. The group supported by the doula experienced significantly fewer labour complications and fewer obstetric interventions.

The physical effects of antenatal care by midwives have also now been investigated in several trials (Table 3). Spira (1986) randomly allocated women in France with complications in pregnancy to antenatal care at home by midwives or to hospital care. No significant differences in gestation or

Table 3. Physical effects of care by midwives.

Reference	Sample size	Intervention	Outcome
Slome et al, 1976	438	Nurse-midwife clinics	↓ forceps delivery
Flint and Poulengeris, 1987	952	Nurse-midwife clinics	↓ instrumental delivery
Spira, 1986	883	Midwife home visits	No effect
Olds et al, 1986	308	Nurse home visits	No effect
R. Bryce et al, unpublished	1977	Nurse-midwife home visits	No effect
A. Oakley et al, unpublished	486	Nurse-midwife home visits	No effect

birthweight were observed between the groups. Olds et al (1986) compared women who received antenatal home visits by nurses, aimed at the reduction of child abuse, to those without the visits in a group of socially disadvantaged young women in New York State. No significant differences in gestation or birthweight were seen, although there were some postnatal psychological advantages for the women who received the visits. Two trials comparing antenatal care and attendance in labour by nurse-midwives to medical care both found significant benefits for the women seen by the midwives in the reduction of intervention in labour. However, there were no significant infant benefits (Slome et al, 1976; Flint and Poulengeris, 1987).

Two trials using the same methodology have recently been completed examining the effects of antenatal midwife home visits, aimed at providing social support, on women thought to be at risk of preterm birth (R. Bryce et al, unpublished data; A. Oakley et al, unpublished data cited in Elbourne et al, 1989). No significant differences in birthweight, gestation or other physical outcomes were found in either trial between women who received the visits and those who did not. Despite enrolling 1077 women, the larger trial still only achieved a 69% power to exclude a 25% relative reduction in preterm birth (R. Bryce et al, unpublished data). The smaller trial had even less power, with 486 participants (A. Oakley et al, unpublished data cited in Elbourne et al, 1989). Part of the reason for the low power was the difficulty that all workers in this area have found in identifying women with a high risk of preterm birth.

Despite the fact that no single trial of increased antenatal social support has had sufficient statistical power to exclude all clinically important reductions in preterm birth or low birthweight for the supported group, the results of the trials have been consistent in that no physical effect or trend was found. Combination of the trial results in a meta-analysis results in an odds ratio and confidence limits close to unity (Elbourne et al, 1989). This appears to constitute sufficient evidence to conclude that antenatal social support interventions do not affect preterm birth or low birthweight.

There are two possible explanations for this lack of effect. One is that effective social support cannot be artificially provided in the antenatal period, regardless of the nature of the provider. Another explanation is that there is not a causal relationship between the support and the outcome, and the observed association is due to confounding. The only trial to compare levels of social support in women who did or did not receive the intervention did not identify any differences in social support between the groups after the intervention (R. Bryce et al, unpublished data). These data support the first explanation that effective social support cannot be provided artificially. There is certainly insufficient evidence to support a change in the type of antenatal care provided to women on the basis of improved infant outcomes.

The data from these trials do suggest, however, that there may be advantages in labour for women who are supported at this time, principally in the form of reduced intervention.

The effects on psychological and behavioural outcomes

In the trials reviewed above, significant adverse effects were not demonstrated in those women receiving non-traditional care, so it is possible that this care could be justified on other grounds. Examples of this could be if the new care provided psychological or behavioural benefits to women, was more satisfying to women, or if it was cheaper than the existing care.

Preparation for childbirth and parenting has been associated with fewer postnatal emotional upsets (Gordon and Gordon, 1960), greater relaxation in labour and fewer complaints in hospital (Shereshefsky and Lockman, 1973), benefits in infant feeding and psychological development (Gutelius et al, 1977), fewer medications in labour (Timm, 1979), less pain in labour (Beck et al, 1980) and improved mother–child interaction (Carter-Jessop, 1981). Other trials showed no psychological or behavioural benefits (Lowe, 1970; Zimmermann-Tansella et al, 1979). Three trials of anti-smoking advice resulted in significant reductions in cigarette smoking (Donovan, 1977; Sexton and Hebel, 1984; MacArthur et al, 1987). Although these benefits from support in the form of antenatal education are modest, antenatal education has been widely adopted into antenatal care. It may be that interventions of this nature which are supplemented to traditional antenatal care, rather than replacing it, and are consequently less threatening to it, require less evidence of benefit in order to be accepted than is required for approaches to antenatal care which require the replacement of existing care.

The principal effect of enhanced antenatal care is an increase in women's satisfaction with the care they have received, indicated by a preference for that care in a future pregnancy. This effect was seen in two trials where women held their own case notes (Elbourne et al, 1987; Lovell et al, 1987). Communication and perceptions of control were increased by holding the notes, although smoking behaviour was unaffected.

The best evidence of psychological and behavioural advantages from supportive care is in the randomized trials of midwife care. Slome et al (1976) found attendance at the clinic to be superior in the nurse-midwife group to the medical group care. The trial by Flint and Poulengeris (1987) of nurse-midwife care by a small team identified several psychological and behavioural benefits in addition to the reduction in intervention in labour that was previously noted. There was a potential for bias in this trial as the analysis was not performed strictly on the basis of randomization. However, assessments of women's perceptions of communication, control and satisfaction all significantly favoured the midwife group. The use of analgesia and epidural anaesthesia was also reduced in the midwife group.

The bias of wishing to please those framing the questions that was previously mentioned needs to be kept in mind when interpreting the data on satisfaction provided by women in trials of new forms of care. In the trial of antenatal midwife social support by R. Bryce et al (unpublished data), women allocated to the nurse-midwife home visits expressed very high levels of satisfaction, yet the results of psychosocial interviews of both groups at approximately 30 weeks of gestation showed no between-group differences in life events, anxiety, locus of control or coping methods. In fact, despite the overtly supportive nature of the home visits and the high level of satisfaction reported, no difference was demonstrated between the groups in levels of social support. This is the only trial to have assessed this. Both the trial by R. Bryce et al and the similar trial of supportive nurse-midwife home visits by A. Oakley et al (unpublished data cited in Elbourne et al, 1989) did not demonstrate significant differences in intrapartum behaviour. The latter trial also failed to demonstrate significant differences in enjoyment of the pregnancy or childbirth, although women receiving visits reported fewer postnatal concerns about their babies.

In summary, antenatal care by a midwife, if part of a small team, is more satisfying to women than medical care, even taking into account possible biases in women's responses. When the midwives also provide care in childbirth, the additional benefits of reduced intervention may accrue. This increase in satisfaction, however, cannot be assumed to equate to increased social support. This could be an explanation for the lack of effect of allegedly supportive interventions on physical outcomes. Whether this increase in satisfaction is enough to justify the expense of setting up an additional style of antenatal care, or the upheaval of dismantling existing services in order to replace them with midwife services, is a decision for health care planners.

INDEPENDENT MIDWIFERY

The preceding evidence clearly supports antenatal care and childbirth by a midwife, acting under supervision by a doctor or acting independently, as an option that should be available to pregnant women. The case for actually replacing the current system of antenatal care with a system provided by independent midwives would be strengthened by the inclusion of a cost-effectiveness analysis in future trials of care by midwives compared with medical care.

There is some difficulty in generalizing the results of the two trials of independent midwifery to all pregnant women (Slome et al, 1976; Flint and Poulengeris, 1987). In the trials, the care was limited to low-risk women, so the results cannot be generalized beyond this group. Such limitations, however, need not necessarily apply to future trials of independent midwifery. It is difficult to accept that the ability of an experienced midwife to recognize complications of pregnancy would necessarily be inferior to that of a doctor training in obstetrics.

Another problem is with generalizing the effects of care in the hands of the small groups of committed midwives involved in the trials to all midwives. Further trials are required to support this generalization. Antenatal care free of the supervision of doctors provides an opportunity for midwives to expand the supportive aspects of their care; however, it is important that one authoritarian figure is not replaced by another! It would be easy to repeat the mistakes of medical antenatal care with impersonal care, talking rather than listening, and paternalism.

Independent midwifery also provides an opportunity to review the effectiveness of traditional antenatal practices such as multiple visits for well women, routine weighing and urine testing, and the provision of gratuitous life-style advice. If ineffective, these practices could be abandoned, allowing more time for listening.

At present the place for independent midwifery is as a safe and satisfactory option for those women dissatisfied with medical care, although, if midwives seize the opportunities to rationally evaluate this practice, in the future independent midwifery may become the usual form of antenatal care.

Acknowledgements

The author acknowledges the contributions to the Pregnancy Home Visiting Programme of Dr Fiona Stanley and Dr Barry Garner of the National Health and Medical Research Council Research Unit in Epidemiology and Preventive Medicine of the University of Western Australia. The research was funded by the Australian Department of Community Services and Health, the Stillbirth and Neonatal Support Group, the King Edward Memorial Hospital Research Fund and the University of Western Australia Department of Medicine.

REFERENCES

Beck NC, Siegel LJ, Davidson P et al (1980) The prediction of pregnancy outcome: maternal preparation, anxiety and attitudinal sets. *Journal of Psychosomatic Research* **22**: 343–351.
Berkowitz GS (1985) Clinical and obstetric risk factors for preterm delivery. *Mount Sinai Journal of Medicine* **52**: 239–247.
Berkowitz GS & Kasl SV (1983) The role of psychological factors in spontaneous preterm delivery. *Journal of Psychosomatic Research* **27**: 283–290.
Boyce WT, Schaefer C, Harrison HR et al (1986) Social and cultural factors in pregnancy complications among Navajo women. *American Journal of Epidemiology* **124**: 242–253.
Bryce R, Cvitanovich A, Hogan J, Monkhouse H & Welch H (1987) Perceptions of antenatal care. *Proceedings of 4th Australian Congress in Obstetrics and Gynaecology*, Perth, p 75.
Canadian Medical Association (1986) Obstetrics '87: a report of the Canadian Medical Association on obstetrical care in Canada. *Canadian Medical Association Journal* **134 (supplement)**: 136.
Carter-Jessop L (1981) Promoting maternal attachment through prenatal intervention. *MCN: American Journal of Maternal Child Nursing* **6**: 107–112.
Chalmers B (1984) Behavioural associations of pregnancy complications. *Journal of Psychosomatic Obstetrics and Gynaecology* **3**: 27–35.
Cohen S (1988) Psychosocial models of the role of social support in the etiology of physical disease. *Health Psychology* **7**: 269–297.
DeVries R (1989) Care givers in pregnancy and childbirth. In Chalmers I, Enkin M & Keirse M (eds) *Effective Care in Pregnancy and Childbirth*, pp 143–161. Oxford: Oxford University Press.

Donovan JW (1977) Randomised controlled trial of anti-smoking advice in pregnancy. *British Journal of Preventive and Social Medicine* **31:** 6–12.

Elbourne D, Richardson M, Chalmers I, Waterhouse I & Holt E (1987) The Newbury Maternity Care Study: a randomized controlled trial to assess a policy of women holding their own obstetric records. *British Journal of Obstetrics and Gynaecology* **94:** 612–619.

Elbourne D, Oakley A & Chalmers I (1989) Social and psychological support during pregnancy. In Chalmers I, Enkin M & Keirse M (eds) *Effective Care in Pregnancy and Childbirth*, pp 221–236. Oxford: Oxford University Press.

Fedrick J & Anderson ABM (1976) Factors associated with spontaneous preterm birth. *British Journal of Obstetrics and Gynaecology* **83:** 342–350.

Flint C & Poulengeris P (1987) *The 'Know Your Midwife' Report*. London: C Flint, 49 Peckerman's Wood.

Garcia J (1982) Women's views of antenatal care. In Enkin M & Chalmers I (eds) *Effectiveness and Satisfaction in Antenatal Care*, pp 81–91. London: Spastics International Medical Publications/Heinemann Medical Books.

Gaskin I (1978) *Spiritual Midwifery*. Summertown: The Book Publishing Company.

Gordon RE & Gordon KK (1960) Social factors in prevention of postpartum emotional problems. *Obstetrics and Gynecology* **15:** 433–438.

Goujon H, Papiernik E & Maine D (1984) The prevention of preterm delivery through prenatal care: an intervention study in Martinique. *International Journal of Gynaecology and Obstetrics* **22:** 339–343.

Gutelius MF, Kirsch AD, MacDonald S, Brooks MR & McErlean T (1977) Controlled study of child health supervision: behavioural results. *Pediatrics* **60:** 294–304.

Hall M, Chng PK & MacGillivray I (1980) Is routine antenatal care worth while? *Lancet* **ii:** 12: 78–80.

Hardy JB, King TM & Repke JT (1987) The Johns Hopkins Adolescent Pregnancy Program: an evaluation. *Obstetrics and Gynecology* **69:** 300–306.

Herron MA, Katz M & Creasy RK (1982) Evaluation of a preterm birth prevention program: a preliminary report. *Obstetrics and Gynecology* **59:** 452–456.

Kaminski M, Goujard J & Rumeau-Rouquette C (1973) Prediction of low birthweight and prematurity by a multiple regression analysis with maternal characteristics known since the beginning of pregnancy. *International Journal of Epidemiology* **2:** 194–204.

Kehrer BH & Wohin CM (1979) Impact of income maintenance on low birthweight: evidence from the Gary experiment. *Journal of Human Resources* **14:** 434–462.

Klaus M, Kennell J, Robertson S & Sosa R (1986) Effects of social support during parturition on maternal and infant morbidity. *British Medical Journal* **293:** 585–587.

Klein M & Zander L (1989) The role of the family practitioner in maternity care. In Chalmers I, Enkin M & Keirse M (eds) *Effective Care in Pregnancy and Childbirth*, pp 181–190. Oxford: Oxford University Press.

Konte JM, Creasy RK & Laroy RK (1988) California North Coast Preterm Birth Prevention Project. *Obstetrics and Gynecology* **71:** 727–730.

Lovell A, Zander LI, James CE et al (1987) The St Thomas' Hospital Maternity Case Notes Study: a randomised controlled trial to assess the effects of giving expectant mothers their own maternity case-notes. *Pediatric and Perinatal Epidemiology* **1:** 57–66.

Lowe ML (1970) Effectiveness of teaching as measured by compliance with medical recommendations. *Nursing Research* **19:** 59–63.

Lumley J (1985) Assessing satisfaction with childbirth. *Birth* **12:** 141–145.

MacArthur C, Newton JR & Know EG (1987) Effect of anti-smoking health education on infant size at birth: a randomized controlled trial. *British Journal of Obstetrics and Gynaecology* **94:** 295–300.

Main DM, Gabbe SG, Richardson D & Strong S (1985) Can preterm deliveries be prevented? *American Journal of Obstetrics and Gynecology* **151:** 892–889.

Nelson NM, Enkin MW, Saigal S, Bennett KJ, Milner R & Sackett DL (1980) A randomised controlled trial of the Leboyer approach to childbirth. *New England Journal of Medicine* **302:** 655–660.

Newton RW & Hunt LP (1984) Psychosocial stress in pregnancy and its relation to low birth weight. *British Medical Journal* **288:** 1191–1194.

Newton RW, Webster PAC, Binu PS, Maskrey N & Phillips AB (1979) Psychosocial stress in pregnancy and its relation to the onset of premature labour. *British Medical Journal* **ii**: 411–413.

Norbeck JS & Tilden VP (1983) Life stress, social support and emotional disequilibrium in complications of pregnancy: a prospective multivariate study. *Journal of Health and Social Behavior* **24**: 30–46.

Nuckolls KB, Cassel J & Kaplan BH (1972) Psychosocial assets, life crisis and the prognosis of pregnancy. *American Journal of Epidemiology* **95**: 431–441.

Oakley A (1979) *Becoming a Mother*. Oxford: Martin Robertson.

Oakley A (1985) Doctors, maternity patients and social scientists. *Birth* **12**: 161–166.

Olds DL, Henderson CR, Tatelbaum R & Chamberlin R (1986) Improving the delivery of prenatal care and outcomes of pregnancy: a randomized trial of nurse home visitation. *Pediatrics* **77**: 16–28.

Papiernik E, Bouyer J, Dreyfus J et al (1985a) Prevention of preterm births: a perinatal study in Hagenau, France. *Pediatrics* **76**: 154–158.

Papiernik E, Maine D, Rush D & Richard A (1985b) Prenatal care and the prevention of preterm delivery. *International Journal of Gynaecology and Obstetrics* **23**: 427–433.

Porter M & MacIntyre S (1984) What is, must be best: a research note on conservative or deferential responses to antenatal care provision. *Social Science and Medicine* **19**: 1197–1200.

Reid M & Garcia J (1989) Women's views of care during pregnancy and childbirth. In Chalmers I, Enkin M & Keirse M (eds) *Effective Care in Pregnancy and Childbirth*, pp 131–142. Oxford: Oxford University Press.

Robinson S (1989) The role of the midwife: opportunities and constraints. In Chalmers I, Enkin M & Keirse M (eds) *Effective Care in Pregnancy and Childbirth*, pp 162–180. Oxford: Oxford University Press.

Rush D, Stein Z & Susser M (1980) A randomized controlled trial of prenatal nutritional supplementation in New York City. *Pediatrics* **65**: 683–697.

Scott KE (1984) Reducing low birth weight by enhanced prenatal care. *Pediatric Research* **18**: 345A (1497).

Sexton M & Hebel R (1984) A clinical trial of change in maternal smoking and its effect on birth weight. *Journal of the American Medical Association* **251**: 911–915.

Shereshefsky PM & Lockman RF (1973) Comparison of counselled and non-counselled groups. In Schereshefsky PM & Yarrow LI (eds) *Psychological Aspects of a First Pregnancy and Early Postnatal Adaptation*, pp 151–163. New York: Raven Press.

Slome C. Wetherbee H, Daly M et al (1976) Effectiveness of certified nurse midwives. A prospective evaluation study. *American Journal of Obstetrics and Gynecology* **124**: 177–182.

Sokol RJ, Woolfe RB, Rosen MG & Weingarden K (1980) Risk, antepartum care, and outcome: impact of a maternity and infant care project. *Obstetrics and Gynecology* **56**: 150–156.

Spencer B (1982) Family Workers in France. *Social Work Service* **30**: 4–8.

Spencer B, Thomas H & Morris J (1989) A randomized controlled trial of the provision of a social support service during pregnancy: the South Manchester Family Worker Project. *British Journal of Obstetrics and Gynaecology* **96**: 281–288.

Spira N (1986) Evaluation de l'intervention prenatale des sages-femmes a domicile. In Papiernick E, Breart G & Spira N (eds) *Prevention of Preterm Birth*, pp 291–308. Paris: INSERM.

Thoits P (1982) Conceptual, methodological, and theoretical problems in studying social support as a buffer against life stress. *Journal of Health and Social Behavior* **23**: 145–159.

Timm MM (1979) Prenatal education evaluation. *Nursing Research* **28**: 338–342.

Zimmermann-Tansella C, Dolcetta G, Azzini V, Bertagni P, Siani R & Tansella M (1979) Preparation courses for childbirth in primipara. A comparison. *Journal of Psychosomatic Research* **23**: 227–233.

6

Screening and surveillance of pregnancy hypertension—an economic approach to the use of daycare

KATHRYN ROSENBERG
SARA TWADDLE

In 1915 the first outpatient antenatal clinics opened in Britain as part of an international movement of concern for maternal and child welfare. By 1935, it was estimated that 80% of pregnant women received some kind of antenatal care (Oakley, 1982). Screening for hypertension as an early detectable sign of 'toxaemia' was seen as an objective of this care from the outset. In 1929, in a report from the Ministry of Health (Memorandum 145/MCW Ministry of Health, 1929) it was stated that 'the detection of early signs of toxaemia is of primary importance, and for this reason there should be frequent and regular testing of urine and observation of blood pressure'. It was in this same report that the pattern of antenatal care was set out: a first visit at 16 weeks, to be followed by visits at 24 and 28 weeks, then fortnightly to 36 weeks and weekly thereafter. Expectations of the efficacy of antenatal care in the management of toxaemia were high. In a textbook of the period (Kerr, 1933) it was stated that 'booked cases, if further divided into those who attended the clinic regularly from the early months of pregnancy and received in consequence complete supervision, and those who attended only casually or late in pregnancy again show very different results. In the former, eclampsia or pre-eclampsia of a grave form is extremely rare; in the latter it is by no means infrequent'. In an editorial in the *Lancet* (Leading article, 1934), it was stated that 'to detect toxaemia in its early stages supervision must be close and continuous' and 'a serious criticism of antenatal care is to be found in our failure to reduce the death rate from toxaemia'.

More recently, Redman (1982) stated, 'No complication of human pregnancy is both so common and potentially so dangerous for mother and child as the syndrome of pre-eclampsia/eclampsia'. However, screening for hypertension as an early sign presents particular problems. The high prevalence of hypertension combined with its dangerous potential (albeit realized in a minority of cases) creates practical difficulties in that screening must be applied to the entire pregnant population and yet be sensitive and frequent enough to detect serious and progressive disease. How this is accomplished and the costs to the women and the health service are the

Baillière's Clinical Obstetrics and Gynaecology—
Vol. 4, No. 1, March 1990
ISBN 0–7020–1476–1

subject of this chapter. In Scotland, national data are available on inpatient and daycare from the standard maternity discharge document, the SMR2 (Cole, 1981), which we will use in the following discussion.

PREGNANCY-INDUCED HYPERTENSION

Definitions

In both epidemiological and clinical studies there are differences and difficulties in the diagnostic criteria used for pregnancy-induced hypertension. These have been widely discussed (Nelson, 1955; Baird, 1977; Redman, 1982, 1987; MacGillivray, 1983; Murnaghan, 1987; Walker, 1987) and include problems with the distinction between essential and pregnancy-induced hypertension and the relative importance of absolute levels of blood pressure or the rise from prepregnancy values. Blood pressure varies at different times of day and at different stages of pregnancy, and is subject to various observer and sampling errors such that isolated recordings are of limited value. In practice, the diagnostic criteria of Nelson (1955) or a diastolic blood pressure of 90 mmHg or greater measured on two or more occasions separated by at least 24 hours is regarded as abnormal. Often, an isolated reading at this level marks the threshold for increased surveillance or other action. When hypertension is defined at this level, it is not a diagnosis of a disease but a marker of an increased risk and an indication for increased monitoring of the fetus and mother (Wallenburg, 1989).

Incidence

Mild pregnancy-induced hypertension as defined by Nelson (1955) is common, particularly in first pregnancies. Population-based incidence among primigravidae in Aberdeen in five-year groupings from 1951 to 1980 varied from 22 to 36% (Hall and Campbell, 1987), while in multiparae the figures were 9 to 21%. Proteinuric hypertension varied from 4 to 7% among primiparae, while among multiparae it was uncommon, occurring in 1 to 2% of pregnancies. Nelson (1955) reported that one fifth of primigravidae in Aberdeen from 1938 to 1953 had a diagnosis of pregnancy-induced hypertension, of which 18.9% were mild and 4.6% severe. It is widely reported (Redman, 1982) that if a diastolic blood pressure of 90 mmHg is accepted as a threshold of hypertensive disease, one quarter of pregnant women would be so classified. Data from the standard statistical document completed for all discharges from Scottish maternity hospitals in 1988 show 13% of pregnancies complicated by hypertension. This national data set covers virtually all deliveries in Scotland but the criteria for coding the complication of hypertension are not as precisely defined or validated as in a research study. Eclampsia is uncommon and reported by various sources (Redman, 1982) to vary between six to ten cases per 10 000 deliveries. Interpretation of these incidence figures must take into account the problems of definition referred to above.

Prediction

Certain factors are related to the risk of developing pregnancy-induced hypertension. These are widely reported and include primiparity and a history of an affected first pregnancy for women expecting their second child (Campbell et al, 1985). Women with essential hypertension are at increased risk of developing superimposed pre-eclampsia. There is no association with social class, but smoking decreases the risk (Redman, 1982). The incidence is increased in multiple pregnancies. There are no biochemical or other predictive clinical signs of proven value (MacGillivray, 1983) and screening and diagnosis are still mainly dependent on careful determination of blood pressure and proteinuria. Because the known risk factors predict poorly and because many patients who present with pregnancy-induced hypertension have no risk factors at all, it is important to be able to identify patients at the mild to moderate stage and select out those who will have a progressive problem and those who will not (Walker, 1987).

Morbidity and mortality

Mild pregnancy-induced hypertension as defined by Nelson (1955) carries little risk to the fetus or mother other than the risk that the disease will progress to a more severe form (Collins and Wallenburg, 1989). Hypertension associated with proteinuria, however, is associated with a marked increase in the incidence of poor fetal outcome (Wallenburg, 1989). Proteinuric hypertension is associated with growth retardation, birth asphyxia, placental abruption and deaths related to immaturity resulting from early, usually elective, delivery in the maternal interest (Redman, 1982). In the mother, severe hypertension with proteinuria and eclampsia are associated with mortality and morbidity resulting from cerebral complications, renal failure and abruption of the placenta.

Turnbull (1987), reporting trends in maternal mortality in England and Wales, stated that for the 30 years studied, from 1952 to 1981, hypertensive diseases remained one of the four main causes of maternal death. Of 36 such deaths from 1979 to 1981, 20 were associated with eclampsia (the majority due to cerebral haemorrhage, oedema or infarction) and 16 with pre-eclampsia (a quarter from cerebral pathology, a quarter from hepatic pathology and a quarter from cardiac failure or arrest). Hypertension ranked sixth, accounting for two of the 27 direct maternal deaths in the period 1981 to 1985 in Scotland (Scottish Home and Health Departments, 1989). Perinatal mortality during the same period classified to the underlying cause of maternal hypertension varied from 0.5 to 0.9 per 1000, the fourth most common cause of perinatal death after unexplained low birthweight, congenital malformation and antepartum haemorrhage.

TREATMENT

A detailed description of the treatment of pregnancy-induced hypertension is beyond the scope of this chapter. There is no convincing evidence, however, that treatment of mild disease with antihypertensive drugs defers or prevents more severe or progressive disease (Collins and Wallenburg, 1989) and the mainstay of care in these cases is frequent observation. In severe hypertension and proteinuric disease, the clinical consensus would be inpatient surveillance, antihypertensives in the maternal interest, anti-convulsant therapy if eclampsia is believed to be imminent and timed delivery. We are concerned here, however, with the use of outpatient, daycare, domiciliary and inpatient facilities to identify those women whose hypertension requires more intensive supervision and intervention.

OBJECTIVES OF ANTENATAL CARE

Frequent outpatient measurement of blood pressure and testing of urine for protein are an accepted part of routine antenatal care. Women who are found to have mildly elevated blood pressure may be further monitored for signs of more severe or progressive disease, while women who are found to have proteinuria or higher levels of hypertension may be admitted for more intense surveillance or treatment. The efficiency of this antenatal screening would be greatest if transient episodes of hypertension were minimal and if severe disease was preceded by mild hypertension of sufficient duration to be detected during routine antenatal care. In a survey of antenatal care in Aberdeen, Hall et al (1980) and Hall and Chng (1982) reviewed the case notes of 1907 women and found that 190 (10%) developed non-proteinuric and 69 (3.7%) proteinuric hypertension as defined by Nelson (1955). Thirty per cent of these cases (70), however, did not show signs of hypertension before labour and were therefore not detectable by antenatal screening. A further 256 women were found to have transient hypertension only (diastolic blood pressure greater than or equal to 90 mmHg on one occasion only). The ratio of 'false positives' to cases of sustained hypertension detected ante-natally was therefore 1.3 to 1. The problem of transient hypertension increased with increasing gestation; more than half the women with raised blood pressure before 36 weeks were found to have sustained hypertension, while after that gestation transient predominated over sustained hyper-tension. The response to this lack of precision in identifying women who will develop established or progressive disease would appear to be a redoubling of effort rather than an acknowledgement of the unpredictability of the disease or the sudden appearance of severe disease. Hall et al (1980) interpreted their findings in terms of the low productivity of antenatal visits in respect of pregnancy-induced hypertension where it exceeded 1% only after 34 weeks' gestation and only in primigravidae. Wallenburg (1989), though accepting the low productivity, stated that antenatal screening had such high potential for prevention of fetal and maternal mortality that the number of second trimester visits for women in their first pregnancy should actually be increased.

Hepburn (1987) examined the case notes of 1302 women, a random one third of all deliveries during one year in a large maternity hospital, in a study of antenatal complications and their management. The study was specifically concerned with the use of antenatal inpatient beds. One half of the women were admitted on at least one occasion antenatally and the majority of these admissions related to four broad categories of complications: abdominal pain, hypertensive disease (defined as a diastolic blood pressure greater than or equal to 90 mmHg), bleeding and suspected poor fetal growth. All of these conditions shared difficulties in diagnosis as well as in identification of the severity or probable ultimate severity and thus the degree of risk for any particular patient. Of the 1284 women with singleton pregnancies, 262 were hypertensive, 228 having pregnancy-induced hypertension and 34 essential hypertension. Of the 228 women with pregnancy-induced hypertension, 173 (76%) presented with mild hypertension (diastolic blood pressure 90–95 mmHg with no proteinuria) and 163 (72%) presented after 35 weeks' gestation. The ratio of sustained to non-sustained cases increased with increasing severity of presenting hypertension. Thus for all women (analysis by parity was not done in this study) with a presenting hypertension of 90–95 mmHg, 65 out of 173 had subsequent readings which were elevated (27 went on to develop a diastolic blood pressure greater than 95 mmHg). Among women whose initial reading was 96–109 mmHg, 22 out of 37 had subsequent raised blood pressure.

Figure 1 illustrates the course of events for the 173 women who presented with mild hypertension and no proteinuria. Although a larger proportion of those women who developed more sustained and severe hypertension were admitted than those with unsustained or mild hypertension, there were 18 admissions among the non-sustained and 16 among the mild group. This use of inpatient facilities to monitor women reflects the unpredictable course and cautious management of this complication.

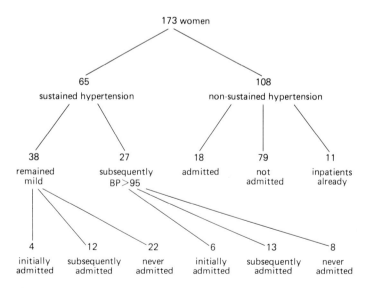

Figure 1. Course of events for 173 women presenting with mild hypertension and no proteinuria (presenting diastolic blood pressure 90–95 mmHg).

Further information on the severity at presentation of hypertension and its progression came from an analysis of women attending daycare after 28 weeks because of a diastolic blood pressure reading greater than 90 mmHg recorded at the antenatal clinic (Walker, 1987). Although the majority of patients remained at the same level of severity of disease as that at the time of their first daycare assessment, this was not always the case. Half of the women finally classified as severe (diastolic blood pressure > 110 mmHg and proteinuria > 0.5 mg/l) were initially less severe, and 7% of the women initially classified as normal progressed to moderate or severe disease. As only percentage figures were given, it is not clear what the numbers studied were.

The use of inpatient facilities to manage hypertension in pregnancy in the four largest Scottish maternity hospitals without daycare facilities is given in Table 1. It is not possible to distinguish between hypertension of different aetiologies or severities when using data from this source, and admissions refer to episodes rather than women. Because the numbers are so far in excess of those expected if only more severe cases were admitted, however, it can be inferred that inpatient beds are used to manage mild cases. These admissions do not include those immediately preceding an induced delivery.

Table 1. Admissions (total and for hypertension) in the four largest Scottish maternity hospitals without daycare.

	Hospital 1		Hospital 2		Hospital 3		Hospital 4	
	1986	1987	1986	1987	1986	1987	1986	1987
Total antenatal inpatient days	3760	3952	10 300	10 487	5287	5299	5139	4264
Antenatal inpatient days for hypertension:								
Number	655	698	1295	1333	1249	1329	639	644
Percentage	17%	18%	12%	13%	24%	25%	12%	15%
Number of admissions for hypertension	237	241	223	208	303	355	176	173
Deliveries	4511	4566	4179	4462	3920	3840	3655	3545

Source of data: Scottish Morbidity Record ad hoc analysis, Information Services Division, Central Services Agency, Scottish Health Service.

Due to the large numbers of women who have transient hypertension and because the progression of mild to more severe forms of the disease is unpredictable, there are large practical and economic consequences associated with the advice, 'when the diastolic pressure is noted to have risen to or above the critical level of 90 mmHg or more in the second half of pregnancy, particularly in a primigravida, it is preferable to admit the woman to hospital for observation and assessment' (MacGillivray, 1983).

As part of the increase in interest in the cost of health care in the United Kingdom, there is a need to evaluate this use of inpatient facilities. In obstetrics, there has been a growth in the use of daycare, which is defined as the use of a designated staffed area to which patients are admitted for observation, monitoring or treatment but from which they are discharged without an overnight stay. It is claimed that the advantage of a daycare assessment unit is that it can exclude women who do not require more intensive monitoring or intervention and it can help to identify patients who are more likely to progress to a more serious form of the disease (Walker, 1987). In a survey of the 24 specialist maternity units in Scotland in 1989, replies from 22 showed that 12 had a designated daycare area. The numbers of admissions varied from 200 to 3883, with assessment of hypertension and fetal monitoring accounting for the majority of admissions.

On clinical grounds, daycare offers advantages over outpatient visits in the supervision of mild hypertension in that it allows repeated blood pressure measurements over a period of time as well as other tests such as cardiotocography and ultrasound examinations not possible during routine antenatal visits. This promise of more thorough assessment of the patient along with the assumption that daycare facilities will reduce costs by avoiding inpatient care has contributed to its growth over the last five years in Scotland.

COST-EFFECTIVE CARE FOR HYPERTENSION IN PREGNANCY

Hypertensive disorders account for a high proportion of inpatient admissions during pregnancy; figures from SMR2 (Table 1) show that between 12 and 24% of all inpatient days in four maternity hospitals in 1986 were a result of this condition. With ever increasing demands on the health service and pressure to reduce or contain health care expenditure, the onus is on finding ways in which to provide equivalent care at a lower cost. This introduces the notion of cost-effectiveness and a need to look at the economic effects of different options of health care provision.

Options for the management of hypertension in pregnancy

Walker (1987) discusses the particular problem associated with hypertension in pregnancy, '. . . that there is not necessarily any progression from the mild to the severe state of the disease'. As a result there can be no single strategy for managing the condition, since there will be a spectrum of severity of hypertension that will present for action. Instead, options will have two elements, one for the care of those with non-progressive disease and another for managing those who progress to severe hypertension. Options for the first element include inpatient care, additional antenatal clinics, a daycare facility, additional general practitioner care, midwife clinics, and domiciliary midwife visits. It is assumed that those with severe or proteinuric hypertension will always be managed as inpatients. In brief, not only is there a spectrum of severity of illness but a spectrum of care options as well.

It is the intention of this section to look at the economic implications of alternatives to inpatient care, with particular regard to Scottish evidence on daycare and domiciliary care in the management of hypertension in pregnancy. A study, currently in progress in two centres in Scotland, is described, along with a discussion of relevant economic issues.

Cost-effectiveness

It is necessary to be clear about the definition of cost-effectiveness. Cost-effectiveness requires that at least two options be compared and the choice of option is based on the lowest cost per unit of outcome. Thus, if we were comparing two ways of managing a given life-threatening condition, such as surgery and drug therapy, then the cost-effective solution would be the alternative that costs the least per life year gained.

The particular form of economic analysis utilized in other studies of daycare is cost minimization analysis, defined by Evans (1980) in the following manner: 'If alternatives to inpatient care are equivalent or superior to inpatient care in their impact on patient health status and satisfaction, then comparing the costs of a care episode provided in the different settings will serve as a conservative estimate of the advantages of such alternatives.' Thus, this requires that outcomes between the two forms of care be equivalent in their impact on health status, an argument that has been advanced for the introduction of daycare.

In all forms of economic evaluation it is necessary to measure both costs and outcomes. Ideally, a societal viewpoint would be adopted when identifying costs and consequences, including the implications for all members of society. This is not possible in most studies however, and instead it is necessary to identify the most important effects of the alternatives and measure these. In looking at various ways of managing hypertension in pregnancy there will be effects on the health service in terms of bed requirements, staff, etc., and effects on the clients of the service. For each group there will be both benefits, such as successful outcomes of pregnancies, reduced requirements for inpatient beds, etc., and costs, both of providing and of using the service.

Evidence of the cost-effectiveness of daycare

There is no published evidence on the cost-effectiveness of daycare in obstetrics; this may reflect its recent introduction into obstetric hospitals. The literature on daycare falls into three main areas: (a) data from daycase surgery; (b) information on day hospitals for the elderly and for rehabilitation; and (c) other forms of daycare. To highlight the most important issues a brief review of these three areas is included below.

Daycase surgery

The studies considered are: Russell et al (1977) in a randomized controlled trial (RCT) of daycare for hernias and haemorrhoids, Prescott et al (1978) in an RCT of daycare for hernias and varicose veins, Evans and Robinson (1980) in a quasi-controlled comparison of the costs of hospital care for medically similar conditions, Pineault et al (1985) in an RCT of daycase surgery for three conditions, and Watts and Pearce (1988) in a study of 40 cataract operations performed as daycase surgery. These all show that potential savings are possible for a majority of the conditions, but that this is only the case if prior selection of patients takes place. This reflects the fact that at least part of the 'savings' result from the caring function of the hospital being transferred to the family or friends of the patient. Another recurrent theme is that potential cost savings can only be realized if the beds freed by a move to daycase surgery are closed with staff numbers falling rather than being redeployed. As one study comments, '. . . as long as facilities exist for inpatient management then their disuse does not offer immediate savings' (Watts and Pearce, 1988). Haworth and Balarajan (1987) address this issue in their review of the evidence in one hospital for four years before and after the introduction of a daycare facility to examine the relationship between inpatient and daycase surgery. They showed that daycare rose from 1.8% to 26.8% of the total surgery, but this was super-imposed on a stable operation and discharge rate. This implies a rise in the total amount of care delivered. The increase in daycare was only associated with a fall in inpatient care for two procedures. The authors conclude that part of the increase in daycase surgery results from a transfer from out-patient surgery, but there is no data available on this matter.

Day hospitals for elderly or rehabilitation patients

The studies considered are MacFarlane et al (1979), Kaplan (1981), Anand et al (1982) and Gerard (1988). In these studies cost-effectiveness is much more difficult to prove than with daycase surgery because of the lack of a single outcome measure upon which to base a comparison. Similarly, costing proves a problem, mainly because of the confusion about which costs should be included, a point which is thoroughly discussed by Hildrick-Smith (1984). The main conclusion from the papers, however, is that cost savings are possible with day hospital care.

Other experiences of daycare

Other forms of daycare have been discussed in the literature, notably daycare for adult diabetics, but there has been no economic component to this. A recent paper on daycare for oncology patients has some economic input. In an RCT of day hospital care for selected adult cancer patients, Mor et al (1988) demonstrate a statistically significant reduction in cost associated with the day unit compared with inpatient care. This is explained both by a reduction in the number of treatment days and by a lower overall cost of treatment in the unit. The study showed no significant difference in outcome and thus concludes that the day unit is cost-effective. Furthermore, sufficient data was available to permit the conclusion that 'hospital cost savings are not offset by higher social costs borne by the family'.

The literature review shows that all forms of daycare can produce potential cost savings when care is transferred from inpatient to daycare. Whether these savings can actually be realized, however, is subject to many factors. Daycare in the management of pregnancy hypertension differs from the cases discussed in the literature in several respects such that extrapolation of the published conclusions is not valid. Daycare for hypertension in pregnancy is not simply a 'one-off' procedure as in daycase surgery; a patient may require several visits to the unit. Outcomes in day surgery i.e. the successful completion of the procedure, are simpler to measure. In the management of pregnancy hypertension, however, the outcome measured is the health and well-being of the mother and baby, which is more difficult to define. In contrast to daycare of the elderly, the amount of care required by any patient is constrained to last a maximum of forty plus weeks; thus the evidence from day hospitals proves fairly limited. Daycare for pregnancy hypertension is unique in that it operates as a form of screening and hence repeated testing of patients is carried out. A reduction in the total number of tests, as compared with inpatient management, is therefore unlikely. In conclusion, the literature on daycare identifies areas of importance, particularly the problems associated with realization of potential savings, but gives little indication of the relative cost-effectiveness of daycare in pregnancy hypertension.

Study description

Although there has been no formal study of the economic impact of daycare for hypertension in pregnancy, it is a widely held belief that it is cost-effective. This belief appears to be an extrapolation from other forms of daycare, even though there are essential differences, as discussed above. Ideally, of course, the economic evaluation would be part of a randomized controlled trial and would precede widespread introduction into the service. In fact, daycare has been growing as an option in obstetrics, and the study design to assess its economic consequences was based on a descriptive comparison of two centres. The two hospitals chosen were Glasgow Royal Maternity, which has had a daycare facility since 1981 but still provides inpatient care for those with severe hypertension, and Aberdeen Maternity, which utilizes a domiciliary midwife service as a secondary screening facility for women who have raised blood pressure and inpatient care for those for whom it is sustained or who have proteinuria. Both centres are similar in numbers of births, teaching hospital status, incidence and treatment of hypertension.

The study aim was to consider the economic consequences of having daycare as an option in the monitoring of hypertension in pregnancy. These economic consequences will be discussed on two levels. First, what is the cost per woman of managing comparable cases of hypertension using daycare or a combination of inpatient care and home visits by a midwife, and second, what are the total costs of managing women with hypertension in a centre with and without daycare facilities?

To answer the first question, comparable groups of women had to be identified at each centre who would be considered suitable for management in daycare. The theoretical guidelines for this group were formulated by the clinicians involved in the study, based on blood pressure measurements and the presence of proteinuria at any time during the entire pregnancy. Only readings of 90 mmHg or above would be considered when grouping was decided. The groups were defined as follows:

1. *Daycare only*: Diastolic blood pressure of 90–99 mmHg, no significant proteinuria. (From this point onwards this group will be referred to as the daycare group, although technically in Aberdeen this should be the 'potential daycare' group.)
2. *Inpatient care only*: Diastolic blood pressure of 100 mmHg or above or significant proteinuria. It is assumed that a woman in this group would be managed as an inpatient regardless of the availability of daycare facilities.
3. *Mixed care*: Those who during their pregnancy were in both groups at some stage.

Thus, a woman with a single reading of 95 would be in the daycare group and one with a single reading of 105 would be in the inpatient group. A woman with a reading of 95 at one point and of 105 at another point would be in the mixed care group.

Study recruitment consisted of 100 consecutive first-time daycare attenders in Glasgow, plus 92 consecutive inpatients admitted for hypertension. Since these groups are not mutually exclusive this resulted in a total of 175 women. In Aberdeen 99 consecutive inpatients and 22 domiciliary patients were recruited during the study period, giving a total of 121 women. Of these, 12 women in Glasgow and six women in Aberdeen were excluded because their diastolic blood pressure never reached 90 mmHg, or because their hypertension only appeared when they were in labour and could not thus be said to constitute an antenatal problem. The groupings of the women at both Glasgow and Aberdeen are shown in Figure 2. From Figure 2 it can be seen

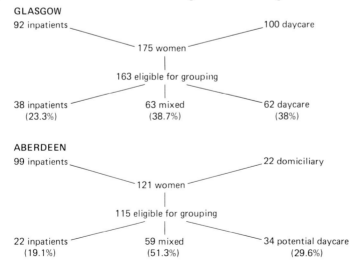

Figure 2. Distribution by theoretical group of study members in Glasgow and Aberdeen.

that the group considered suitable for daycare management has 62 members in Glasgow and 34 in Aberdeen. We will first consider, for this group, both the outcomes and the resources used by each woman during her pregnancy for all hypertension-related care in Aberdeen and in Glasgow Royal Maternity. The groups in the two centres were compared for age, parity, obstetric and medical history, and social class. As was discussed above, if outcomes were found to be achieved to the same degree by the two options then the appropriate form of economic evaluation is cost minimization.

Data collection was retrospective, with the main source of information being the patient case record. Hypertension-related care was defined as being all admissions, daycare attendances, domiciliary midwife visits and tests, such as ultrasound, where the sole or major reason for instigation was a raised blood pressure recording or the presence of proteinuria. Any procedures that were carried out for research purposes were recorded but will not be included as part of the main resource implications. Additionally, admissions for antepartum haemorrhage, after a diagnosis of hypertension had been made, were included because of the strong association between the two conditions. Furthermore, women were asked to complete questionnaires at daycare, during domiciliary visits and during inpatient stays about the costs they had incurred, including travel, time and childcare costs. Data was coded and analysed using a spreadsheet package and the Statistical Package for the Social Sciences Personal Computer (SPSSPC).

The final results of the study will be presented as average cost per pregnancy for each group in each centre. As costings have not been ascertained at this stage, resource consumption, e.g. number of inpatient days, number of cardiotocographs (CTGs) and ultrasounds, will be compared in this interim discussion.

Interim results for daycare groups

Groups description. The groups in the two centres were compared for age, parity, hypertension in a previous pregnancy, number of hospital antenatal clinic attendances and mode of delivery. None of these were found to be significantly different. There were very few chronic medical conditions. The conclusion from this description is that there is no significant difference between the two daycare groups.

Outcomes. Comparisons of outcomes between the two centres based on singleton-only births reduces the sample size in Glasgow to 61 women, but leaves the number in Aberdeen unchanged. As has been noted before, for cost minimization to be appropriate outcomes must be the same under the two options.

The outcome measures used for comparing the two groups were birthweight, proportion of low birthweight babies, i.e. those less than 2500 g, gestation at delivery, Apgar scores at one and five minutes, complication rate, and necessity for admission to the special care unit. Table 2 summarizes the results.

Outcomes were compared between the two centres and none were found

Table 2. Measures of outcome.

	Aberdeen	Glasgow
Mean birthweight	3420 g	3520 g
Birthweight < 2500 g	2	0
Gestation at delivery (weeks)	40	39.5
Mean Apgars	8.4/9.5	8.0/9.5*
Complications	0	2
Admissions to SCBU	2	3

* Excludes an outlier with Apgars of 0 and 0, following a delivery complicated by shoulder dystocia.
SCBU = special care baby unit.

to be significantly different. Thus, it is acceptable to proceed with a cost minimization analysis.

Resource implications. The resource use associated with the two groups is shown in Table 3. The average figures can be interpreted as the expected number of each resource consumed by a woman in each centre.

To give some idea of the relative resource use, a brief description of what happens during daycare and domiciliary visits is useful. A visit to daycare generally lasts about five hours. Blood pressure is measured five times, urinalysis is performed and samples for biochemistry and haematology testing are taken. All patients are reviewed by an obstetrician. CTGs and ultrasound examinations are used where appropriate. The patients receive lunch.

The domiciliary visit, of approximately 20 minutes, is made by a midwife to check blood pressure and perform urinalysis. If the blood pressure remains raised, or protein is present, then the midwife will refer the patient

Table 3. Total and average resource use by groups of women suitable for daycare.

	Aberdeen total	Glasgow total	Aberdeen average	Glasgow average
Number of women	34	62	—	—
Domiciliary visits	89	0	2.6	—
Daycare visits	0	126	—	2.0
CTGs at daycare	0	89	—	1.4
USGs at daycare	0	93	—	1.5
Hypertensive admissions	18	6	0.5	0.1
Inpatient days	55	25	1.6	0.4
Inductions for raised BP	9	13		
Inpatient tests				
FBC	17	7	0.9	0.1
Clotting screens	3	0	0.08	0
Clinical chemistry	15	6	0.8	0.1
MSSU	7	2	0.5	0.03
USG	1	2	0.03	0.03
CTG	26	14	1.4	0.2
24-hour urine	0	6	0	0.1

CTG = cardiotocograph; USG = ultrasonograph; BP = blood pressure; FBC = full blood count; MSSU = mid-stream specimen of urine.

for inpatient care. This contrasts with daycare where if the pressure is still raised the woman will be asked to return to daycare, although if significant protein or severe hypertension is present she will be admitted.

Based on existing knowledge of NHS costs, the single most expensive element above is the inpatient day. Glasgow is more cost-effective if 1.6–0.4 inpatient days + 2.6 domiciliary visits is more expensive than two daycare visits. Preliminary results indicate that this is the case, implying that Glasgow has the more cost-effective system when hospital costs per patient are considered. There will be a point, however, at which there will be no difference between the costs of the two options or indeed where the Glasgow approach would become more expensive if the average number of admissions and daycare visits were to rise. In the final evaluation a sensitivity analysis will be conducted to check the robustness of the final result to these figures.

On the assumption that the daycare and inpatient approach is more cost-effective per patient than the domiciliary and inpatient approach, does this allow the conclusion that a move to daycare represents an overall cost-effective use of resources? This depends on many factors which will be discussed below.

Discussion

Even with the implication that Glasgow is more cost-effective on a cost per patient basis, this alone can say little about the final 'savings' from adopting daycare elsewhere for several reasons: (a) any cost generated will be the 'steady state' cost of systems that are already in operation, (b) the criteria defined for the groups might not actually apply in practice, (c) the existence of a daycare unit may generate additional non-inpatient workload, and (d) the inpatient beds freed by daycare may not be closed but used for other purposes. It is important that these factors be considered in some depth as their existence will lead to an erosion of the potential savings.

The problem of using two systems which have been in operation for some time, such as is the case in this study, is that there will be no indication of the 'upheaval' costs associated with moving from one option to another. The inpatient beds freed could be used for daycare patients, but most financial benefits of daycare arise from the reduced requirement for 24-hour nursing; nursing costs are the single largest element in hospital costs. In order to obtain this reduction, a separate unit is required, capable of being closed at nights and weekends. This has resulted in purpose-built units being opened or the conversion of whole wards, as was the case in Glasgow Royal Maternity. There will be no measure, therefore, of the type of costs expected in conversion, which will have an effect on any predicted savings in the short term. The difference in cost per woman between the two systems must thus be taken as a maximum estimate of the potential savings that could arise by moving from one system to the other.

Inclusion in the daycare only group required that the woman's diastolic blood pressure never rose above 99 mmHg during her entire pregnancy, and she had no significant proteinuria. The above analysis assumes that practice follows theoretical guidelines and that women with a diastolic blood pressure less than 90 mmHg or that women with more severe forms of hypertension are not managed in daycare (in the latter case the outcome side of the cost analysis may not remain the same). In the Glasgow daycare group, six of the 62 theoretical members were admitted for raised blood pressure, and hence are actually in the mixed care group. Similarly, there are some members of both the theoretical mixed and inpatient groups who, in practice, were seen only in daycare. The data above illustrates that the guidelines do not hold strictly in practice and thus, once again, it is important to stress that any estimated savings will be the maximum possible.

Whether or not the existence of a daycare unit actually generates its own demand was the question addressed by Haworth and Balarajan (1987). For this to be the case in Glasgow, more women would have to receive attention, in this case a visit to daycare, than would be the case if there was solely an inpatient facility. Likewise there may be some demand generated by the domiciliary service. Some data is available on this, arising from the manner in which the study members were recruited. In Glasgow there were ten women who were referred to daycare having never had a diastolic measurement of 90 mmHg nor any proteinuria, and in Aberdeen there were four such women. The reason for the care these women received was given as 'hypertension' in all cases. Thus, it would appear that at least some of the workload associated with both the daycare unit and the domiciliary midwife service arises because of its mere existence. From SMR2 data (Table 4) we can see the change in inpatient admissions for hypertension after the establishment of a daycare facility in two large Scottish maternity hospitals. There was a decrement in inpatient days of 1156 which accompanied the addition of 2072 day admissions for hypertension, but there remains a significant number of inpatient days attributed to this complication. To look at this more thoroughly would require a 'before and after study' of the introduction of a daycare unit. This has been undertaken at the Queen Mother's Hospital in Glasgow, the conclusion being that 'the PADU (Pregnancy Assessment Day Unit) has increased the overall hospital workload despite decreasing the number of days each patient is admitted' (McGregor, 1987). Once again

Table 4. Inpatient bed use for hypertension following the introduction of a daycare facility in two large Scottish maternity hospitals.

	Hospital 5			Hospital 6		
	Births	Daycare admissions	Inpatient days	Births	Daycare admissions	Inpatient days
1980	3817	0	1066			
1981	3733	45	1197			
1982	3585	110	921			
1983	3937	331	776			
1984	3991	779	790			
1985	4233	951	736	3595	4	1140
1986	4301	1134	370	3642	285	958
1987	4308	1059	434	3468	1013	616

Source of data: SMR2 ad hoc analysis, Information Services Division.

this will have an effect on any potential savings.

A crucial aspect of estimating the potential savings associated with a change in policy is the use made of the resources freed. If fully-staffed beds are not closed and staff levels reduced, then the potential savings will be completely erased. Another option is to redeploy the beds for other uses, either in obstetrics or in other specialties. This would, however, require a separate evaluation of the benefits associated with the change.

We thus reiterate that the study will estimate the maximum potential savings; this will be reduced by any or all of the above factors.

Women's costs and views

Costs to women. Data on the cost to women of attending the different care settings has been collected. There will be time costs, including travel and lost work or leisure time, travel costs such as bus fares, and childcare costs for multiparous women. This data was collected to elicit whether the lower health service costs associated with a daycare facility arise alongside higher costs to women.

Women's views. This too is a vitally important component. It has been illustrated above that in medical terms outcomes are the same between the two centres. It may be, however, that women prefer to be inpatients and by concentrating solely on medical outcomes we are ignoring other benefits to the women. This is especially important if a higher cost to women is found to be associated with one of the options. In centres where the women actually have a choice of where they receive their care, this would not be a problem since their 'revealed preference', the mode of care they choose, is assumed to be the result of an informed decision, encompassing the woman's perceptions of all costs and benefits. Thus, if the woman were to choose a location which is more costly in time and travel terms, this implies her perceived benefit is at least equal to the cost involved. Analysis of women's costs and views will be available in the final report of the study.

Conclusion

The preliminary results of the study appear to indicate that daycare is a cost-effective option for the care of women with non-proteinuric mild hypertension when compared with a package of domiciliary and inpatient care. However, this is based on resource use and not on actual costs. There is also as yet no indication of the effect that a daycare policy has on costs to women.

One finding of the study is the similarity of outcomes under the two settings, which suggests that daycare is at least as efficacious as inpatient care for this particular group of women.

The above results, however, do not actually imply that there will be cost savings associated with a move to daycare for the NHS. The realization of any potential savings depends on several factors, the most important of which is the use to which any freed resources will be put.

SUMMARY

Frequent measurement of blood pressure is an accepted part of routine outpatient antenatal care. Women found to have mild hypertension may be further monitored for signs of progressive disease, while women with proteinuria or severe hypertension may be admitted for more intensive surveillance or treatment. In practice, the course and ultimate severity of this disorder are unpredictable and women with mild hypertension are frequently admitted. Recently, daycare has grown as an option for assessing women with hypertension as it offers the advantage of more extensive evaluation than is possible at an outpatient clinic and is widely assumed to be more cost-effective than conventional management. However, its use in obstetrics has not been subject to a formal economic appraisal. Such an evaluation is currently being carried out in two hospitals in Scotland, one of which uses daycare and inpatient admissions in the management of hypertension and one of which uses domiciliary midwife visits as well as hospital beds. Preliminary results suggest that the pregnancy outcome in terms of birthweight, gestation at delivery, admission to a special unit, etc., are the same in the two units for women with mild hypertension (diastolic 90–99 mmHg, no proteinuria). The costs per patient were less in the hospital with a daycare unit. These lower individual costs, however, do not mean that the overall costs to the health service are less in a hospital with daycare. This will depend on the average number of visits to daycare for women with mild hypertension, the proportion of hypertensive women receiving daycare, whether freed inpatient beds are closed or redeployed, and the capital costs of establishing a day unit. Data has also been collected on women's costs and views which will ultimately be presented and should play a part in any decision to implement or continue daycare.

Acknowledgements

Sara Twaddle is supported by the Health Services Research Committee, Chief Scientist's Office, Scottish Home and Health Department. The authors thank Dr Valerie Harper, Sister Helen Cheyne and Dr Susan Cole for their assistance, and Dr Gillian McIlwaine for her helpful comments on earlier drafts of this chapter.

REFERENCES

Anand KB, Thomas JH, Osborne KL & Osmolski R (1982) Cost and effectiveness of a geriatric day hospital. *Journal of the Royal College of Physicians of London* **16:** 53–56.
Baird D (1977) Epidemiological aspects of hypertensive pregnancy. *Clinics in Obstetrics and Gynaecology* **4:** 531–547.
Campbell DM, MacGillivray I & Carrhill R (1985) Pre-eclampsia in a second pregnancy. *British Journal of Obstetrics and Gynaecology* **92:** 131–140.
Cole S (1981) Scottish maternity and neonatal records. In Chalmers I & McIlwaine GM (eds) *Perinatal Audit and Surveillance.* Proceedings of the Eighth Study Group of the Royal College of Obstetricians and Gynaecologists.
Collins R & Wallenburg HCS (1989) Pharmacological prevention and treatment of hypertensive disorders in pregnancy. In Chalmers I, Enkin M & Keirse MJNC (eds) *Effective Care in Pregnancy*, pp 512–533. Oxford: Oxford University Press.

Evans RG (1980) Alternatives to traditional care at Children's Hospital, Vancouver: the economic studies of cost savings. In Robinson GC & Clarke HF (eds) *The Hospital Care of Children*, pp 170–196. New York: Oxford University Press.

Evans RG & Robinson GC (1980) Surgical day care: measurements of the economic payoff. *Canadian Medical Association Journal* **123:** 873–880.

Gerard K (1988) An appraisal of the cost-effectiveness of alternative day care settings for frail elderly people. *Age and Ageing* **17:** 311–318.

Hall M & Chng PK (1982) Antenatal care in practice. In Enkin M & Chalmers I (eds) *Effectiveness and Satisfaction in Antenatal Care*, pp 60–68. London: Spastics International Medical Publications/William Heinemann Medical Books.

Hall M & Campbell D (1987) Geographical epidemiology of hypertension in pregnancy. In Sharp F & Symonds EM (eds) *Hypertension in Pregnancy*. Proceedings of the Sixteenth Study Group of the Royal College of Obstetricians and Gynaecologists, pp 33–50. New York: Perinatology Press.

Hall M, Chng PK & MacGillivray I (1980) Is routine antenatal care worthwhile? *Lancet* **ii:** 78–80.

Haworth EA & Balarajan R (1987) Day surgery: does it add to or replace inpatient surgery? *British Medical Journal* **294:** 133–135.

Hepburn M (1987) *The role of antenatal inpatient care in obstetric practice*. MD thesis, University of Edinburgh.

Hildrick-Smith M (1984) Geriatric day hospitals—changing emphasis in costs. *Age and Ageing* **13:** 95–100.

Kaplan M (1981) Day care experiment proves cost-effective. *Hospitals* **55:** 101–104.

Kerr JMM (1933) *Maternal Mortality and Morbidity. A Study of Their Problems*. London: WB Saunders.

Leading article (1934) Eclampsia and antenatal care. *Lancet* **ii:** 364–365.

MacFarlane JPR, Collings T, Graham K & MacIntosh JC (1979) Day hospitals in modern clinical practice—cost benefit. *Age and Ageing* **8 (supplement):** 80–86.

MacGillivray I (1983) *Pre-eclampsia: the Hypertensive Disease of Pregnancy*. London: WB Saunders.

McGregor EM (1987) *An assessment of day care management in obstetric practice*. Undergraduate project, University of Glasgow.

Memorandum 145/MCW Ministry of Health (1929) *Maternal Mortality in Childbirth. Antenatal Clinics: Their Conduct and Scope*. London: HMSO.

Mor V, Stalker MS, Gralla R et al (1988) Day hospital as an alternative to inpatient care for cancer patients: a random assignment trial. *Journal of Clinical Epidemiology* **41:** 771–785.

Murnaghan GA (1987) Methods of measuring blood pressure variability. In Sharp F & Symonds EM (eds) *Hypertension in Pregnancy*. Proceedings of the Sixteenth Study Group of the Royal College of Obstetricians and Gynaecologists, pp 19–28. New York: Perinatology Press.

Nelson TR (1955) A clinical study of pre-eclampsia. *Journal of Obstetrics and Gynaecology of the British Empire* **62:** 48–66.

Oakley A (1982) The origins and development of antenatal care. In Enkin M & Chalmers I (eds) *Effectiveness and Satisfaction in Antenatal Care*, pp 1–21. London: Spastics International Medical Publications/William Heinemann Medical Books.

Pineault R, Contandriopoulos AP, Valois M, Bastian ML & Lance JM (1985) Randomized clinical trial of one-day surgery. *Medical Care* **23:** 171–182.

Prescott RJ, Cuthbertson C, Fenwick N, Garroway WM & Ruckley CV (1978) Economic aspects of day care after operations for hernia or varicose veins. *Journal of Epidemiology and Community Health* **32:** 222–225.

Redman C (1982) Screening for pre-eclampsia. In Enkin M & Chalmers I (eds) *Effectiveness and Satisfaction in Antenatal Care*, pp 69–80. London: Spastics International Medical Publications/William Heinemann Medical Books.

Redman C (1987) The definition of pre-eclampsia. In Sharp F & Symonds EM (eds) *Hypertension in Pregnancy*. Proceedings of the Sixteenth Study Group of the Royal College of Obstetricians and Gynaecologists, pp 3–13. New York: Perinatology Press.

Russell IT, Devlin HB, Fell M, Glass NJ & Newell DJ (1977) Day-case surgery for hernias and haemorrhoids. *Lancet* **i:** 844–847.

Scottish Home and Health Department (1989) *Report on Maternal and Perinatal Deaths in Scotland*. Edinburgh: HMSO.

Turnbull AC (1987) Maternal mortality and present trends. In Sharp F & Symonds EM (eds) *Hypertension in Pregnancy*. Proceedings of the Sixteenth Study Group of the Royal College of Obstetricians and Gynaecologists, pp 135–144. New York: Perinatology Press.

Walker JJ (1987) The case for early recognition and intervention in pregnancy-induced hypertension. In Sharp F & Symonds EM (eds) *Hypertension in Pregnancy*. Proceedings of the Sixteenth Study Group of the Royal College of Obstetricians and Gynaecologists, pp 289–299. New York: Perinatology Press.

Wallenburg HCS (1989) Detecting hypertensive disorders of pregnancy. In Chalmers I, Enkin M & Keirse MJNC (eds) *Effective Care in Pregnancy*, pp 382–402. Oxford: Oxford University Press.

Watts MT & Pearce JL (1988) Day-case cataract surgery. *British Journal of Ophthalmology* **72:** 897–899.

7

Multiple pregnancy

DORIS M. CAMPBELL

INCIDENCE

In reviewing the antenatal management of multiple pregnancies it is relevant to consider twin pregnancies separately from higher multiples. Throughout the world, the prevalence of twin births varies considerably, with low rates of between 2 and 7 per 1000 in Hawaii, Japan and Taiwan, an intermediate prevalence between 9 and 20 per 1000 in Europe and many of the African, American and Asian countries, and a particularly high prevalence in parts of Africa, particularly Nigeria, the Seychelles, Transvaal and Zimbabwe, and American countries into which migration from West Africa has occurred, with twinning rates in excess of 20 per 1000 births. Most of the geographical variation in twin births is considered to be due to the variation in dizygotic twinning rates, with monozygotic twinning rates being remarkably constant at around 3.5 per 1000 maternities (Little and Thompson, 1988).

With respect to higher multiple pregnancy rates, Hellin's Rule (Hellin, 1895), namely the frequency of higher multiple births may be expressed as a power function of the twinning rate, has been shown to be applicable in most places throughout the world for naturally occurring multiple pregnancies. Recently, however, the use of ovulation-inducing drugs such as clomiphene or gonadotrophins and assisted reproductive programmes have greatly increased higher multiple pregnancy rates, the incidence of higher multiple births increasing with the number of embryos replaced in in vitro fertilization programmes.

OUTCOME

Multiple pregnancy is recognized as having an increased risk for both maternal and fetal morbidity and mortality (Newton, 1986). The increase in pregnancy complications, in particular pre-eclampsia, antepartum and postpartum haemorrhage, along with problems during labour and delivery are frequently associated with increased maternal morbidity and occasionally mortality. Perinatal mortality is much higher in twins than in singletons and is even greater for higher multiples (Campbell and MacGillivray, 1988a). The perinatal mortality rate in most studies is four to five times greater in twin pregnancies compared with singleton pregnancies. This is perhaps not surprising in view of the increased incidence of complications of pregnancy, early delivery and relatively low birthweight. When the causes of perinatal death in twin pregnancy are examined in detail, the complications of early delivery account for between two thirds and three quarters of all baby deaths (Ellis et al, 1979; Medearis et al, 1979; Patel et al, 1984; Campbell and MacGillivray, 1988a). For these reasons, antenatal care in multiple pregnancy requires additional surveillance over and above that which is routine in singleton pregnancy.

DIAGNOSIS OF MULTIPLE PREGNANCY

The diagnosis of twin pregnancy is now generally made by ultrasonic scanning after clinical suspicion. In cases of greater multiples, however, ultrasonic examination may not detect all the fetuses because of their mobility in early gestation and because of fetal shadowing of one fetus by another in late pregnancy. Radiography can confirm the number of fetuses from mid-pregnancy onwards.

The diagnosis of multiple pregnancy as soon as possible is important, not only because of the greater frequency and early onset of complications compared with a singleton pregnancy, but also to assist in the accurate assessment of gestational age. Early diagnosis is also important so that arrangements can be made for booking for delivery in a specialist centre equipped to deal with twin deliveries and their neonatal care.

Failure to diagnose multiple pregnancy can lead to serious problems for both mothers and babies. In the United States of America it is estimated that 12–20% of twin pregnancies are identified after the onset of labour (Newton, 1986). This rate of undiagnosed twins prior to labour is higher, however, than that quoted by the Scottish Twin Study (Patel et al, 1984), where the total population of 650 twin pregnancies for Scotland in 1983 were reviewed and 95% were diagnosed antenatally.

Ultrasonic scanning

Although altogether 559 (86%) of the twin pregnancies in the Scottish Twin Study (Patel et al, 1984) were confirmed by ultrasound, 44 of these were not identified at the first scan. When the ultrasonic scan was carried out before 12 weeks, 28 out of 128 twin pregnancies (21.9%) were not diagnosed, whereas when the scan was after 20 weeks, only two out of 68 (2.9%) were missed.

Routine ultrasonic scanning at booking has been advocated for all pregnant women with several aims, one of which is the identification of twin or multiple pregnancy. This is unlikely to detect all multiple pregnancies as the gestation at time of scanning/booking may not be optimal to the diagnosis of multiple pregnancy, and twin pregnancy may be missed when one fetus of appropriate size for gestation is seen and the ultrasonographer does not look for a second.

Clinical signs and symptoms

It is still important therefore to look out for other clinical evidence of multiple pregnancies. The most notable feature is the greater size of the uterus in multiple pregnancy compared with singleton pregnancy, but clinical suspicion of multiple pregnancy should be aroused by increased weekly rate of weight gain, particularly in the first half of pregnancy, and by abdominal palpation when a suspiciously large number of fetal parts may be found. Additionally, sometimes a head is clearly felt which seems to be small in relation to the size of the uterus.

Clinical suspicion may also be aroused by the demonstration of two fetal hearts by Doppler ultrasound, when a difference of ten beats per minute between two fetal hearts is suggestive of twin pregnancy. Maternal perception of size and indication of more movements (Malmstrom and Malmstrom, 1988) or unexpected anaemia or increase in nausea or vomiting in early pregnancy may also lead the obstetrician to consider multiple pregnancy. Ultrasonic scanning can then be used to confirm a diagnosis with safety.

Hormone levels

Because of the increased placental and fetal mass in multiple pregnancies, higher levels of pregnancy hormones are found in plasma. The determination of human chorionic gonadotrophin, human placental lactogen and serum α-fetoprotein have all been claimed to be useful in the early detection of multiple pregnancies (Grennert et al, 1976; Vandekerckhove et al 1984). When these are considered separately, human placental lactogen appears to be the most useful indicator of multiple gestation, identifying approximately 95% of multiple pregnancies. Vandekerckhove et al (1984) found that when all three hormones were considered together, all twin pregnancies were detected between 14 and 24 weeks of pregnancy.

Routine screening programmes for the identification of patients with neural tube defects by maternal serum α-fetoprotein between 16 and 18 weeks is practised in many centres. This will identify a significant number of twins at that gestation. Thom et al (1984) considered 88 twin pairs identified from such a screening programme: only 36 had a mean serum α-fetoprotein concentration of more than twice the multiple of the median, and 52 out of the 88 twin pregnancies (59%) would not have been identified by this means.

Conclusion

In summary, while routine screening programmes such as ultrasonic scanning and hormone measurements would detect the majority of twin pregnancies, some will be missed and it is important for the clinician to be alert to the detection of multiple pregnancy later in gestation.

FETAL ABNORMALITIES

Problems in multiple pregnancies

Congenital anomalies in multiple births provide a wider range of problems than those in singleton births. If more than one of the infants is affected, parents have to care for more than one handicapped child. If, as is more common, only one child is affected, the parents have to cope with balancing their attention between children of the same age but with different mental and physical needs.

Recent advances in prenatal diagnosis have created new opportunities but have also posed new problems for women expecting twins. Selective intra-uterine killing of the abnormal fetus, known as selective fetocide or selective birth, is a technique that is now available but the risks to the surviving twin when such a procedure is performed have not yet been evaluated. Careful counselling is therefore important for all parents before they embark on prenatal diagnosis for fetal anomalies when a multiple pregnancy is present. They must be clearly aware of the options available to them if one fetus is found to be abnormal, i.e. the continuation of the pregnancy, termination of the pregnancy or selective fetocide.

The risks of a particular abnormality are different in multiple pregnancy (Little and Bryan, 1986, 1988). In the majority of the studies reviewed by Little and Bryan, malformations were found to be commoner in twins than in singletons. Some of the differences in prevalence rates of anomalies associated with multiple births relate to difficulties in ascertainment of anomalies, length and detail of follow-up, and obtaining the appropriate control population.

Anomalies specific to multiple births

Some abnormalities occur only with multiple pregnancy. These include acardia, fetus-in-fetu and conjoined twins. However, these are very rare: acardia, which only occurs with monochorionic placentation, has been estimated at about one in 35 000 births or one in 100 monozygotic twins (Little and Bryan, 1988). It has been noted to occur more frequently in triplet pregnancy (James, 1978; Schinzel et al, 1979). The prevalence of conjoined twins resulting from very late and imperfect division of the embryo has been quoted at one in 200 monozygotic twins (Hanson, 1975). Again, triplet pregnancy carries an increased risk of this condition (Schinzel et al, 1979).

In the past, the diagnosis of such monsters was rarely made antepartum and outcome was very poor. Ultrasonic scanning of multiple pregnancy has the potential to improve this by earlier detection, allowing for appropriate perinatal management after careful counselling of the patients (D'Alton and Dudley, 1986). There are several reports in the literature of such cases (Filler, 1986).

Abnormalities not specific to multiple pregnancy

Abnormalities that have been noted to be increased in twin pregnancies

(Kallen, 1986) include neural tube defects, in particular anencephaly and hydrocephalus, cardiac defects (Burn and Corney, 1984), gut atresias and kidney malformation (Little and Bryan, 1986).

With respect to chromosomal abnormalities, Down's syndrome does not occur more commonly in twin pregnancy (MacGillivray, 1975) and may even be decreased in like sex twinning (Hay and Wehrung, 1970; Layde et al, 1980; Windham and Bjerkedal, 1984), even in women of the older age group. On the other hand, disorders of the sex chromosomes (Turner's and Klinefelter's syndromes) seem in excess in multiple births (Little and Bryan, 1988).

Concordance

Risks

The chances of both twins having a congenital anomaly, either the same or different, are small. Even when twin fetuses have been exposed to teratogens such as drugs, intrauterine infections or alcohol, discordance for anomalies has often been reported (Little and Bryan, 1988). Such differences may be due to differences in the susceptibility of individual fetuses to insults, perhaps due to upset in the blood supplies or to slightly different stages of embryonic development at the critical time. Other explanations why discordance is the norm include differences in gene penetration, cytoplasmic inheritance and occurrence of post-cleavage mutation in only one twin (Gericke, 1986).

Zygosity

Prior to counselling parents when one fetus in a multiple pregnancy has been found to have a specific anomaly, it would be useful to be able to determine the risk of anomaly to the others. Knowing the zygosity might help, e.g. Down's syndrome is more likely to affect both in a monozygotic twin pregnancy, and this has been attempted using ultrasound to determine the thickness of the membranes or lack of membrane between the fetuses. While promising, this as yet has not been confirmed as being of value in an individual case (D'Alton and Dudley, 1986) when zygosity has been determined by genetic markers.

Amniocentesis

Genetic amniocentesis has been performed in multiple pregnancy and is more complicated than in singleton pregnancies (D'Alton and Dudley, 1986). The success rate varies from 68% (Librach et al, 1984) to 93% (Pijpers et al, 1988). Although the risks of a failed pregnancy after amniocentesis has not been determined in a controlled manner, it has been estimated as being between 3% and 5%.

Librach and colleagues (1984) considered there was an increased risk of spontaneous abortion compared with singleton pregnancies and the degree of risk was dependent on a number of technical factors. They cautioned against using more than two needle insertions to sample both sacs. Pijpers et al (1988), however, found no relation between fetal loss and the number of needle insertions. The success of such a procedure has also been related to the experience of the operator, posterior placentation and a gestational age of more than 17 weeks.

Pijpers et al (1988) reported difficulties in interpretation of results, particularly of elevated α-fetoprotein levels as α-fetoprotein diffuses across the amniotic membranes between the two sacs. They found two pregnancies with elevated amniotic fluid α-fetoprotein levels in both sacs when only one twin showed an abnormality, which in each case was in the renal tract.

Fetal blood sampling

This technique has been developed by Rodeck and Wass (1981) in twin pregnancy but is not without risk and should only be used in pregnancies suspected to have a severe handicapping abnormality from previous obstetric or family history.

Selective fetocide

Technique

Techniques such as hysterotomy and removal of the defective fetus (Beck et al, 1981; Gigon et al, 1981), the injection of air into the umbilical vein (Rodeck, 1984) or cardiac puncture (Aberg et al, 1978; Redwine and Hays, 1986) have all been used to effect intrauterine death of a twin diagnosed with a specific abnormality, e.g. trisomy-21, Tay–Sachs disease, haemophilia, Duchenne muscular dystrophy, microcephaly, spina bifida or epidermolysis bullosa letalis.

Problems

Most of these anomalies are ones associated with a severe handicap in later life. When the abnormality present is a lethal abnormality, e.g. anencephaly, it is probably best to counsel continuation of the pregnancy although parents may require extra support for the remainder of the pregnancy and additional help following delivery of one live and one dead twin (Bryan, 1983). Although there is a theoretical risk of intravascular coagulopathy in the surviving twin after selective fetocide, this would be limited to monochorionic and therefore monozygotic twins. It is, however, a risk to be considered over and above that of infection, preterm delivery and abortion when counselling.

ROUTINE ANTENATAL CARE

As women with multiple pregnancies fall into the category of being at high risk of complications, particularly pre-eclampsia, polyhydramnios, antepartum haemorrhage and preterm labour (MacGillivray and Campbell, 1988), they should routinely be seen more frequently for antenatal care. It is not necessary that women expecting twins should be undressed and examined abdominally any more frequently than singletons provided they are feeling adequate fetal movements, and antenatal care should therefore concentrate on the detection of commonly occurring asymptomatic problems. Early delivery and low birthweight are the main features of multiple pregnancy associated with increased morbidity and mortality for the baby and antenatal care should concentrate on the detection and prevention of such problems.

Education/antenatal classes

Additionally, women expecting twins may need more support and advice and usually have more questions to be answered than women with singleton pregnancies. Antenatal education specific to multiple pregnancy may be of value in highlighting and allaying worries, both with respect to the antenatal period and to labour and delivery. This is particularly useful when women expecting twins can meet women who have already had multiple births (e.g. from twin clubs), when practical advice can be given as to preparation for more than one baby.

PRE-ECLAMPSIA

It is well-known that there is a greater frequency of pre-eclampsia in twin pregnancy compared with singleton pregnancy, although the actual incidence from different centres varies, in part due to variation in the definition of this condition. In women with a twin pregnancy MacGillivray and Campbell (1988) showed a five- to ten-fold increase in the rate of severe pre-eclampsia in primigravid and multiparous women respectively. Eclampsia was also commoner in twin pregnancies.

Because of the increased frequency of severe pre-eclampsia and its association with growth retardation, this is a very serious condition for the mother and babies. Special vigilance over mothers expecting twins is needed, with more frequent routine blood pressure checking and urine testing, especially after 30 weeks when weekly checks may be indicated. Any single sign of developing pre-eclampsia, e.g. proteinuria alone or a mild rise in blood pressure, should be considered as a reason for hospital admission as the progression of the disease may be very rapid in multiple pregnancy. Once hospitalized the management of this condition is similar to singleton pregnancy, with frequent monitoring of the mother and the babies' well-being to enable optimum timing of delivery. Elective early delivery may often be necessary for the mother's health. In the MacGillivray and Campbell (1988) series of preterm twin deliveries for the Grampian region 1969–1983, 35 out of 46 (76.1%) of twin pregnancies electively delivered before 37 weeks were on account of severe pre-eclampsia, indicating how much this condition contributes to both maternal and perinatal mortality and morbidity.

PRETERM LABOUR

Risk factors

Predicting those multiple pregnancies at risk of preterm labour or the impending onset of preterm labour has proved difficult. Weekes et al (1977) found that low maternal age, low parity and monozygosity were significantly related to preterm labour in twin pregnancies. This was confirmed in Aberdeen with respect to parity and zygosity (MacGillivray and Campbell, 1988), but it is not easy to determine zygosity when the twins are in utero unless babies can be identified on ultrasound as being of the opposite sex, and thus dizygotic. In contrast to singleton pregnancy, low socio-economic status and smoking have not proved to be useful in identifying women with twin pregnancies at risk of early delivery and low birthweight (MacGillivray and Campbell, 1988).

Cervical scoring

Houlton et al (1982) advocated weekly routine examination of the cervix from about 28 weeks onwards to determine the length and dilatation of the cervix. The cervical score was determined by subtracting the dilatation from the length in centimetres. They found a significant association between this score and the onset of labour within the next two weeks, with a predictive value of 60% and a false-positive rate of 20% overall, but these rates improved to 80% and 5% respectively when only primiparous women were studied. Neilson et al (1986), in a controlled trial of 172 patients with twin pregnancies, found that a cervical score of less than -2 before 34 weeks predicted spontaneous delivery, with a sensitivity of 42%, specificity of 84% and predictive value of 71%. On the other hand, O'Connor et al (1981) and MacGillivray and Campbell (1988) found that cervical assessment was not helpful in predicting preterm labour. MacGillivray and Campbell (1988), however, commented that although a closed cervix does not ensure that preterm labour will not occur, dilatation to more than 2 cm at 28–38 weeks' gestation indicates that the onset of labour is very likely and admission to hospital should therefore be considered. The use of vaginal ultrasound in the detection of cervical dilatation is as yet in its infancy but may prove to be of some value in the early detection of a dilating cervix in multiple pregnancy.

Prophylaxis

β-Sympathomimetic drugs

β-Sympathomimetic drugs have been used prophylactically from first detection of multiple pregnancy to try to prevent the onset of preterm labour. Although Tamby Raja et al (1978) showed that the mean gestation length was significantly greater in the 42 women treated with ritodrine compared with the 42 controls, matched for age and parity only, most controlled trials have found no beneficial effect of routine prophylaxis using such drugs in multiple pregnancies (Cetrulo and Freeman, 1976; Marivate et al, 1977; O'Connor et al, 1979; Skjaerris and Aberg, 1982; Gummerus and Halonen, 1987). Currently the majority of evidence does not seem to provide any clear indication of benefit of routine administration of β-adrenergic stimulants in women with twin pregnancies.

Cervical cerclage

In the belief that cervical incompetence is a factor in the aetiology of preterm labour in multiple pregnancy, cervical cerclage has been suggested. Weekes et al (1977) showed no difference in the onset of spontaneous preterm labour, mean gestation at delivery or mean birthweights of twins between three groups of women, one where a cervical suture was inserted routinely as soon as possible after diagnosis, a group treated by bedrest, and a third group with no specific treatment. Sinha et al (1979) compared a group where a cervical suture was inserted prophylactically in the first trimester with a matched control group and found that preterm labour was more likely in those where cervical sutures had been inserted and concluded that cervical cerclage was possibly harmful in multiple pregnancies.

Exercise

In view of the fact that heavy physical exercise and work have been proposed as risk factors for preterm labour, Heluin et al (1979) suggested that women expecting multiple births should avoid physical activity. Papiernik et al (1985) reviewed the impact of such a prenatal programme and considered it to be beneficial in avoiding early delivery. Their work, however, was suspect because they compared their selected group with a group of multiple pregnancies referred late in gestation to their centre and no controlled studies to support this view have been done. Schneider et al (1985) presented some evidence that the standing position was associated with premature contractions in a very small group of women. Women with a multiple pregnancy may, however, find it more difficult to carry on their usual daily activities because of the extra burden of increased size, body weight and oedema in later pregnancy.

Coitus

Coitus has often been suggested as a precipitating factor for preterm labour, and Rayburn and Wilson (1980) recommended that normal sexual activity should be limited in situations of high risk for preterm delivery such as multiple pregnancy. Neilson and Mutambira (1989) questioned women in Harare expecting twin pregnancies on the frequency of coitus. There were no significant differences in the frequency of positive responses between those who went into labour before term when compared with those who delivered at term. They concluded that coitus was not an important precipitant of preterm labour in women with twin pregnancies.

FETAL GROWTH

Clinical assessment

As in singleton pregnancy, poor weight gain in twin pregnancies may indicate a poor pregnancy response and a greater risk of poor fetal growth. Clinically, fetal growth of twins can be assessed approximately by measuring the fundal height and abdominal girth of the mother. Charting of these has been reported to be of value both in the early detection of multiple pregnancy and in the assessment of fetal growth (Schneider et al, 1978; Leroy et al, 1982). This has been confirmed recently by Neilson et al (1988), who found the symphysis–fundal height to be useful in the detection of small for gestational age babies. The sensitivity of their prediction when both babies were small ranged from 40 to 67% and when one baby was small from 15 to 30%. Specificity ranged from 87 to 93%, depending on the gestation when the measurement was made. Although they postulated that symphysis–fundal height measurement might reflect overdistension of the uterus and early delivery, this was not confirmed in their studies.

Ultrasonic scanning

Twin growth charts

Regular assessment of fetal growth by ultrasound scanning has been advocated in twin pregnancies (D'Alton and Dudley, 1986). Consideration should be given to the derivation of intrauterine growth curves of fetal size for multiple pregnancies as the birthweight of twins is generally accepted to be less than singletons. Although this is not agreed by all (Neilson, 1988), it would seem appropriate in view of the fact that in all series birthweight-specific perinatal mortality is less in twin pregnancy than in singleton pregnancy for birthweights up to 2500 g, but thereafter the rates are very similar (Campbell and MacGillivray, 1988a).

Several groups have now determined growth standards for the measurement of biparietal diameter (BPD) and abdominal circumference (AC) by ultrasonic examination in multiple pregnancy (Keuly and Goldberg, 1988), but most of these have been cross-sectional in nature (e.g. Crane et al, 1980; Socol et al, 1984; Grumbach et al, 1986). Recently fetal growth as assessed by measurement of BPD and AC has been examined longitudinally in multiple pregnancy (Smith et al, 1989). It is now possible to determine the appropriateness of fetal growth in multiple pregnancies relative to known standards and detect whether there is poor fetal growth for an individual twin.

Estimation of fetal weight

The estimation of fetal weight derived from ultrasonic measurements of the fetus in utero has been applied to multiple pregnancies (Storlazzi et al, 1987; Yarkoni et al, 1987). Campbell et al (1989), using 60 pairs of twins, evaluated several models of birthweight derived from BPD and AC measurement and concluded that the differences between actual baby weight and estimated fetal weight are greater in twin pregnancy than in singleton pregnancy. Additionally it is not possible always to derive an estimated fetal weight from formulas using both BPD and AC as the BPD was unobtainable in 40% of twin 1 and 25% for twin 2. There are differences in the rates of over- and under-estimation of fetal weight of twin 1 and twin 2, namely an over-estimation of twin 2 and under-estimation of twin 1 when AC only is used. This may be due to the relative position of twins in the uterus; in particular a greater degree of flexion of twin 2 may lead to difficulty in assessing the AC. Overall, at the present time the rate of growth of AC is likely to be of greater value in determining whether twins are small for gestational age or not.

Discordant fetal growth

Ultrasonic scanning is of use in detecting twins with discordant intrauterine growth as substantial difference in the measurements between twins can be noted. There are several published guidelines for diagnosing discordant fetal growth in twin pregnancy by ultrasound (D'Alton and Dudley, 1986), but only rarely has the pregnancy outcome other than low birthweight been assessed. Indeed, Socol et al (1984) concluded that the predictive value of a difference in either BPD or AC for the diagnosis of aberrant growth was poor and did not affect perinatal outcome. Recently a combination of ultrasonic assessment and umbilical artery velocimetry (Divon et al, 1989) has been used for the prediction of discordancy defined as a birthweight difference of more than 15%. Again the relevance of intrapair differences in birthweight between twins has not been considered with respect to perinatal mortality and morbidity. Diagnosing discordant fetal growth may not be of much value other than to alert medical staff to the possibility of twin-to-twin transfusion.

Twin-to-twin transfusion

An imbalance in blood flow between twins can produce the relatively rare disorder known as twin transfusion syndrome, resulting in one anaemic and one polycythaemic twin (Burn and Corney, 1988). The placentation of such twins is usually monochorionic and placental vascular anastomoses can generally be demonstrated. The generally accepted diagnostic criterion is a haemoglobin difference between the twins of 5 g/100 ml as this is unusual in dichorionic twin pregnancy. Others have suggested that in the chronic form this syndrome will result in large birthweight differences, although no definite diagnostic criteria have been agreed. Danskin and Neilson (1989) have recently challenged the diagnosis of this syndrome as they found as many dichorionic as monochorionic pregnancies in their defined group using the above criterion. Ultrasonic studies of fetal growth and studies of umbilical artery waveforms (Giles et al, 1985) may alert staff to suspect such a problem and notify paediatricians at delivery.

HOSPITALIZATION AND BEDREST

Routine hospital admission

Review of clinical trials

Hospitalization and bedrest have been widely advocated in the antepartum management of multiple pregnancies. It was believed that bedrest would reduce the incidence of pre-eclampsia, improve fetal growth and prevent preterm labour. MacGillivray and Campbell (1988) reviewed the literature on clinical trials of bedrest in twin pregnancies published from 1960 onwards and, although many studies have considered bedrest to be beneficial, there are an equal number showing no effect; in particular, the randomized controlled studies of hospitalization of women with twin pregnancies from Finland (Hartikainen-Sorri and Jouppila, 1984) and from Zimbabwe (Saunders et al, 1985) have shown no evidence of prolongation of pregnancy by hospitalization. Recently Crowther et al (1989) reported the results of their randomized control trial of hospitalization in a group of high-risk women in Harare and once again have been unable to demonstrate any benefit either in the prolongation of the pregnancy or in the improvement in perinatal outcome from bedrest in hospital.

Social and financial cost

Additionally, there are considerable disadvantages in adopting a policy such as routine admission to hospital in multiple pregnancy because of the disruption that this causes in the life of the woman and her family (Powers and Miller, 1979; Tresmontant et al, 1983) coupled with the considerable financial cost involved in such a management; for example, Patel et al (1984) assessed the cost of a single admission for bedrest to hospital to be over £2000 per patient.

Non-routine hospital admission

Although routine hospitalization of women with twin pregnancies is therefore not indicated, it is essential that women with twin pregnancies should be admitted to hospital for surveillance as soon as any specific indication is present, such as the development of pre-eclampsia, antepartum haemorrhage or threatened preterm labour.

Onset of preterm labour

Onset of preterm labour may be insidious. As part of their study into the mode of onset of preterm delivery MacGillivray and Campbell (1988) scrutinized the notes of all twin pregnancies from the Grampian region of Scotland from 1969–1983. Cervical dilatation on admission was noted, if vaginal examination had been performed, along with the time of onset of labour. The findings are presented in Table 1. Although 35% of women did

Table 1. Distribution of cervical dilatation on admission in preterm labour in twin pregnancies, Grampian region of Scotland 1969–1983, by type of onset of labour.

Cervical dilatation on admission (cm)	Spontaneous rupture of membranes		Contraction and retraction		Total	
	%	n	%	n	%	n
0–1	7.5	10	6.2	8	6.8	18
2–3	27.6	37	22.3	29	25.0	66
4–5	11.2	15	22.3	29	16.7	44
6–7	3.0	4	8.5	11	5.7	15
8–9	4.5	6	4.6	6	4.5	12
10	4.5	6	7.7	10	6.1	16
Not known	41.8	56	28.5	37	35.2	93
Total	100.1	134	100.1	130	100.0	264

not have a vaginal assessment on admission, overall 33% were admitted at cervical dilatation of more than 4 cm and 11% at 8 cm or more. Consequently, many of these women delivered very soon after admission. As it is not possible to predict those with an asymptomatic onset of labour, in some areas it may be necessary to admit women with twin pregnancies to hospital from about 30 weeks onwards because of the distance they reside from the central unit. In this way the babies will be delivered under the best possible circumstances and can receive any urgent paediatric care that may be required.

Fetal monitoring

Movements. Following the admission for pregnancy complications, monitoring the condition of the mother and baby is essential. Fetal movement charts may be of value but it has to be remembered that the movements are greater in twin pregnancies than in singleton pregnancies and even greater in triplets (Samueloff et al, 1983). Counting the number of movements may therefore be of limited use.

Cardiotocography. Antepartum fetal heart rate monitoring is possible in multiple pregnancies, but is more technically difficult than in singleton pregnancies. Bailey et al (1980) in 50 cases of multiple pregnancy found non-stress cardiotocography to be of value in predicting adverse fetal outcome when the cardiotocogram was non-reactive. This was confirmed by Lenstrup (1984) and Blake et al (1984). Newton et al (1983) commented that most often there is an abnormal test in only one of the two fetuses. This presents difficulty in management as early delivery on behalf of the affected twin may result in complications of preterm delivery in the healthy co-twin. Clearly other risk factors such as pre-eclampsia or antepartum haemorrhage have to be considered along with, most importantly, the gestational age as a predictor of problems of prematurity.

MODE OF DELIVERY

During the antenatal period the mode of delivery and attendant personnel should be discussed with the mother who is expecting a multiple birth.

Elective caesarean section

In twin pregnancies elective caesarean section is a highly controversial topic, especially if there has been a previous birth by caesarean section. Recently the need to always perform a caesarean section in a twin pregnancy where there has been a previous lower segment caesarean scar has been questioned. No advantage in terms of neonatal morbidity or mortality has been detected, although considerable maternal morbidity following repeat caesarean section has been demonstrated (Gilbert et al, 1988; Strong et al, 1989).

Elective caesarean section for fetal reasons in twin pregnancy is highly controversial. Two main factors dominate the argument, namely length of gestation, in particular a very short gestation, and malpresentation of either twin. Many workers in North America (Farroqui et al, 1973; Taylor, 1976; Cetrulo et al, 1980; Kelsick and Minkoff, 1982) have suggested that caesarean section be performed for all twin pregnancies where the presentation is other than cephalic/cephalic, particularly at gestations of less than 34 weeks. Such a policy has resulted in caesarean section rates of about 80% of deliveries at less than 34 weeks. Others, particularly in Europe and the UK, have taken a more conservative approach, with vaginal delivery unless there is a clear indication for caesarean section such as the development of fetal distress or obstructed labour. Such an approach does not appear to have resulted in poorer outcomes (MacGillivray and Campbell, 1981; Olofsson and Rydhstrom, 1985; Rydhstrom and Ohrlander, 1985). Recently this has also been reported from North America (Bell et al, 1986; Chervenak, 1986).

Counselling

During the antenatal period a mother expecting a multiple birth will be anxious about labour and delivery. This should be discussed at a suitable point, either by the obstetrician in charge or at an antenatal class where more general points can be raised. The issues that women raise include the conduct of labour, pain relief, intravenous fluids, fetal monitoring and the delivery of the second twin.

HIGHER MULTIPLES

With the advent of assisted reproduction in the form of ovulation induction and in vitro fertilization programmes the number of higher multiple pregnancies has increased, leading to concern about the management and perinatal outcome of such pregnancies.

Although the complication rate is generally considered to be greater in higher order multiples, there are no rates quoted for specific problems. Harrison and Rossiter (1985) comment that none of the women with a triplet pregnancy in Northern Nigeria who had booked for antenatal care were free of complications. However, none were hospitalized.

Most reviews of the management of triplet pregnancy concentrate on outcome relative to mode of delivery (Campbell and MacGillivray, 1988b). In Western countries delivery is usually by elective caesarean section rather than allowing the onset of labour and vaginal delivery. Only those women with very early onset of preterm labour are allowed to deliver vaginally. It is difficult to reach a valid conclusion therefore about the merits of one method of delivery versus the other. Harrison and Rossiter (1985) allowed all six booked women with triplets to have vaginal delivery with a perinatal mortality of 277 per 1000. Comparable perinatal mortality rates have been found from other centres for vaginal delivery, but lower rates (approximately 60 per 1000) have been noted for caesarean section deliveries.

It is because of the increased risks both to mothers and fetuses of high order multiple pregnancies that selective reduction in the first trimester has been suggested as an alternative management in high order multiple pregnancy after assisted reproduction (Berkowitz et al, 1988). However, this raises difficult legal and ethical issues (Howie, 1988). Prevention of high order multiple pregnancies is clearly the best option and staff practising such techniques as induction of ovulation and multiple embryo or oocyte replacement in in vitro fertilization or gamete intrafallopian transfer have an obligation to strive to limit the numbers of higher order multiples to a minimum.

SUMMARY

Most multiple pregnancies are diagnosed, but early diagnosis still presents some problems. Congenital malformation is commoner in multiple pregnancies, usually without concordance, which complicates decisions about pregnancy termination.

Because of the higher perinatal mortality rates, women with multiple pregnancies should be offered extra antenatal care, with the specific objectives of early diagnosis and timely treatment of pre-eclampsia, preterm labour and growth retardation. If growth retardation affects only one fetus, intervention must be carefully judged.

Measures such as bedrest, fetal monitoring and elective operative delivery are reviewed, and no evidence of benefit is found from their routine use. However, such interventions are valuable in selected cases.

REFERENCES

Aberg A, Mitelman F & Cantz M (1978) Cardiac puncture of fetus with Hurler's disease avoiding abortion of unaffected co-twin. *Lancet* ii: 990–991.

Bailey D, Flynn AM, Kelly J & O'Connor M (1980) Antepartum fetal heart monitoring in multiple pregnancy. *British Journal of Obstetrics and Gynaecology* **87**: 561–564.

Beck L, Terinde R, Röhrborn G et al (1981) Twin pregnancy, abortion of one fetus with Down's syndrome by sectio parva, the other delivered mature and healthy. *European Journal of Obstetrics, Gynecology and Reproductive Biology* **100**: 276–282.

Bell D, Johansson D, McLean FH & Usher RH (1986) Birth asphyxia, trauma and mortality in twins: has caesarean section improved outcome? *American Journal of Obstetrics and Gynecology* **154**: 235–239.

Berkowitz RL, Lynd L, Chitkara U et al (1988) Selective reduction of multifetal pregnancies in the first trimester. *New England Journal of Medicine* **318**: 1043–1047.

Blake GD, Knuppel RA, Ingardia CJ, Lake M, Aumann G & Hanson M et al (1984) Evaluation of nonstress fetal heart rate testing in multiple gestation. *Obstetrics and Gynecology* **63**: 528–532.

Bryan EM (1983) *The Nature and Nurture of Twins*, pp 36–37, 156–165. London: Baillière Tindall.

Burn J & Corney G (1984) Congenital heart defects and twinning. *Acta Geneticae Medicae et Gemellologiae* **33**: 61–69.

Burn J & Corney G (1988) Zygosity determination and the types of twinning. Twin transfusion syndrome. In MacGillivray I, Campbell DM & Thompson B (eds) *Twinning and Twins*, pp 37–66. Chichester: John Wiley and Sons.

Campbell DM & MacGillivray I (1988a) Outcome of twin pregnancies. In MacGillivray I, Campbell DM & Thompson B (eds) *Twinning and Twins*, pp 179–205. Chichester, New York, Brisbane, Toronto, Singapore: John Wiley and Sons.

Campbell DM & MacGillivray I (1988b) Management of labour and delivery: higher multiples. In MacGillivray I, Campbell DM & Thompson B (eds) *Twinning and Twins*, pp 158–160. Chichester, New York, Brisbane, Toronto, Singapore: John Wiley and Sons.

Campbell DM, Smith AP & Wilson AW (1989) Estimating fetal weight in twin pregnancy— how good are we? *Acta Geneticae Medicae et Gemellologiae* (in press).

Cetrulo CL & Freeman RK (1976) Ritodrine HC1 for the prevention of premature labour in twin pregnancies. *Acta Geneticae Medicae et Gemellologiae* **25**: 321–324.

Cetrulo CL, Ingardia CJ & Sbarra AJ (1980) Management of multiple gestations. *Clinics in Obstetrics and Gynaecology* **23**: 533–548.

Chervenak FA (1986) The controversy of mode of delivery in twins: the intrapartum management of twin gestation (part II). *Seminars in Perinatology* **10**: 44–49.

Crane JF, Tamich PG & Kapla M (1980) Ultrasonic growth patterns in normal and discordant twins. *Obstetrics and Gynecology* **55**: 678–683.

Crowther CA, Neilson JP, Verkuyl DAA et al (1989) Preterm labour in twin pregnancies: can it be prevented by hospital admission? *British Journal of Obstetrics and Gynaecology* **96**: 850–853.

D'Alton ME & Dudley DKL (1986) Ultrasound in antenatal management of twin gestation. *Seminars in Perinatology* **10(1)**: 30–38.

Danskin FH & Neilson JP (1989) Twin-to-twin transfusion syndrome: what are appropriate diagnostic criteria. *American Journal of Obstetrics and Gynecology* **161**: 365–369.

Divon MY, Girz BA, Sklar A, Guidetti DA & Langer O (1989) Discordant twins—a prospective study of the diagnostic value of real-time ultrasonography combined with umbilical artery velocimetry. *American Journal of Obstetrics and Gynecology* **161**: 757–760.

Ellis RF, Berger GS, Keith L & Depp R (1979) The Northwestern University Multihospital Twin Study. II Mortality of first versus second twin. *Acta Geneticae Medicae et Gemellologiae* **28**: 347–352.

Farroqui MD, Grossman JH & Shauman RA (1973) A review of twin pregnancies and perinatal mortality. *Obstetrical and Gynecological Survey* **28**: 144–145.

Filler RM (1986) Conjoined twins and their separation. *Seminars in Perinatalogy* **10(1)**: 82–91.

Gericke GS (1986) Genetic and teratological consideration in the analysis of concordant and discordant abnormalities in twins. *South African Medical Journal* **69**: 111–114.

Gigon U, Moser H & Aufdermauer P (1981) Twin pregnancy with operative removal of one fetus with chromosomal mosaicism 46XX/45XO and term delivery of a healthy baby. *Zeitschrift für Geburtshilfe und Perinatologie* **185**: 365–366.

Gilbert L, Saunders N & Sharp F (1988) The management of multiple pregnancy in women with a lower segment caesarean scar. Is a repeat caesarean section really the safe option? *British Journal of Obstetrics and Gynaecology* **95:** 1312–1316.

Giles WB, Trudinger BJ & Cook CM (1985) Umbilical waveforms in twin pregnancy. *Acta Geneticae Medicae et Gemellologiae* **34:** 233–237.

Grennert L, Gennser G, Persson P et al (1976) Ultrasound and human placental lactogen screening for early detection of twin pregnancies. *Lancet* **i:** 4–6.

Grumbach K, Coleman BG, Arger PH et al (1986) Twin and singleton growth patterns compared using ultrasound. *Radiology* **158:** 237–241.

Gummerus M & Halonen O (1987) Prophylactic longterm oral tocolysis of multiple pregnancies. *British Journal of Obstetrics and Gynaecology* **94:** 249–251.

Hanson JW (1975) Incidence of conjoined twinning. *Lancet* **ii:** 1257 (letter).

Harrison KA & Rossiter CE (1985) Multiple pregnancy. *British Journal of Obstetrics and Gynaecology* **92(supplement 5):** 49–60.

Hartikainen-Sorri AL & Jouppila P (1984) Is routine hospitalization needed in antenatal care of twin pregnancy. *Journal of Perinatal Medicine* **12:** 31–34.

Hay S & Wehrung DA (1970) Congenital malformations in twins. *American Journal of Human Genetics* **22:** 662–678.

Hellin D (1895) Die Ursache der Multiparitat der Unipaeren. *Tiere Uberhaupt und der Zwillingsschwangerschaft beim Menschen Insbesondere.* Munich: Seltz and Schaner.

Heluin G, Bessis R & Papiernik E (1979) Clinical management of twin pregnancies. *Acta Geneticae Medicae et Gemellologiae* **28:** 333.

Houlton MC, Marivate M & Philpott RH (1982) Factors associated with pre-term labour and changes in the cervix before labour in twin pregnancy. *British Journal of Obstetrics and Gynaecology* **89(3):** 190–194.

Howie PW (1988) Selective reduction in multiple pregnancy. Legal confusion and ethical dilemmas. *British Medical Journal* **297:** 433–434.

James WH (1978) A note on the epidemiology of acardiac monsters. *Teratology* **15:** 211–216.

Kallen B (1986) Congenital malformations in twins: a population study. *Acta Geneticae Medicae et Gemellologiae* **35:** 167–178.

Kelsick F & Minkoff J (1982) Management of the breech second twin. *American Journal of Obstetrics and Gynecology* **144:** 783–786.

Keuly AB & Goldberg BB (1988) *Obstetrical Measurements in Ultrasound. A Reference Manual*, pp 202–210. Chicago: Year Book Medical Publishers.

Layde PM, Erickson JO, Falek A & McCarthy BJ (1980) Congenital malformations in twins. *American Journal of Human Genetics* **32:** 69–78.

Lenstrup C (1984) Reactive value of antepartum non-stress test in multiple pregnancies. *Acta Obstetrica et Gynecologica Scandinavica* **63(7):** 597–601.

Leroy B, Lefort F & Jeny R (1982) Uterine height and umbilical perimeter curves in twin pregnancies. *Acta Geneticae Medicae et Gemellologiae* **31:** 195–198.

Librach CL, Doran TA, Benzie RJ & Jones JM (1984) Genetic amniocentesis in seventy twin pregnancies. *American Journal of Obstetrics and Gynecology* **148:** 585–591.

Little J & Bryan E (1986) Congenital anomalies in twins. *Seminars in Perinatology* **10(1):** 50–64.

Little J & Bryan EM (1988) Congenital anomalies. In MacGillivray I, Campbell DM & Thompson B (eds) *Twinning and Twins*, pp 207–240. Chichester: John Wiley and Sons.

Little J & Thompson B (1988) Descriptive epidemiology. In MacGillivray I, Campbell DM & Thompson B (eds) *Twinning and Twins*, pp 37–66. Chichester: John Wiley and Sons.

MacGillivray I (1975) Malformations and other abnormalities in twins. In MacGillivray I, Nylander PPS & Corney G (eds) *Human Multiple Reproduction*, pp 165–175. London: WB Saunders.

MacGillivray I & Campbell DM (1981) The outcome of twin pregnancies in Aberdeen. In Gedda L, Parisi P & Nance WE (eds) *Twin Research 3, Part A, Twin Biology and Multiple Pregnancy*, pp 203–206. New York: Alan R Liss.

MacGillivray I & Campbell DM (1988) Management of twin pregnancies. In MacGillivray I, Campbell DM & Thompson B (eds) *Twinning and Twins*, pp 111–139. Chichester: John Wiley and Sons.

Malmstrom PEM & Malmstrom EJ (1988) Maternal recognition of twin pregnancy. *Acta Geneticae Medicae et Gemellologiae* **37:** 187–192.

Marivate M, de Villiers KQ & Fairbrother P (1977) Effect of prophylactic outpatient administration of fenoterol on the time and onset of spontaneous labour and fetal growth rate in twin pregnancy. *American Journal of Obstetrics and Gynecology* **128:** 707–708.

Medearis AL, Jonas HS, Stookbauer JW et al (1979) Perinatal deaths in twin pregnancy. A five-year analysis of statistics in Missouri. *American Journal of Obstetrics and Gynecology* **134:** 413–418.

Neilson JP (1988) Fetal growth in twin pregnancies. *Acta Geneticae Medicae et Gemellologiae* **37:** 35–39.

Neilson JP & Mutambira M (1989) Coitus, twin pregnancy and preterm labour. *American Journal of Obstetrics and Gynecology* **160:** 416–418.

Neilson JP, Crowther C, Verkuyl DAA & Bannerman C (1986) Cervical assessment in the management of twin pregnancy. *Acta Geneticae Medicae et Gemellologiae* **35:** 68 (abstract).

Neilson JP, Verkuyl DAA & Bannerman C (1988) Tape measurement of symphysis–fundal height in twin pregnancies. *British Journal of Obstetrics and Gynaecology* **95:** 1054–1059.

Newton ER (1986) Antepartum care in multiple gestation. *Seminars in Perinatology* **10(1):** 19–29.

Newton ER, Genest DR et al (1983) Management of non reactive non stress test in a twin gestation. *Obstetrics and Gynecology* **68:** 345–350.

O'Connor MC, Murphy H & Dalrymple IJ (1979) Double blind trial of ritodrine and placebo in twin pregnancy. *British Journal of Obstetrics and Gynaecology* **86:** 706–709.

O'Connor MC, Arias E, Royston JP & Dalrymple IJ (1981) The merits of special antenatal care for twin pregnancies. *British Journal of Obstetrics and Gynaecology* **88:** 222–230.

Olofsson P & Rydhstrom H (1985) Twin delivery: how should the second twin be delivered? *American Journal of Obstetrics and Gynecology* **153:** 479–481.

Papiernik E, Mussy MA, Vial M & Richard A (1985) A low rate of perinatal deaths for twin births. *Acta Geneticae Medicae et Gemellologiae* **34:** 201–206.

Patel N, Bowie W, Campbell DM et al (1984) *Scottish Twin Study, 1983 Report.* Glasgow: Social Paediatric and Obstetric Research Unit, University of Glasgow and Greater Glasgow Health Board.

Pijpers L, Jahoda MGJ, Vosters RPL et al (1988) Genetic amniocentesis in twin pregnancies. *British Journal of Obstetrics and Gynaecology* **95:** 323–326.

Powers WF & Miller TC (1979) Bed rest in twin pregnancy: identification of a critical period and its cost implications. *American Journal of Obstetrics and Gynecology* **134(1):** 23–30.

Rayburn WF & Wilson AE (1980) Coital activity and premature delivery. *American Journal of Obstetrics and Gynecology* **137:** 972–974.

Redwine FO & Hays PM (1986) Selective birth. *Seminars in Perinatology* **10:** 73–81.

Rodeck CH (1984) Fetoscopy in the management of twin pregnancies discordant for a severe abnormality. *Acta Geneticae Medicae et Gemellologiae* **33:** 57–60.

Rodeck CH & Wass D (1981) Sampling pure fetal blood in twin pregnancies by fetoscopy using a single uterine puncture. *Prenatal Diagnosis* **1:** 43–49.

Rydhstrom H & Ohrlander S (1985) Twin deliveries in Sweden 1973–1981. The value of an increasing caesarean section rate. *Archives of Gynecology* **237:** 168.

Samueloff A, Evron S & Sadovsky E (1983) Fetal movements in multiple pregnancy. *American Journal of Obstetrics and Gynecology* **146:** 789–792.

Saunders MC, Dick JS, Brown I et al (1985) The effects of hospital admission for bed rest on the duration of twin pregnancy. *Lancet* **ii:** 793–795.

Schinzel AAGL, Smith DW & Miller JR (1979) Monozygotic twinning and structural defects. *Journal of Pediatrics* **95:** 921–930.

Schneider KTM, Huch A & Huch R (1985) Premature contractions: are they caused by maternal standing? *Acta Geneticae Medicae et Gemellologiae* **34:** 175–178.

Schneider L, Bessis R, Hajeri H & Papiernik E (1978) On twin care: early detection of twin pregnancies with the use of charts of normal uterine height and waist measurements. In Nance WE, Allen G & Parisi P (eds) *Twin Research: Clinical Studies,* pp 143–146. New York: Alan R Liss.

Sinha DP, Nandakumar VC, Brough AK & Beebeejaum MS (1979) Relative cervical incompetence in twin pregnancy. Assessment and efficacy of cervical suture. *Acta Geneticae Medicae et Gemellologiae* **28:** 327–331.

Skjaerris J & Aberg A (1982) Prevention of prematurity in twin pregnancy by orally administered Terbutaline. *Acta Obstetricia et Gynecologica Scandinavica Supplement* **108:** 39–40.

Smith APM, Campbell DM & Lemon J (1989) Growth patterns in preterm and term twin deliveries. *Acta Geneticae Medicae et Gemellologiae* (in press).

Socol ML, Tamura RK, Sabbagha RE et al (1984) Diminished biparietal diameter and abdominal circumference growth in twins. *Obstetrics and Gynecology* 64: 235–238.

Storlazzi E, Vintzileos AM, Campbell WA et al (1987) Ultrasonic diagnosis of discordant fetal growth in twin gestations. *Obstetrics and Gynecology* 69: 363–367.

Strong TH, Phelan JP, Myong GA & Sarno AP (1989) Vaginal birth after caesarean delivery in the twin gestation. *American Journal of Obstetrics and Gynecology* 161: 29–32.

Tamby Raja RL, Atputharajah V & Slamon Y (1978) Prevention of prematurity in twins. *Australian and New Zealand Journal of Obstetrics and Gynaecology* 18: 179–183.

Taylor EW (1976). Editorial. *Obstetrical and Gynecological Survey* 31: 535.

Thom H, Buckland C, Campbell AGM et al (1984) Maternal serum alpha-feto-protein in monozygotic and dizygotic twin pregnancy. *Prenatal Diagnosis* 4(5): 341–346.

Tresmontant R, Heluin G & Papiernik E (1983) Cost of care and prevention of preterm births in twin pregnancies. *Acta Geneticae Medicae et Gemellologiae* 32: 99–103.

Vandekerckhove F, Dhont M, Thiery M & Derom R (1984) Screening for multiple pregnancy. *Acta Geneticae Medicae et Gemellologiae* 33(4): 571–574.

Weekes ARL, Menzies DN & de Boer CH (1977) The relative efficacy of bed rest, cervical suture and no treatment in the management of twin pregnancy. *British Journal of Obstetrics and Gynaecology* 84: 161–164.

Windham GC & Bjerkedal T (1984) Malformations in twins and their siblings, Norway, 1967–1979. *Acta Geneticae Medicae et Gemellologiae* 33: 87–95.

Windham GC, Bjerkedal T & Sever LE (1982) The association of twinning and neural tube defects: studies in Los Angeles, California and Norway. *Acta Geneticae Medicae et Gemellologiae* 31: 165–172.

Yarkoni S, Reece EA, Holford T et al (1987) Estimated fetal weight in the evaluation of growth in twin gestations. A prospective longitudinal study. *Obstetrics and Gynecology* 69: 636–639.

8

Medical complications in pregnancy

MICHAEL MARESH

The aim of this chapter is to describe how antenatal care is modified for women with pre-existing and newly diagnosed medical conditions. Only the more common conditions will be covered and the underlying pathophysiology will only be discussed briefly. However, understanding the physiological changes in a system such as the cardiovascular system is critical for the correct management of the cardiac patient. Similarly, it is important to appreciate the natural history of the condition; for instance, chronic renal failure may deteriorate significantly during the nine months of pregnancy.

DIABETES

The incidence of insulin-dependent diabetes mellitus (IDDM) is in the order of one in 500 pregnancies. Non-insulin-dependent diabetes mellitus (NIDDM) is usually less frequent, apart from in certain areas with a high prevalence of obesity and certain ethnic groups (e.g. Indians). Accordingly, the average UK obstetrician will only look after about two to three diabetic pregnancies a year. The centralizing of the care of diabetic pregnant women onto one obstetrician allows the development of a multidisciplinary clinical team comprised of an obstetrician, physician, midwife and dietician.

The most recent perinatal mortality survey of diabetic pregnancy in the UK was in 1980 (Beard and Lowy, 1982), when the overall perinatal mortality rate in IDDM was 60 per 1000 and 50% of the losses were unexplained stillbirths. The results from large centralized units are very encouraging. The perinatal mortality rate at St Mary's, Manchester, in IDDM is six per 1000 (one neonatal death from multiple malformations in the last ten years), which is similar to that published by Brudenell and Doddridge (1989).

Impaired glucose tolerance (IGT) in pregnancy is more common, but disagreement as to what definition to use gives different prevalence rates. However, a large European study has now been reported by Lind (1989) and from it recommendations can now be made (see Chapter 2). There is controversy as to whether the excess perinatal morbidity and mortality is caused by the condition or is associated with the other variables of increased age and obesity usually found in these women. The subject has been recently reviewed (Maresh, 1988).

The underlying message in the management of diabetic pregnancy is that

Baillière's Clinical Obstetrics and Gynaecology—
Vol. 4, No. 1, March 1990
ISBN 0–7020–1476–1

normoglycaemia must be achieved throughout. This means that plasma glucose concentrations should be less than 6 mmol/l apart from in the immediate postprandial period.

Preconceptional care

To obtain normoglycaemia during embryogenesis requires attention to diabetic control before conception. The development of preconceptional clinics has in general not been that successful, with the less motivated, who need more help, not attending. An exception has been in East Germany (Fuhrmann et al, 1983). Accordingly, different strategies need to be used. The most successful in the UK has been in Edinburgh where the same physician runs the adolescent and pregnancy service and this, combined with other initiatives, results in 75% of women obtaining specific prepregnancy advice (Steel et al, 1989). The increasing use of computerized diabetic registers allows age–sex searches to be performed and non-attenders to be visited at home, one of the strategies we are using with a specific community midwife. In order to achieve good results all medical and paramedical workers involved with women with diabetes must stress the need for good diabetic control prior to conception. Furthermore they should arrange for a prepregnancy medical evaluation for the women, which ideally should take place in the combined diabetic/antenatal clinic. Apart from checking that normoglycaemia is being obtained and satisfactory capillary blood testing is being performed, and measuring the glycated (glycosylated) haemoglobin (an indicator of long-term control), a number of other objectives can be achieved. The retina should be inspected and any treatment initiated. Renal function should be documented, and body mass index is assessed and if outside the accepted range dietary measures should be implemented. Smoking should be actively discouraged and rubella immunity checked. Women on the contraceptive pill should be advised to stop and change to a barrier method prior to attempting to conceive. There is also an opportunity for the obstetrician to outline pregnancy care and to explain how the women can arrange to be seen immediately pregnancy is suspected.

First trimester

The endocrinological changes of early pregnancy cause resistance to insulin action and this coupled with nausea may cause significant problems with diabetic control during embryogenesis. Thus the pregnant woman with diabetes must be seen as soon as she thinks she is pregnant. Hospital admission may be helpful to try and ensure normoglycaemia and gives the opportunity for thorough diabetic assessment and education which may not have occurred preconception. For the woman with NIDDM not being treated with insulin admission for assessment is best at this stage since insulin will usually be required in the first or early second trimester. An ultrasound scan should be performed at seven weeks to check on viability and repeated after a week if there is doubt. Whether there is an increased risk of spontaneous abortion remains controversial, but there does appear to be a relationship with poor diabetic control (Mills et al, 1988b).

Second trimester

Continued attention to diabetic control is mandatory, with multiple self-monitoring of capillary blood glucose concentrations, ideally four to six times a day every day. Assessing the results on the reagent strips is best done by meter rather than the naked eye, assuming the accuracy of the meter is regularly checked. Home capillary glucose concentrations can also be measured by collecting samples into capillary tubes or impregnating special paper, allowing the hospital to verify results. Glycated haemoglobin should be estimated monthly. If normoglycaemia is not being obtained rapidly through adjustments of insulin dosage or regimen, then hospital admission should not be delayed. Weight gain should be monitored carefully to try to prevent fat deposition which will antagonize insulin action. This is of particular importance for the obese woman with NIDDM or IGT. Skilled dietetic advice is often critical for achieving the tight control required.

Screening for congenital malformations should be offered to all women who had diabetes in the first trimester because of the threefold increase in malformations. A number of studies have shown a relationship with poor control during embryogenesis, e.g. glycated haemoglobin more than 10% at 12 weeks, the most recent being Stubbs et al (1986). That the recent large American study of Mills et al (1988a) did not find this does not refute the hypothesis since most of the women had good control. The risk is also increased in those with diabetic vascular disease, although a recent report suggests that with improvements in control this difference is no longer significant (Damm and Molsted-Pedersen, 1989). α-Fetoprotein results need careful interpretation in view of the tendency for them to be lower in diabetic pregnancy; this was first reported by Wald et al (1979) and has been subsequently confirmed. Specific anomalies are found in association with diabetes and these were confirmed in the 1980 UK survey (Lowy et al, 1986). Accordingly, ultrasound screening at 18–20 weeks should specifically look for:

1. Neural tube defects—anencephaly, microcephaly, holoprosencephaly.
2. Cardiac lesions—transposition of the great vessels, ventricular septal defects.
3. Caudal regression syndrome—sacral anomalies, short femurs, cloacal anomalies.

Screening is not just for the purpose of discussing termination of pregnancy, but in the case of cardiac anomalies in particular arranging for appropriate perinatal care. Further cardiac screening for anomalies may be repeated later in pregnancy when visualization may be easier. Chromosomal anomalies are not more frequent and so amniocentesis is not specifically indicated.

Women with nephropathy and retinopathy need to have these assessed regularly for any signs of deterioration.

Third trimester

Towards the end of the second and into the third trimester there are obstetric markers of diabetic control, namely fetal growth rate and liquor volume. Accordingly, apart from maintaining tight diabetic control (as outlined above), there is a need for careful serial assessment, preferably by the same experienced clinician, of fundal height, uterine size and liquor volume. This should be supplemented by two-weekly ultrasound measurements, particularly of abdominal circumference and liquor volume. These should start by 24–26 weeks to act as a baseline for subsequent assessment of growth rate. This clinical and ultrasound regimen should be applied to all cases, whether with IDDM, NIDDM or IGT. Abnormalities of fetal growth are best managed by admission and monitoring of the diabetic control and fetal condition. The role of Doppler blood flow velocity waveform measurements in diabetic pregnancy has not been satisfactorily evaluated. Biochemical tests of placental function no longer appear to have any role (Dooley et al, 1984).

If fetal growth is normal and diabetic control satisfactory, then routine weekly clinic visits should continue up until 35 weeks. From then on it is advisable to perform cardiotocographs two to three times weekly. Since asphyxia is the final precursor of the unexplained fetal deaths, cardio-tocography is the best test available. It should be started earlier if:

1.   There is an abnormality of fetal growth (growth acceleration or retar-dation).
2.   Diabetic control is poor.
3.   There are vascular complications (nephropathy or retinopathy).
4.   There is likely to be vascular disease (diabetes for >20 years).

Although this approach may be regarded as controversial, the results at St Mary's, Manchester, support this approach, whereas in the results published by Drury (1986) routine cardiotocography was not performed and a number of deaths in utero were reported.

Biophysical profile scoring has been recommended in diabetic pregnancy, but there is no evidence that the use of the additional parameters (fetal breathing, fetal tone and movement) is beneficial (Johnson et al, 1988). More relevant would be careful scanning for early signs of heart failure associated with the cardiomegaly resulting from fetal hyperinsulinaemia secondary to suboptimal diabetic control.

Despite the frequent claims that women with diabetes have an increased risk of almost all pregnancy complications, a recent review found little evidence to support this (Cousins, 1987).

Timing and route of delivery

Controversy still exists between the policy of routine delivery at 38 weeks and the conservative approach of continued close monitoring whilst awaiting spontaneous labour (Drury, 1986; Molsted-Pedersen and Kuhl, 1986). For the diabetic woman with no complications the conservative approach can be adopted with outpatient monitoring. For those with complications, induction of labour should be considered by 38 weeks (if not indicated earlier); if the cervix is unfavourable, admission to hospital is wisest whilst awaiting a change. Uncomplicated mild hypertension does not necessarily require intervention. The onset of growth retardation demands admission and early recourse to delivery since the fetus of the diabetic mother may be particularly prone to asphyxia due to one or more of the following:

1. Undetected maternal vascular disease.
2. Inefficient oxygen release if glycated haemoglobin raised.
3. Placental lesions decreasing oxygen transfer.
4. Increased oxygen demand by hyperinsulinaemic fetus.
5. Increased lactate associated with fetal hyperglycaemia.

Growth acceleration poses another problem because of the risk of traumatic delivery. This applies to women with NIDDM and IGT as well. If the fetus is grossly macrosomic then a caesarean section will be required. If contemplated before 38 weeks this will be one of the few occasions when the lecithin–sphingomyelin ratio and phosphatidylglycerol concentration should be checked first. Milder cases of macrosomia should be evaluated for vaginal delivery by ultrasound measurement of thoracic circumference and radiological pelvic assessment. Computed tomographic radiography is probably the ideal since fetal shoulder and maternal pelvic measurements can be obtained without excessive radiological exposure (Kitzmiller et al, 1987).

It must be emphasized that the strategy of trying to achieve a high rate of spontaneous labour and vaginal delivery must be undertaken with meticulous care by an experienced team; this also applies to intrapartum management, which is not considered here. If not, there will be an increase in unexplained stillbirth and traumatic delivery.

CARDIAC DISEASE

Cardiac disease in pregnancy is associated with a heterogeneous and changing set of conditions. Rheumatic mitral valve disease, with which formerly the average obstetrician had considerable experience, is now rare. Extrapolating from the English data of de Swiet and Fidler (1981) it is likely to occur now only in the order of two per 1000 pregnancies, even in a referral unit. Congenital heart disease is increasing, partly due to improved investigative techniques diagnosing minor abnormalities, but more importantly due to the developments in paediatric cardiac surgery allowing children with major abnormalities to survive and thus be able to become pregnant. The most recent maternal mortality figures in England and Wales show a rate of about ten deaths per million maternities (Department of Health, 1989). Nearly all deaths occurred after delivery or abortion. About half of the deaths were associated with coronary arterial disease.

This wide range of problems which may be of varying severity makes it impossible to discuss antenatal management of specific problems in any detail, so most of this section will cover only general points which are not necessarily applicable to all cases. The management of a number of specific conditions has been recently reviewed by de Swiet (1989).

Preconceptional care

Women with either Eisenmenger's syndrome or with pulmonary hypertension should be advised not to conceive because of the high maternal mortality. Although experience is limited in women who have had a myocardial infarction, it does not appear to be a strong contraindication to pregnancy. Those with artificial heart valves should be counselled with regard to anticoagulation problems (see below).

Early antenatal care

Women with the serious conditions just mentioned may have become pregnant deliberately against medical advice and usually will not contemplate termination of pregnancy. However, they must still be counselled.

It is traditional to assess the cardiovascular system of all women at their first antenatal attendance. Whilst the school and employer's medical checks will have detected most cases of significant heart disease, this will not apply to recent immigrants. The haemodynamic changes present even in early pregnancy make diagnosis difficult. However, symptoms which require a cardiac opinion include severe dyspnoea, paroxysmal nocturnal dyspnoea, syncope with exertion, haemoptysis and chest pain on exertion. Relevant signs include cyanosis, clubbing, arrhythmias, loud harsh systolic murmurs and any diastolic murmur. The traditional investigations of chest X-ray and electrocardiography (ECG) are of limited value in pregnancy (due to the pregnancy-associated cardiovascular changes) unless there is a marked derangement. Echocardiography is the investigation of choice.

A definitive cardiac diagnosis must be made as soon as possible (if not already known) so that the behaviour of the lesion with the haemodynamic changes of pregnancy can be predicted. Many congenital lesions are trivial and it is important to reassure the women since otherwise she may become very alarmed by the normal dyspnoea of pregnancy. The problems associated with rheumatic heart disease are harder to predict and there is an extensive literature on the subject (Szekely et al, 1973). The unreliability of classification of severity on the basis of symptoms is exemplified by a report where of those who developed heart failure, 39% were initially classified as normal (Sugrue et al, 1981). However, with improvements in cardiac imaging techniques such complications should become more predictable.

Although it may be difficult to justify a combined cardiac/antenatal clinic in a typical district hospital, it is important that the women can be seen by the two specialists at one visit and that good communication occurs. The mainstay of management is to prevent additional stress on the heart which might cause heart failure by:

1. Avoiding excessive activity with early recourse to hospital admission.
2. Iron therapy to avoid anaemia.
3. Treating any possibility of infection vigorously.
4. Treating even mild hypertension.
5. Avoiding excessive weight gain.

Regular cardiac assessment is aimed at detecting any signs of heart failure.

In addition, arrhythmias must be looked for and in those with rheumatic mitral valve disease digitalization considered. Any sign of pulmonary oedema must be treated vigorously with diuretics. Cardiac surgery is rarely performed in pregnancy. In the past, closed mitral valvotomy was regularly performed with good results (Szekely et al, 1973), but in developed countries the condition is likely to have been diagnosed before and corrected. Open heart surgery is usually only indicated for refractory pulmonary oedema and the fetal loss rate associated with bypass surgery is about 20% (Becker, 1983).

Women with congenital cardiac disease should be offered a detailed fetal cardiac ultrasound assessment at about 20 weeks' gestation since there is a 5–10% risk of the fetus having a lesion (Burn, 1987). This is not just for consideration of termination of pregnancy, which with the advances in paediatric cardiac surgery is probably occurring less often, but also to allow for immediate post-delivery neonatal assessment.

Late antenatal care

General measures as outlined above should continue. Fetal growth retardation is likely to occur if there is chronic maternal hypoxia and so all women who appear to have significant heart disease need careful clinical and ultrasound evaluation of fetal growth from 24 weeks. Evidence of growth retardation should lead to admission and regular antenatal cardiotocography.

Premature contractions should not be treated with β-sympathomimetic agents without careful consideration of the effects the resultant tachycardia and vasodilatation will have on the cardiac dynamics in each case. Some of the cases of pulmonary oedema which have been noticed in association with treatment with β-sympathomimetic drugs and corticosteroids may have been precipitated by underlying cardiac lesions.

Preparation for delivery

It is important for obstetricians, cardiologists and anaesthetists to have an agreed plan well in advance. Decisions need to be made with regard to place of delivery (delivery unit or intensive care), whether Swan–Ganz central catheterization is going to be attempted, whether there are any haemodynamic contraindications to epidurals and whether antibiotic prophylaxis is needed (Working Party of the British Society for Antimicrobial Chemotherapy, 1982). Induction of labour should not be performed as a routine, but obviously may be indicated for fetal or maternal reasons. However, with the high success rates of current methods it is appealing, as it facilitates a planned management routine for the very high risk case.

THROMBOEMBOLISM

About one in 200 000 pregnant women die in the antenatal period from thromboembolism, deaths from postpartum thromboembolism being about twice as common (Department of Health, 1989). The incidence of non-fatal antenatal thromboembolism is less accurately known, but is likely to be between one and three per 1000 pregnancies. Increased age and parity are independent risk factors, along with obesity, immobility and a past history of thromboembolism.

Preconceptional care

Women with artificial heart valves are usually considered to need permanent anticoagulation with warfarin. If contemplating pregnancy they need to be warned of the slight risk of teratogenesis from warfarin. The typical syndrome involves abnormal bone and cartilage formation. However, a study looking at precisely this group (Chen et al, 1982) found no evidence of this. Accordingly, women can be reassured that they are not subjecting the fetus to a very high risk, but they should be advised to have their warfarin regimen monitored closely to avoid possible harmful effects from high dosages.

Antenatal prophylaxis

There has been much discussion over the last few years about the management of the woman with a previous venous thrombosis or embolism. It has been claimed that the incidence of a repeat episode is about 12% (Badaracco and Vessey, 1974), but this was a retrospective postal survey and is likely to be an overestimate. A survey of British obstetricians in 1979 (de Swiet et al, 1980) showed that 88% would use anticoagulants for a woman who had had a thromboembolic episode in a previous pregnancy and that most would use a regimen of warfarin up until about 36 weeks' gestation, when they would change to heparin to try and avoid the fetal risk of intracerebral bleeding should labour start whilst fully anticoagulated. However, apart from possible teratogenesis and these late pregnancy risks, there is a concern about effects at other times, Warfarin crosses the placenta and might cause small intracerebral haemorrhages throughout pregnancy. This could cause optic atrophy, microcephaly and mental retardation, which have been described with warfarin (Shaul and Hall, 1977). The risk of these is probably small and in a controlled follow-up study of 20 infants exposed to warfarin in the second and third trimesters no intellectual difference was noted at four years of age (Chong et al, 1984). These concerns about warfarin in pregnancy have caused a re-evaluation of therapy. However, whilst long-term prophylaxis with subcutaneous heparin appeared attractive because of no placental transfer, maternal effects on bone have been noticed. Demineralization of bone has been reported in patients on long-term heparin therapy (Jaffe and Willis, 1965) and this has now been reported in pregnancy (Wise and Hall, 1980). Further studies have shown this to occur without symptoms (de Swiet et al, 1983). In addition, this change may be irreversible, which augurs poorly for the postmenopausal period.

In view of these problems with prophylactic therapy and the probable low risk of recurrence a more selective management is recommended. Prophylactic drug therapy is withheld after the problem has been discussed with the pregnant mother. She is advised about the symptoms of thromboembolism and told to report immediately to the hospital if she suspects any of them. Prolonged bedrest, whether in or out of hospital, should be covered by subcutaneous heparin, a dosage of 7500 units twice a day being recommended. If elective caesarean under general anaesthetic is planned then subcutaneous heparin can be safely used pre- and postoperatively without affecting blood loss. However, if the option of regional analgesia for labour and delivery is to remain then dextran can be infused which offers some thromboembolic protection without interfering with clotting, thus permitting epidural anaesthesia.

Diagnosis of thromboembolism in pregnancy

All staff involved with maternity care must be aware that minor respiratory symptoms such as cough, chest pain, dyspnoea or a slight pyrexia may be indicative of small pulmonary emboli. Major pulmonary emboli are usually obvious, with chest pain, dyspnoea, cyanosis, hypotension and a raised jugular venous pressure.

Deep venous thrombosis occurs more commonly in the left leg and has the classic signs of a hot, tender, swollen limb. However, in the non-pregnant patient no underlying thrombosis is found in over 50% of classic cases (Sandler et al, 1984) and the same is likely to be found in pregnancy. In view of the implications for management in the rest of the pregnancy, future pregnancies and contraceptive practice, the diagnosis must be confirmed or refuted by investigations. The method of choice is venography of the femoral and distal system with shielding of the uterus. This is gradually being replaced by ultrasound Doppler flow studies as radiologists increasingly have access to and the expertise with the appropriate equipment (Whitehouse, 1987). Simple investigations for confirmation of pulmonary embolism such as chest X-ray and ECG are not usually helpful unless there has been a major embolus since pregnancy changes may mimic the minor signs (e.g. inverted T wave in lead III of the ECG). Accordingly all suspected cases should have ventilation/perfusion lung scans performed, which are perfectly safe in pregnancy. If there is any delay in obtaining the definitive test the patient should be anticoagulated with heparin whilst waiting, since the risks of such treatment are negligible and it should minimize the risk of clot extension and new emboli.

Once the diagnosis of a thromboembolism has been made, treatment should be by a slow continuous intravenous infusion of heparin in normal saline, at a starting rate of 40000 units per day. The dose can then be adjusted according to the laboratory results (protamine sulphate neutralization test, partial thromboplastin test). After about seven days the heparin can be given subcutaneously, lower doses of about 10000 units twice daily being usually advised. These do not affect the whole blood clotting system and should be continued until six weeks postpartum. The management with regard to preparation for delivery is the same as for those on routine prophylaxis (see above).

RENAL DISEASE

A number of general comments will be made about the management of renal disease in pregnancy; more details can be obtained from a recent edition in this series devoted to the subject (Lindheimer and Davison, 1987).

Preconceptional advice

Women with severe renal impairment (plasma creatinine > 250 μmol/l) are generally infertile. Consideration of pregnancy should be postponed until after transplantation, when it is clear that the graft has not been rejected and only low-dose maintenance immunosuppressives are needed. Even then the question of long-term maternal survival and bringing up a child has to be discussed. Women with moderate renal damage used to be advised against pregnancy. A more recent series showed a relatively good fetal outcome in women with plasma creatinine concentrations between 150 and 240 μmol/l (Hou et al, 1985), but there was a suggestion of accelerated renal impairment. Accordingly advice must be guarded in this group in particular if there have been problems with hypertension. Women with plasma creatinine concentrations < 125 μmol/l usually have a successful fetal outcome without acceleration of their disease (Davison, 1989) provided correct antenatal care is given.

Anti-hypertensive therapy should be reviewed. In view of uncertainties about captopril and teratogenesis (Editorial, 1989), women needing treatment should preferably be controlled on β-blockers or methyldopa prior to pregnancy, since there appear to be no detrimental effects on development with these drugs.

Antenatal maternal assessment

The keynote to management is obsessional monitoring. Renal function should be assessed by 24-hour urine estimation of creatinine clearance and protein excretion as well as by measuring plasma concentrations of urea, electrolytes, creatinine and urate. This should be done at four-weekly intervals up to 32 weeks' gestation, unless there is evidence of any deterioration in which case it should be assessed more frequently. After 32 weeks it is wise to measure these parameters every one to two weeks, depending on the severity of the condition. Plasma albumin concentrations and full blood count and platelets should also be measured.

Blood pressure should be monitored at two-weekly intervals up to 32 weeks and then weekly. If already on antihypertensive treatment, increases in dosage are usually best managed on an inpatient basis, and this is essential for the proper assessment of those with newly diagnosed hypertension. β-Blockers and methyldopa again are the preferred agents in view of their wide usage in obstetrics.

Asymptomatic bacteriuria should be looked for at all visits and treated to minimize possible deterioration in renal function.

The renal patient is not immune to superimposed pre-eclampsia and eclampsia and accordingly deterioration in hypertension or protein excretion demands very careful inpatient assessment looking for any symptoms or signs of impending eclampsia.

Antenatal fetal assessment

Moderate and severe renal disease is usually associated with severe fetal growth retardation so that a good baseline ultrasound scan is mandatory. Detailed anomaly scanning should be offered to all, not because of a specific increase in anomalies, but in view of the maternal risks being taken during the pregnancy. Subsequently serial ultrasound scanning for growth should commence by 24–26 weeks and continue two-weekly. Any suggestion of a decreasing growth rate requires inpatient admission and regular antenatal cardiotocographs. Abnormalities in these should be managed in the normal way. Whilst widely practised, there is no specific reason to induce labour if the condition of the mother and fetus is being monitored and is satisfactory. Premature delivery is common either through preterm labour, which is more common with renal disease, or through medical intervention for fetal or maternal indications.

Management of the renal transplant patient

There is now wide experience in management and this has recently been reviewed (Davison, 1987). There appears to be no increased risk of teratogenesis from immunosuppressive therapy. It is wisest to follow the protocol outlined above so that any deterioration and possible transplant rejection can be detected early. Fetal growth retardation is again more common even in the absence of renal impairment, as is premature delivery. A renal transplant on its own is not an indication for caesarean delivery.

Diagnosis of renal disease in pregnancy

In view of the changes in plasma volume and glomerular filtration rate in pregnancy, plasma creatinine concentrations $>75\,\mu mol/l$ and urea $>4.5\,mmol/l$ should be regarded as suspicious of underlying renal impairment. Accordingly these women should be managed as outlined above.

The most common time for consideration of renal disease is in the differential diagnosis of pre-eclampsia. The distinction is not academic since with renal disease continuing fetal growth may occur, whilst with pre-eclampsia this is unlikely. These cases usually require permanent hospitalization with careful monitoring of maternal renal function and blood pressure and fetal evaluation with ultrasound and cardiotocography. It has been claimed that 90% of cases of 'pre-eclampsia' diagnosed before 37 weeks are likely to be of renal origin (Ihle et al, 1987). This figure appears very high, but emphasizes that attempts at making a definitive diagnosis should be made. Current opinion is that renal biopsy in pregnancy is only indicated if there is a strong suggestion that the underlying lesion may be steroid-responsive or renal function is deteriorating rapidly (Lindheimer and Davison, 1987). After pregnancy attempts must be made to make a definitive diagnosis in all cases.

EPILEPSY

Epilepsy occurs in about five in 1000 pregnant women and thus is a potential problem met regularly by obstetricians.

Preconceptional care

There is generally considered to be a twofold increase in the incidence of congenital malformations (in particular facial clefts) in infants born to mothers with epilepsy. Mothers taking anticonvulsant drugs have a higher incidence of congenital anomalies than those not taking drugs. Paternal epilepsy does not appear to increase the risk (Friis et al, 1986). Accordingly it is important that therapy is reviewed by a physician prior to pregnancy. If no fits have occurred for three years then consideration should be given to stopping therapy well in advance of conception. If the woman is having multiple drug therapy then attempts should be made to reduce to one drug only. Also, the lowest acceptable dosage should be used.

In terms of specific drugs, all are likely to increase the risk of congenital malformations. Sodium valproate is associated with neural tube defects, although the risk has subsequently been thought to be only in the order of 1% (Lindhout and Schmidt, 1986). Phenytoin does appear to be associated with a slight increase in facial clefts (Meadow, 1968) and the 'fetal hydantoin syndrome', i.e. growth retardation, microcephaly, abnormal facies and mental retardation (Hanson and Smith, 1975). Carbamazepine has been specifically recommended for young women because of its lack of teratogenic effects. However, a decrease in head circumference at birth was noted by Hiilesmaa et al (1981). A subsequent report (Jones et al, 1989) found no such decrease, but did observe some of the features of the 'fetal hydantoin syndrome'. Accordingly, in view of the potential problems of all drugs, it is important that the general principles mentioned above are followed.

Early pregnancy

Once conception has occurred the actual drugs used should not be altered, but the serum levels should be determined and the dosage adjusted to ensure a therapeutic concentration is being obtained. There are many reasons why this may not be occurring. The woman may not be taking her therapy because of concern about effects on fetal development. If this is happening she should be reassured that the risk of having an abnormal baby are only slightly increased and advised to take the medication. There are also pharmacokinetic reasons for subtherapeutic concentrations. Absorption may be decreased and clearance increased, and the increase in plasma volume will lower the concentration. However, phenytoin is bound to plasma proteins and the bound proportion may alter during pregnancy, but it is the free component which is active. Thus total serum concentrations may not be totally reliable; measuring salivary concentrations, which appear to correlate well with unbound phenytoin, has been suggested as a better alternative (Knott et al, 1986). Regular measurement of drug concentrations are needed throughout pregnancy.

Since phenytoin may result in a lowering of serum folic acid concentrations, supplementary folic acid is advisable, but the dosage present in the conventional haematinic supplements (350–500 µg) should suffice.

Any woman who has been taking sodium valproate should be offered antenatal screening for neural tube defects by α-fetoprotein measurement in the mother and detailed ultrasound scanning with or without amniotic fluid determination of α-fetoprotein concentration. With the excellent results obtained by paediatric surgeons it is unusual to consider termination of pregnancy for facial clefts, but a regional obstetric unit is likely to have the expertise and equipment available to make this diagnosis early enough. More difficult is the antenatal diagnosis of the full hydantoin syndrome with microcephaly. This is helped by scanning as early as possible for gestational assessment based on gestational sac size or crown–rump length and then second trimester measurements of femur length as well as head measurements on at least two occasions. Exactly what measurements constitute microcephaly are uncertain, but values above the mean minus three standard deviations should be regarded as normal. The uncertainties about the diagnosis make counselling difficult.

Late pregnancy

Clinical estimation of fetal growth is best aided by routine ultrasound growth measurements. This should distinguish between a symmetrical growth retardation pattern, which may be associated with epilepsy and is unlikely to require any intervention, and an unrelated asymmetrical pattern which may well do so.

The occurrence of a first ever fit in pregnancy demands a thorough neurological assessment assuming that it was clear that it was not an eclamptic fit. Pregnancy does not appear to be epileptogenic so tumours need to be excluded by computed tomographic brain scanning. Arteriovenous malformations may also cause complications precipitating fits. It is not usual to commence antiepileptic therapy unless the fits are recurrent.

There is little evidence of any increased incidence of obstetric complications in association with epilepsy unless there is status epilepticus. Similarly epilepsy is not an indication for elective delivery.

THYROID DISEASE

Thyroid disease in pregnancy has not attracted as much research as the other complications already discussed. This is no doubt because risks to the mother in pregnancy are rare. However, there are some fetal risks and these are described below. Estimates of the incidence vary due to the difficulties in diagnosing the condition because of the alterations in thyroid function tests in pregnancy (see below). Figures often quoted are nine in 1000 pregnancies being associated with hypothyroidism and two in 1000 with hyperthyroidism (Niswander et al, 1972). Goitre does not appear to be more common in pregnancy in areas where there is adequate dietary iodine (Crook et al, 1967; Levy et al, 1980). An American study in pregnant teenagers (Long et al, 1985) found a 6% incidence, which was similar to their control group.

Preconceptional care

Thyroid dysfunction may be associated with subfertility. Treatment of hyperthyroidism may result in return of fertility, so that contraception must be discussed at the same time. Ovulatory dysfunction in hypothyroidism may be caused by hyperprolactinaemia. Whilst hypothyroidism is said to be associated with miscarriage, women with recurrent miscarriages rarely show thyroid dysfunction. For those women with hyperthyroidism due to Graves' disease, subtotal thyroidectomy may be considered prior to pregnancy as this may result in avoiding drugs in pregnancy. In practice this is rarely performed unles thyroid control is unsatisfactory.

It has been suggested that propylthiouracil is the treatment of choice for hyperthyroidism during pregnancy. This is based on three considerations:

1. Evidence for teratogenesis with antithyroid drugs is slight. However, scalp defects have been reported to be associated with carbimazole and methimazole (Milham, 1985).
2. Propylthiouracil is likely to cross the placenta less readily than the imidazole drugs. However, this appears to be of little relevance, as in a recent report there was no discernible difference in the effects of propylthiouracil and methimazole on fetal or maternal thyroid function (Momotani et al, 1986).
3. Imidazoles appear to be concentrated more in the breast milk than propylthiouracil. However, normal thyroid function has been reported in breast-fed infants whose mothers were taking no more than 15 mg carbimazole daily (Lamberg et al, 1984). Thyroid function should be monitored in all breast-fed infants of hyperthyroid mothers anyway.

Accordingly there appears little evidence to recommend changing therapy prior to pregnancy in a thyrotoxic woman who is well controlled.

Assessment of thyroid function in pregnancy

Whilst the two active thyroid hormones thyroxine (T_4) and triiodothyronine (T_3) are both produced by the thyroid gland, most of the T_3 is produced peripherally from T_4. Almost all of the circulating thyroid hormones are bound, mostly to thyroxine-binding globulin (TBG), leaving less than 1% circulating as free active hormone (Ramsay et al, 1983).

In pregnancy the increased glomerular filtration rate is likely to be responsible for the greater urinary iodide loss and decreased plasma concentration. Accordingly thyroid uptake of iodine increases. If there is a deficiency of dietary iodine, thyroid hypertrophy occurs and a goitre may be palpable. As for most binding globulins, pregnancy results in an increased synthesis and avidity of TBG so that more T_4 and T_3 are bound with an overall increase in total thyroid hormone concentrations in the blood. The actual concentration of free hormone is usually derived, but with these pregnancy changes this is not that precise. However, assays are now available for measuring the free hormones and longitudinal studies have shown that in normal pregnancy both free T_4 and T_3 decrease in concentration with increasing gestation (Parker, 1985; Rodin et al, 1989). Thus interpretation of results not only has to allow for pregnancy, but also for gestational age. Thyrotrophin (thyroid-stimulating hormone; TSH) can now be measured by a highly sensitive assay, but these results confirm earlier findings of no specific changes with pregnancy and gestation (Rodin et al, 1989). However, suppression of TSH production has been reported in the first trimester (Chan and Swaminathan, 1988).

Hypothyroidism in pregnancy

Women with a previously diagnosed disorder who are being adequately treated with T_4 maintenance therapy should not need dosage adjustment during pregnancy since the requirements do not alter. Free T_4 should be in the upper range of normal and the TSH concentration should be low, indicating suppression.

The diagnosis of hypothyroidism in pregnancy for the first time may be difficult since symptoms such as weight gain will be masked. However, the other symptoms and signs such as cold intolerance, decreased appetite, skin roughening and a slow pulse may be more obvious. The T_4 concentration may be within the normal range for the non-pregnant, but will be low for pregnancy. If there is uncertainty then the free T_4 and TSH concentrations should be measured. Once diagnosed, thyroxine replacement therapy should be commenced and T_4 concentrations measured monthly in order to achieve a suitable dosage.

Since maternal hypothyroidism may be associated with antibodies which cross the placenta, fetal hypothyroidism may occur in inadequately treated women. The simplest indicator of fetal thyroid status is the heart rate which should be counted at each antenatal assessment and should be within the normal range. Maternal serum and amniotic fluid thyroid measurements can not be used to assess fetal status, and fetal blood sampling for this is not widely available and not without risk. Fetal hyperthyroidism (see below) can occur in the presence of maternal hypothyroidism if the original problem had been Graves' disease (which had been treated surgically with resultant hypothyroidism), with stimulating antibodies still circulating and passing to the fetus.

Hyperthyroidism in pregnancy

Most cases of hyperthyroidism are associated with Graves' disease. Other causes include a toxic nodular goitre, a toxic adenoma, acute transient thyroiditis and in association with Hashimoto's disease. The diagnosis of hyperthyroidism for the first time in pregnancy is rare due to its association with subfertility. If suspected in early pregnancy a hydatidiform mole should be excluded immediately, since the β-subunit of human chorionic gonadatrophin has a thyroid-stimulating effect with resultant raised T_4 concentrations. The symptoms and signs which would make one suspect hyper-thyroidism are no different in pregnancy, but the palpitations and heat intolerance may be confused as pregnancy symptoms. A high index of suspicion is needed since untreated thyrotoxicosis is associated with a poor pregnancy outcome and congenital malformations (Momotani et al, 1984). The diagnosis is confirmed by the presence of a T_4 concentration elevated even for pregnancy. If there is any doubt then the free T_4 level should be measured. Treatment with either carbimazole or propylthiouracil should be commenced. Supplementation with β-blockers is not routinely required unless there is concern about maternal or fetal signs such as a marked tachycardia.

Monitoring of the pregnant woman with treated hyperthyroidism is best done by monthly clinical evaluation and estimations of T_4 and TSH. There is a tendency for Graves' disease to improve during pregnancy, so efforts should be made to have the woman on the minimum dosage required of antithyroid drugs. There is probably no need to give additional thyroid hormone to try to prevent fetal hypothyroidism since more antithyroid drug will be needed by the mother and little T_4 crosses to the fetus. This aspect has been reviewed by Ramsay et al (1983).

Monitoring of the fetus in maternal hyperthyroid disease is important because of the slight possibility of fetal thyrotoxicosis. A 50% perinatal mortality has been reported with this condition (Pekonen et al, 1984). In addition, there is a risk of subsequent neurological impairment and cranio-synostosis (Daneman and Howard, 1980; Cove and Johnston, 1985). Although detection of maternal thyroid-stimulating antibodies may be pre-dictive of fetal thyrotoxicosis, direct fetal parameters are more relevant. The fetal growth rate should be monitored since the thyrotoxic fetus will be underweight. More importantly the fetal heart rate should be counted precisely. A persistent baseline fetal tachycardia should be treated by maternal antithyroid therapy. β-Blocker drugs are likely to be needed only if there is a high risk of imminent fetal death.

CONCLUSIONS

A medical disorder in pregnancy can only be managed satisfactorily if there is a clear understanding of the physiological changes of pregnancy in that system and the natural progress of the disease process.

Whilst a number of obstetricians may be able to give appropriate prepreg-nancy advice, few women will actually present to them. Accordingly it is important that the principles are conveyed to all health workers and obste-tricians are freely available to discuss cases in more detail.

A normal outcome to pregnancy is most likely to be obtained if obste-tricians and physicians work closely together, preferably in combined clinics. This is becoming even more important as women's expectations for a successful pregnancy outcome are increasing, even with severe medical disorders.

REFERENCES

Badaracco MA & Vessey MP (1974) Recurrence of venous thromboembolic disease and use of oral contraceptives. *British Medical Journal* **i:** 215–217.

Beard RW & Lowy C (1982) The British survey of diabetic pregnancies. *British Journal of Obstetrics and Gynaecology* **89:** 783–786.

Becker RM (1983) Intracardiac surgery in pregnant women. *Annals of Thoracic Surgery* **36:** 453–458.

Brudenell JM & Doddridge MC (1989) *Diabetic Pregnancy*, p 90. London: Churchill Livingstone.

Burn J (1987) The next lady has a heart defect. *British Journal of Obstetrics and Gynaecology* **94:** 97–99.

Chan BY & Swaminathan R (1988) Serum thyrotrophin concentration measured by sensitive assays in normal pregnancy. *British Journal of Obstetrics and Gynaecology* **95:** 1332–1336.

Chen WWC, Chan CS, Lee PR, Wang RYR & Wong VCW (1982) Pregnancy in patients with prosthetic heart valves: an experience with 45 pregnancies. *Quarterly Journal of Medicine* **51:** 358–365.

Chong MKB, Harvey D & de Swiet M (1984) Follow-up study of children whose mothers were treated with warfarin during pregnancy. *British Journal of Obstetrics and Gynaecology* **91:** 1070–1073.

Cousins L (1987) Pregnancy complications among diabetic women: review 1965–1985. *Obstetrical and Gynecological Survey* **42:** 140–149.

Cove DH & Johnston P (1985) Fetal hyperthyroidism: experience of treatment in four siblings. *Lancet* **i:** 430–432.

Crooks J, Tulloch MI, Turnbull AC et al (1967) Comparative incidence of goitre in pregnancy in Iceland and Scotland. *Lancet* **ii:** 625–627.

Damm P & Molsted-Pederson L (1989) Significant decrease in congenital malformations in newborn infants of an unselected population of diabetic women. *American Journal of Obstetrics and Gynecology* **161:** 1163–1167.

Daneman D & Howard NJ (1980) Neonatal thyrotoxicosis: intellectual impairment and craniosynostosis in later years. *Journal of Pediatrics* **97:** 257–259.

Davison JM (1987) Pregnancy in renal allograft recipients: prognosis and management. *Baillière's Clinical Obstetrics and Gynaecology* **1(4):** 1027–1045.

Davison JM (1989) Renal disease. In de Swiet M (ed.) *Medical Disorders in Obstetric Practice* 2nd edn, pp 306–407. London: Blackwell.

Department of Health (1989) *Report on Confidential Enquiries into Maternal Deaths in England and Wales 1982–1984.* London: HMSO.

de Swiet M (1989) Heart disease in pregnancy. In de Swiet M (ed.) *Medical Disorders in Obstetric Practice* 2nd edn, pp 198–248. London: Blackwell.

de Swiet M & Fidler J (1981) Heart disease in pregnancy: some controversies. *Journal of the Royal College of Physicians of London* **15:** 183–186.

de Swiet M, Bulpitt CJ & Lewis PJ (1980) How obstetricians use anticoagulants in the prophylaxis of thromboembolism. *Journal of Obstetrics and Gynaecology* **1:** 29–32.

de Swiet M, Ward PD, Fidler J et al (1983) Prolonged heparin therapy in pregnancy causes bone demineralization. *British Journal of Obstetrics and Gynaecology* **90:** 1129–1134.

Dooley SL, Depp R, Socol ML, Tamura RK & Vaisrub N (1984) Urinary estriols in diabetic pregnancy: a reappraisal. *Obstetrics and Gynecology* **64:** 469–475.

Drury MI (1986) Management of the pregnancy diabetic patient—are the pundits right? *Diabetologia* **29:** 10–12.

Editorial (1989) Are ACE inhibitors safe in pregnancy? *Lancet* **ii:** 482–483.

Friis ML, Holm NV, Sindrup EH, Fogh-Andersen P & Hauge M (1986) Facial clefts in sibs and children of epileptic patients. *Neurology* **36:** 346–350.

Fuhrmann K, Reiher H, Semmler K et al (1983) Prevention of congenital malformations in infants of insulin dependent diabetic mothers. *Diabetes Care* **6:** 219–223.

Hanson JW & Smith DW (1975) The fetal hydantoin syndrome. *Journal of Pediatrics* **87:** 285–290.

Hiilesmaa VK, Teramo K, Granstrom ML & Bardy AH (1981) Fetal head growth retardation associated with maternal antiepileptic drugs. *Lancet* **ii:** 165–167.

Hou SH, Grossman SD & Madias NE (1985) Pregnancy in women with renal disease and moderate renal insufficiency. *American Journal of Medicine* **78**: 185–194.

Ihle BU, Long P & Oats J (1987) Early onset pre-eclampsia: recognition of underlying renal disease. *British Medical Journal* **294**: 79–81.

Jaffe MD & Willis PW (1965) Multiple fractures associated with long-term sodium heparin therapy. *Journal of the American Medical Association* **193**: 152–154.

Johnson JM, Lange IR, Harman CR, Torchia MG & Manning FA (1988) Biophysical profile scoring in the management of the diabetic pregnancy. *Obstetrics and Gynecology* **72**: 841–846.

Jones KL, Lacro RV, Johnson KA & Adams J (1989) Pattern of malformations in the children of women treated with carbamazepine during pregnancy. *New England Journal of Medicine* **320**: 1661–1666.

Kitzmiller JL, Mall JC, Gin GD et al (1987) Measurement of fetal shoulder width with computed tomography in diabetic women. *Obstetrics and Gynecology* **70**: 941–945.

Knott C, Williams CP & Reynolds F (1986) Phenytoin kinetics during pregnancy and the puerperium. *British Journal of Obstetrics and Gynaecology* **93**: 1030–1037.

Lamberg B-A, Ikonen E, Österlund K et al (1984) Antithyroid treatment of maternal hyperthyroidism during lactation. *Clinical Endocrinology* **21**: 81–87.

Levy RP, Newman DM, Rejali LS & Barford DAG (1980) The myth of goiter in pregnancy. *American Journal of Obstetrics and Gynecology* **137**: 701–703.

Lind T (1989) A prospective multicentre study to determine the influence of pregnancy upon the 75 g oral glucose tolerance test (OGTT). In Sutherland HW, Stowers JM & Pearson DWM (eds) *Carbohydrate Metabolism in Pregnancy and the Newborn IV*, pp 209–226. Berlin: Springer–Verlag.

Lindheimer MD & Davison JM (eds) (1987) Renal disease in pregnancy. *Baillière's Clinical Obstetrics and Gynaecology* **1(4)**.

Lindhout D & Schmidt D (1986) In-utero exposure to valproate and neural tube defects. *Lancet* **i**: 1392–1393.

Long TJ, Felice ME & Hollingsworth DR (1985) Goiter in pregnant teenagers. *American Journal of Obstetrics and Gynecology* **152**: 670–674.

Lowy C, Beard RW & Goldschmidt J (1986) Congenital malformations in babies of diabetic mothers. *Diabetic Medicine* **3**: 458–462.

Maresh M (1988) Gestational diabetes. In Chamberlain G (ed.) *Contemporary Obstetrics and Gynaecology*, pp 185–198. London: Butterworths.

Meadow SR (1968) Anticonvulsant drugs and congenital abnormalities. *Lancet* **ii**: 1296.

Milham S (1985) Scalp defects in infants of mothers treated for hyperthyroidism with methimazole or carbimazole during pregnancy. *Teratology* **32**: 321.

Mills JL, Knopp RH, Simpson JL et al (1988a) Lack of relation of increased malformation rates in infants of diabetic mothers to glycemic control during organogenesis. *New England Journal of Medicine* **318**: 671–676.

Mills JL, Simpson JL, Driscoll SG et al (1988b) Incidence of spontaneous abortion among normal women and insulin-dependent diabetic women whose pregnancies were identified within 21 days of conception. *New England Journal of Medicine* **319**: 1617–1623.

Molsted-Pederson L & Kuhl C (1986) Obstetrical management in diabetic pregnancy: the Copenhagen experience. *Diabetologia* **29**: 13–16.

Momotani N, Ito K, Hamada N et al (1984) Maternal hyperthyroidism and congenital malformation in the offspring. *Clinical Endocrinology* **20**: 695–700.

Momotani N, Jaeduk N, Oyanagi H et al (1985) Antithyroid drug therapy for Graves' disease during pregnancy. *New England Journal of Medicine* **315**: 24–28.

Niswander RR, Gordon M & Berendes HW (1972) The women and their pregnancies. *The Collaborative Perinatal Study of the National Institute of Neurologic Disease and Stroke*, vol. 1, pp 246–249. Philadelphia: WB Saunders.

Parker JH (1985) Amerlex free triiodothyronine and free thyroxine levels in normal pregnancy. *British Journal of Obstetrics and Gynaecology* **92**: 1234–1238.

Pekonen F, Teramo K, Makinen T et al (1984) Prenatal diagnosis and treatment of fetal thyrotoxicosis. *American Journal of Obstetrics and Gynecology* **150**: 893–894.

Ramsay I, Kaur S & Krassas G (1983) Thyrotoxicosis in pregnancy: results of treatment by antithyroid drugs combined with T_4. *Clinical Endocrinology* **18**: 73–85.

Rodin A, Mashiter G, Quartero R et al (1989) Thyroid function in normal pregnancy. *Journal of Obstetrics and Gynaecology* **10:** 89–94.

Sandler DA, Martin JF, Duncan JS et al (1984) Diagnosis of deep-vein thrombosis: comparison of clinical evaluation, ultrasound, plethysmography and venoscan with X-ray venogram. *Lancet* **ii:** 716–719.

Shaul WL & Hall JG (1977) Multiple congenital anomalies associated with oral anticoagulants. *American Journal of Obstetrics and Gynecology* **127:** 191–198.

Steel JM, Johnstone FD & Smith AF (1989) Pre-pregnancy preparation. In Sutherland HW, Stowers JM & Pearson DWM (eds) *Carbohydrate Metabolism in Pregnancy and the Newborn (Aberdeen, 1988)*, pp 129–139. Berlin: Springer–Verlag.

Stubbs SM, Doddridge MC, John PN, Steel JM & Wright AD (1986) Haemoglobin A_1 and congenital malformation. *Diabetic Medicine* **4:** 156–159.

Sugrue D, Blake S & MacDonald D (1981) Pregnancy complicated by maternal heart disease at the National Maternity Hospital, Dublin, Ireland, 1969 to 1978. *American Journal of Obstetrics and Gynecology* **139:** 1–6.

Szekely P, Turner R & Snaith L (1973) Pregnancy and the changing pattern of rheumatic heart disease. *British Heart Journal* **35:** 1293–1303.

Wald NJ, Cuckle HS, Boreham J, Stirrat G & Turnbull A (1979) Maternal serum alpha-fetoprotein and diabetes mellitus. *British Journal of Obstetrics and Gynaecology* **86:** 101–105.

Whitehouse G (1987) Radiological diagnosis of deep vein thrombosis. *British Medical Journal* **295:** 801–802.

Wise PH & Hall AJ (1980) Heparin-induced osteopenia in pregnancy. *British Medical Journal* **281:** 110–111.

Working Party of the British Society for Antimicrobial Chemotherapy (1982) The antibiotic prophylaxis of infective endocarditis. *Lancet* **ii:** 1323–1326.

9

Social problems

MARY HEPBURN

THE DEVELOPMENT OF ANTENATAL CARE

In Britain, antenatal care was effectively introduced during the First World War to improve maternal health, initially because of its relevance to infant welfare and latterly as an end in itself. Its value was not immediately acknowledged universally. The eugenicists, having argued that infant welfare work which might save weak or unfit children was inadvisable, considered that any antenatal intervention should be directed towards education of the mother (Pearson, 1913); any adverse effect of poverty on infant welfare was seen as being an indirect one and attributable to maternal ignorance, poor habits and inefficiency which could be overcome by education.

When it was introduced, antenatal care was uncritically viewed as conferring an unspecified benefit on mother and baby which was 'dose dependent'. In a study of maternal mortality in the Glasgow Royal Maternity Hospital from 1926 to 1930, the primary cause of death in 35% of cases was stated to be inadequate or absent antenatal care (Kerr, 1933).

The objectives of antenatal care, in addition to lowering the death rate among mothers and babies, largely centred on improvement of health antenatally by detection of general health problems and early diagnosis of pregnancy complications, and preparation or education of women for labour with consequent improved outcome (Browne, 1932; Kerr, 1933); more recently the preventive aspects of education have received greater emphasis.

Outpatient care

Antenatal outpatient care was initially delivered by hospital clinics and later also by community-based local authority clinics, with the development of a system of shared care between these two agencies. Subsequently the local authority clinics played a progressively smaller part and ultimately closed, while the role of the general practitioner expanded and the system of hospital/general practitioner shared care became established, dominated and controlled by the hospital.

A largely arbitrary regime for outpatient antenatal care was outlined by the Ministry of Health (1930) and was adhered to without question for many years. Only recently has this system been evaluated (Hall et al, 1980) and, with the identification of reasonable objectives, a more rational regimen proposed; nevertheless in many areas the system has remained essentially unchanged in terms of timing and content of consultations. Outpatient care is usually divided between community-based general practitioners and/or midwives and hospital-based obstetricians and/or midwives. The Royal College of Obstetricians and Gynaecologists Working Party Report on Antenatal and Intrapartum Care (Royal College of Obstetricians and Gynaecologists, 1982), in addition to recommending greater flexibility in individual provision of antenatal care, also recommended increased community-based care and increased provision of care by midwives. There are wide inter- and intraregional variations in both the extent and the type of community-based antenatal care which is provided, and this is further complicated by the continued debate over the precise roles of the three groups of carers—obstetricians, midwives and general practitioners—with the areas of overlap providing a source of considerable contention.

Inpatient care

More or less coincidental with the introduction of outpatient antenatal care was the allocation of maternity hospital beds for inpatient antenatal care. Ballantyne (1901) originally envisaged such beds would be used for women with pre-existing problems, either pregnancy-related or intercurrent maternal disease, for women whose need arose during their pregnancy as a pregnancy complication, or for essentially healthy women simply in need of rest in later pregnancy. These views were subsequently echoed by Munro Kerr (Kerr, 1933). In a study in Glasgow Royal Maternity Hospital in 1983, however, pre-existing problems contributed little to antenatal admission, 77% of which were due to current pregnancy problems (Hepburn, 1987). The need envisaged by Ballantyne for rest by healthy women, or indeed social problems in general, was rarely cited as a reason for admission; in those cases where such factors might have been relevant, a contributory role was not acknowledged and indeed, the belief is widespread that social admissions would represent an unjustifiable use of medical resources. The value of antenatal care as a therapeutic measure has been studied for only a very small number of conditions (Enkin and Chalmers, 1982) and, with the exception of a few serious complications, there is no consensus of opinion on grounds for antenatal admission to hospital, far less evaluation of this method of treatment. In many areas there is increased use of daycare facilities for observation and monitoring of suspected abnormalities with the objective of reducing inpatient care. Such services require evaluation to see whether this is in fact always the case or whether it may, on occasions, merely involve investigations with no corresponding decrease in admissions.

EFFECTS OF SOCIO-ECONOMIC DEPRIVATION ON HEALTH AND HEALTH CARE

The health of all, including the unborn fetus, is affected by social and economic factors. Both deprivation in its widest context, whether material, physical or psychological, and life-style or behaviour associated with deprivation adversely affect health; in reproductive terms the consequent adverse pregnancy outcome is reflected in higher rates of perinatal and infant mortality and morbidity, including fetal malformations, low birthweight, preterm delivery and childhood illness. These effects have been widely reported individually and collectively (Baird and Wyper, 1941; Baird, 1945; Oakley et al, 1982; Townsend and Davidson, 1982; Ilsley, 1983). While initially this association was considered either to be non-existent (McKinlay, 1929) or of minimal significance (Kerr, 1933), it is now recognized that not only is this association consistently present but the magnitude of the gradient between social classes has remained depressingly constant (Enkin and Chalmers, 1982; Townsend and Davidson, 1982); moreover, any adverse effects of such social disadvantage may be manifest in successive generations (Baird, 1985). It has been suggested that social class differences in health are the result of associated life-styles and behaviours such as cigarette smoking (Brooke et al, 1989; Morrison et al, 1989; Najman et al, 1989). While these factors undoubtedly make a very significant contribution, it is well established that they are not amenable to change by simple advice and provision of information, and, moreover, there is evidence that they merely act as indicators of adverse maternal factors from which they are inseparable and which remain of primary importance (Blane, 1985). Nevertheless, treatment of social problems is widely regarded as being outside the remit of antenatal care, while the harmful aspects of life-style associated with social disadvantage are viewed as being under the control of and therefore the responsibility of the individual concerned.

Not only do social problems directly affect health, but they also exert an indirect effect; service provision is often poorer in poor areas (Tudor Hart, 1971) and the existence of class differentials in provision and utilization of health care services means that working class people are less likely than middle class people to use the services available. Thus, for whatever reason, those from lower socio-economic groups are less likely to receive adequate health care, and, in particular, women are less likely to receive antenatal care (Townsend and Davidson, 1982). When considering provision of antenatal care for women who have special social needs or who come from backgrounds of social deprivation, it is therefore essential to consider the siting and format of such care as well as its content.

ANTENATAL CARE FOR WOMEN WITH SOCIAL NEEDS

Outpatient care

The Possilpark pilot scheme

In February 1986, a clinic was established as a pilot scheme in a health centre in Possilpark, an area of North Glasgow characterized by very high levels of multiple deprivation: according to the 1981 census more than half the population aged 16–24 years were unemployed; one third of children were living in single adult families; the heads of 46% of households were on low income (including unemployment); one third of households were classified as overcrowded and almost two thirds of children lived in overcrowded conditions; and 93% of households did not own a car. By 1986, almost one third of all households were made up of single adults with children, and, in 1987, 55% of the population were living at or below Supplementary Benefit level.

The clinic could not aim to care for all women in the area, but the objective was to provide a comprehensive, multidisciplinary service to those women identified as having special needs or problems; in almost half the cases these transpired to relate to drug use either by the woman or her partner. The remainder included girls aged under 16 years, women with problems such as alcoholism, mental handicap or psychiatric illness, and women with a past history either of problems in coping for which support was required or of persistent non-attendance for antenatal care in previous pregnancies. There were also a very few women with no major problems who attended the clinic after hearing about it from other women. Referrals came from a number of sources including various members of the primary care team, the Social Work Department, other hospital specialities and services, community- and hospital-based drug services, the prostitutes' drop-in centre and various other voluntary and statutory agencies. Self referrals also became increasingly common, not only among women with no problems, but also among women with a wide range of difficulties, especially drug abuse. Thus numbers rose gradually so that in its first three years the clinic was attended by 250 women, almost half of whom attended in the third year. Twenty per cent of the women were married and 15% had a partner who was employed. Among these women there were three perinatal deaths, 7% of babies delivered preterm (<37 completed weeks' gestation), and 13% of babies had birthweights less than 2500 g. Such numbers are too small to be significant; nevertheless in a group of high-risk women, they are encouraging in their comparability with statistics for the rest of the City.

The ultimate aim is to extend this type of community-based service for women with special needs to all areas of the City; as an interim measure, in June 1988, an antenatal clinic was established in the Glasgow Royal Maternity Hospital to provide the same comprehensive type of care for women with problems relating to drug use by themselves or their partners. In the first 16 months, 120 women attended the clinic; by that time from the combined clinic populations, 113 women who were themselves intravenous (i.v.) drug users had delivered. There were two first trimester spontaneous abortions, one termination of pregnancy for fetal anomaly, one non-lethal fetal anomaly and no perinatal deaths. Seven per cent of babies were delivered preterm, while 10% had birthweights less than 2500 g. As in the case of the Possilpark clinic, pregnancy outcome for this group of i.v. drug-using women is gratifyingly average. Much of the following discussion derives from experience gained in the establishment and running of these two clinics.

Community-based services in general

To be effective, antenatal care must consider women in the context of their whole families and their home environment. Reference has already been made to the recommendations of the Royal College of Obstetricians and Gynaecologists Working Party for increased community-based services, and the benefits of such clinics have been demonstrated in terms of acceptability to women (Parboosingh and Kerr, 1982; Reid et al, 1983) and in terms of obstetric outcome (Parboosingh and Kerr, 1982). Community-based clinics are of value not only in reducing travelling time, but also in making attendance financially possible; it is often more expensive to travel to a hospital at some distance, but the practice of retrospective reimbursement of travelling expenses is of little benefit to the woman who does not possess sufficient money to travel to the hospital in the first place.

We have found an additional benefit in the case of those women who, despite living close to the clinic, nevertheless fail to attend as a result of their various problems. Arrangements can be made either to have such women escorted to the clinic or simply visited before or during the clinic to encourage them to attend. We find such home visiting of great value, but rarely use it to carry out routine examinations, for which the women are strongly encouraged to attend the clinic.

Clinics may be sited anywhere within the community, but where health centres are available, these provide additional benefits by having a wide range of services and expertise on one site. Regardless of their situation, however, these clinics should provide ample space and facilities for women to bring with them not only their children, but also partners, relatives or friends whom they might wish to have involved in their care.

Services provided. The care provided should not relate exclusively to the pregnancy but the opportunity provided by this contact should be used to deal with other issues, including not only those relating to general health but also those of a social rather than medical nature. Many women are unable to attend the antenatal clinic because social deprivation leads to other more pressing demands on their time; attendance to claim unemployment or social security benefits, or attendance at the Social Work or Housing Departments may be of greater practical importance and take priority over attendance at the antenatal clinic. The provision within the clinic setting of information regarding welfare rights, and counselling about or help with social problems, or even simply the adoption by clinic staff of a liaison role with the appropriate agencies, may ease such difficulties, relieve much stress and facilitate attendance at the clinic. Provision of such services also affords the opportunity for social workers to develop, from early in the pregnancy, relationships with the women which are perceived by the women as supportive; this contrasts with the more commonly held view of social workers in such circumstances as having a more punitive role providing crisis intervention against the women's interests. Such close collaboration with the Social Work Department has, for women attending our clinic, undoubtedly contributed to the high level of success in keeping babies in the care of mothers who might otherwise have failed to cope. A further factor is the recognition by the Social Work Department that maternal drug use is not a reason to remove a child from the mother's custody.

Women with drug- or alcohol-related problems benefit from the services of trained counsellors who can provide long-term support; in the case of i.v. drug use there is also the need for counselling about specific associated health risks, in particular infection with the human immunodeficiency virus (HIV), with the offer of an HIV screening service for those who wish it. The specific services required by women with problems of drug or alcohol abuse will be discussed in greater detail later in this chapter.

While attendance for antenatal care poses problems, attendance for parentcraft classes poses even greater problems! In our service, when largely traditional parentcraft classes were initially provided on a different day from the antenatal clinic, attendance rates were negligible. When parentcraft was provided as an integral part of a clinic which women attended on a weekly basis from 30 to 34 weeks and which was re-scheduled to avoid clashing with a popular television programme, attendance rates rose to virtually 100%! This reorganization followed a survey of the views and wishes of women attending the clinic, the results of which were in agreement with a study in the east end of Glasgow which suggested that, while women did not find special classes acceptable, they still wanted parentcraft information (Williams, 1989). In providing such parentcraft advice, however, it is essential to ensure the content and emphasis is appropriate for the population at which it is targeted.

While it is important to get maximum benefit from attendance at the antenatal clinic by provision of as many additional services as possible, it is also vital to ensure that women do not have unwanted services forced upon them, since this might deter them from attending the clinic.

One further service which we have found less popular has been the provision in the clinic of dental care. The incidence of dental problems among the women who attend our clinic is extremely high, particularly among women who use drugs; such women have the additional problem that withdrawal from drugs often precipitates severe toothache which requires immediate attention. Many of the women have never or rarely attended a dentist, however, and the presence of a dental nurse in the clinic area proved quite threatening to many. In any event very few women followed up this initial contact, and encouragement to attend a dental service in a rather more distant part of the health centre has proved more rewarding.

The timing of services is also important. Women admitted that the common local practice of carrying out cervical smears at postnatal review caused increasing apprehension during pregnancy and discouraged some from attending postnatally. We have found most women with gentle persuasion will accept cervical cytology antenatally; most then express relief that their apprehension was groundless and an additional and possibly the greatest benefit is the opportunity for treatment of the minor disorders and infections which are often present.

As well as allowing provision of services directly relating to the health of the pregnant woman, attendance at the antenatal clinic can be used to provide more general health care or even, on occasions, treatment of other members of the family; one such example has been the opportunity for immunization of other children in a family where previous attempts had failed.

Providers of care. The association between social deprivation and poor pregnancy outcome is well documented; such women therefore have high-risk pregnancies which merit care by an obstetrician. As a result of their social problems, however, they have a need for long-term care of the whole family which is most appropriately met by the general practitioner. Despite the increased risk of poor outcome, their obstetric management is often very straightforward and, as discussed, their obstetric risk may be more effectively managed by addressing their social problems. A significant part of their antenatal care can therefore fall within the remit of the midwife; a community midwife working in a particular area where she becomes well known can provide supportive care in the home, can encourage women to attend earlier and can reinforce the vital link between obstetrician and general practitioner, promoting continuity of care. Most discussions on provision of antenatal care tend to argue in favour of one professional at the expense of the other two; lists of advantages and disadvantages are used to support the case for one individual having a principal role in preference to the others. Such an attitude is, however, counterproductive; the range of problems faced by these women requires the skills of all three who, in collaboration not competition, make contributions of equal importance as members of a larger multidisciplinary team.

In our experience it is often desirable to have two people present at consultations to maintain consistency, especially in the case of women with drug problems who may be very manipulative; antenatal care is therefore provided by a single obstetrician and a midwife, or a general practitioner and the same midwife or, where unavoidable, one of these three alone. Most aspects of antenatal care are equally undertaken by all participants; because of the small number of staff involved, continuity of care is excellent and close relationships with the women can be established. Continuity of care is extremely important. Circumstances sometimes demand service modification; for example, some women, particularly those with drug problems, can only obtain general practitioner care on a three-monthly basis with compulsory rotational allocation by the Health Board. Nevertheless, regardless of who provides care or how responsibility is allocated, it is vital that all workers contributing to the care of the women liaise closely and regularly and it is helpful if they do not see their individual roles as being rigidly defined.

In our service, weekly meetings are held and regularly attended by medical, midwifery, health visiting and social work staff as well as a representative from the adjacent drugs project. At these meetings, with the women's knowledge, consent, and on many occasions at their request, referrals are made, problems are raised and dealt with and progress is reported.

Efficiency of service provision. The need for an accessible and immediately available service is largely incompatible with a rigidly structured clinic. One unsatisfactory aspect in the running of this clinic is therefore the potential for long waiting times by the women. Waiting times, while often quite short, vary enormously and delays can occur. This is due to a number of factors. While women do attend with gratifying regularity, they often do not keep to their appointment times or even their appointment day. Those who attend on the wrong day often do so because they have a problem with which they require help; this may prove to be very time-consuming and can lead to quite lengthy delays in the clinic. While women obliged to wait often protest, those who do so are also those most likely to use the service in this way themselves, and most express the view that the opportunity for immediate help outweighs the disadvantage of delay; the frequently made offer of a more rigid appointment system with a reduction in delays at the cost of some flexibility is repeatedly rejected by most women. The range of other services available helps to reduce waiting times or at least ensure they are used more productively. Women with different types of problem tend to arrive at different times. Thus those women who would prefer a more rigid appointment system and many of the very young girls usually attend at the beginning of the clinic, enabling them to be seen quickly and without delay. Women with drug problems, on the other hand, tend to arrive much later in the clinic. To some extent, therefore, the clinic regulates its own format, but nevertheless this is an area which requires continual assessment and an ongoing search for ways of overcoming the problem of waiting times.

Inpatient care

Antenatal inpatient care, as already noted, was originally envisaged as being indicated for three groups of women: those whose problems predated the pregnancy either as previous pregnancy problems or as intercurrent disease (now relatively rare in obstetric practice in Britain), those whose complications developed during the current pregnancy, and those essentially healthy women who, because of social or domestic factors, might benefit from admission to hospital for rest (Ballantyne, 1901). Thus, despite the reluctance to recognize the association between deprivation and poor obstetric outcome, it was conceded at a very early stage that inpatient care might have a role in the management of non-medical problems. The study of the use of antenatal inpatient care in Glasgow already referred to was carried out in a sample of 1302 women, being a random one third of the women delivering in Glasgow Royal Maternity Hospital in 1983 (Hepburn, 1987). In this study, 49% of women were admitted antenatally at least once and, as noted, 77% of admissions were due to current pregnancy complications; of these the majority were due to a relatively small number of conditions covered by the headings of hypertension, bleeding, abdominal pain and suspected poor fetal growth. Each of these conditions covered a broad spectrum of severity. It was apparent that for all these conditions there were difficulties not only in making the diagnosis, but also in assessing the degree of severity of the condition. Moreover, since serious conditions were not necessarily preceded by mild disorder, it was difficult to make an assessment of prognosis or identify those pregnancies at risk. Such difficulties no doubt contributed to the fact that even such little information as exists regarding the natural history of these conditions was largely ignored; selection of women for admission appeared random, as did subsequent management and, although no firm conclusions regarding benefit could be drawn from such a study, little benefit from admission was discernible.

Social problems were rarely cited as a reason for admission or even acknowledged as a contributory factor, despite the fact that 35% of the women were in social classes IV or V or had husbands who were unemployed and a further 15% were unmarried. It is possible clinicians did not regard social problems as a valid reason for admission. Alternatively, while recognizing such a need, they might have felt under pressure to attribute the admission to strictly medical grounds. A third possibility is that clinicians' decision-making was affected by social problems, but only at a subconscious level with a consequent lowering of threshold for admission, but the data did not support this hypothesis. While the study related to practice in one hospital only, it seems likely that the situation in other hospitals and other areas is not too dissimilar.

Women from areas of social deprivation commonly experience difficulties with housing or domestic relationships, often with financial problems as a contributory or causative factor. Caring for their families under such circumstances may place women under considerable stress. Stress itself can be harmful and has, for example, been implicated as a cause of preterm labour (Newton et al, 1979). Admission to hospital may break a vicious cycle and allow an opportunity for involving other agencies in an attempt to resolve some of the problems. At an even more basic level, one or more brief admissions may allow women a breathing space and some relief from the relentless pressure of their home environment. For some women, admission to hospital may provide the most effective opportunity for treating minor disorders or pregnancy complications. Admission can also be invaluable in helping women with specific social problems such as drug or other substance abuse; these will be considered in more detail later.

Admission to hospital may thus be justified in the management of non-medical problems. Conversely, however, for many women, admission to hospital might itself cause stress by separating them from their families; difficulty in finding someone to care for the family in their absence could further add to their anxieties. The lack of proven benefit from hospital admission for most pregnancy complications should therefore be borne in mind when making such a recommendation. It would appear many hospital admissions are instigated largely to reassure staff and, if there is an absence of proven benefit, women should not be pressurized into agreeing to such admissions nor should they be made to feel guilty if they are unable to accept such a recommendation.

Antenatal bed requirements are arbitrarily calculated on the basis of a constant relationship with postnatal bed requirements (Department of Health, Scotland, 1959; Ministry of Health, 1959; Department of Health and Social Security. Central Health Services Council Standing Midwifery and Maternity Advisory Committee, 1970; House of Commons Social Services Committee, 1980) and on the assumption that current practices are correct. Since there is a lack of data describing current practices and since admission for most of the conditions for which it is used has yet to be evaluated, such an assumption is questionable. The link between social deprivation (with its associated stresses) and adverse pregnancy outcome has been well documented. While the benefits of hospital admission for social problems have not been established either, such admissions would appear to be no less justified than those in current practice; hospital admission simply for rest, mental or physical, should be seen as a valid form of management and one on which the woman's views should be taken into account when making any decision.

ANTENATAL CARE FOR WOMEN WITH PROBLEMS OF ADDICTION

The term 'drugs' as commonly used does not include alcohol; while there are many similarities between drugs and alcohol there are also differences in patterns and trends of use and in legal and social acceptability. The drugs which are commonly subject to abuse are usually either illegal to possess or illegally obtained, and use of such drugs, particularly in Scotland, correlates very closely with social deprivation (Standing Committee on Drug Abuse, 1985); while there is drug use among the upper socio-economic groups, it is in magnitude much less significant, involves different drugs and is associated with a different range of problems. Whatever the social background, however, those people who use drugs cannot be distinguished as a separate pathological entity and are no different from other non-drug-using people in the same community.

Unlike drugs, alcohol consumption is legal and its use does not show the same social class distribution—if anything, the reverse trend is true (Office of Population Censuses and Surveys, 1984)—although there may be a small subgroup of women from lower socio-economic groups who drink heavily and also smoke heavily (Heller et al, 1988).

Patterns of use of both drugs and alcohol are changing. Consumption levels in women, particularly young women, are increasing in both relative and absolute terms. In the case of drugs there have also been changes in the type of drugs used, with a decline in heroin use and an increase in consumption of pharmaceutical drugs, especially buprenorphine (Temgesic) and benzodiazepines (notably temazepam). These changes have been particularly marked in Scotland.

Both drugs and alcohol are similar, however, in having a wide range of levels of consumption; many of those who use either substance have their use under control, maintain a normal life-style, and do not have a major problem of addiction. Antenatal care for women with problem drug or alcohol use must address not only the problem of addiction and any consequent health problems, but also any social problems present either as cause or effect of the problems of addiction.

Alcohol consumption during pregnancy

Problem alcohol consumption does not correlate with socio-economic deprivation and if anything, the reverse trend is true; however, the majority of people in Britain drink alcohol, with only 7% of men and 13% of women in 1984 claiming to be abstainers (Office of Population Censuses and Surveys, 1984). Information regarding drinking habits is obtained by self-reporting. Since consumption of alcohol is legal and socially acceptable, only causing problems when it becomes 'excessive', information regarding numbers of people who drink is likely to be more accurate than information regarding individual levels of consumption. Whatever the source of inaccuracy, such self-reported information would suggest levels of drinking in the general population lower than those suggested by alcohol sales (Office of Population Censuses and Surveys, 1984). Since drinking is common and acceptable there may be an unwillingness, either conscious or subconscious, on the part of the woman, her partner, her friends or her family to acknowledge when such a problem exists. While women who have alcohol problems are not especially likely to have backgrounds of material deprivation, they may have other underlying social problems and may ultimately have additional problems as a result of their drinking. Specialist help from trained counsellors should be offered to pregnant women with alcohol problems as an integral part of their antenatal care; the aim should be to help such women to reduce or stop their drinking, to help modify and stabilize their life-style, to provide long-term support, both to the women and their partners or families should they wish it, and to try to resolve any other social problems present for whatever reason.

The precise risks to the fetus of maternal drinking during pregnancy remain controversial. The relative risks of different patterns of drinking, either in binges or on a regular basis, of different types of alcohol, whether spirits or beer, and of different doses of alcohol at different stages of pregnancy remain a source of debate, as indeed are the nature, if any, of any possible effects which alcohol may have on the fetus. The most severe postulated effect is that spectrum of abnormalities termed the 'fetal alcohol syndrome' (Jones and Smith, 1973). Although it is claimed this syndrome is seen only in children of alcoholics (Hill and Tennyson, 1986), conversely not all alcoholic women have children who exhibit such abnormalities, and even among women who drink heavily this 'syndrome' is rare. It has also been suggested that the spectrum of defects is not peculiar to children of alcoholics and merely represents damage by a non-specific agent at a particular stage of pregnancy (Zuckerman and Hingson, 1986). Others report simply a reduction in birthweight in babies of women who drink, but this effect is variously observed with high, moderate or low levels of consumption; some have observed no such association (Little, 1977; Marbury et al, 1983; Wright et al, 1983; Mills et al, 1984; Zuckerman and Hingson, 1986; Halmesmaki et al, 1987). Other adverse features of the mother's life-style, including smoking, use of other drugs and poor nutrition, make assessment of risk even more difficult.

To be absolutely certain of avoiding any possible damage to the fetus from alcohol, the only safe policy to advocate is one of total abstinence from before the time of conception. Even if such advice is considered appropriate, however, it should never be included in information given verbally or in leaflets at antenatal clinics where many women, already pregnant, will have consumed alcohol at around the time of conception; such advice will therefore be not only irrelevant but potentially harmful. From the information currently available, however, total abstinence may be considered unreasonable for the individual and low levels of drinking should not constitute an unacceptable risk for the fetus (Royal College of Obstetricians and Gynaecologists, 1985). Again, total abstinence might not be attainable for all; for those who drink heavily any reduction in intake is worthwhile in gross terms and the subtleties of assessing risk with low level consumption become less relevant.

Provision of information alone is not sufficient. Help is needed to achieve behaviour modification; as already noted, help in dealing with alcohol problems should be provided by trained professionals and such treatment can be given on an outpatient or inpatient basis as necessary. While inpatient treatment for alcoholism is usually provided in a psychiatric hospital, there may be occasions when the maternity hospital is more appropriate, allowing, among other things, monitoring of fetal well-being while the mental health team helps to care for the mother in close liaison with maternity staff.

Drug misuse in pregnancy

There are no accurate data on numbers of women who use drugs or on details of their habit. As with alcohol, information regarding the taking of drugs and the timing, dosage and identity of drugs taken is self-reported; since drug use involves illegal activities, such data is unreliable. Anxiety about possible child-care repercussions may also deter women from admitting such a history, and unfortunately on occasions such fears have been shown to be well founded. That so many women volunteer such information despite the risks demonstrates the very strong sense of responsibility the women feel towards their unborn child. Drug use *per se* is not incompatible with adequate child care; the problem arises when drug use leads to a chaotic life-style and no baby should ever be removed from the mother's care solely on the grounds of maternal drug use. The relevant authorities must not only recognize this fact but must reassure women that they recognize it so that drug-using women will feel free to seek help without fear of retribution.

Pregnant women who use drugs will, especially in Scotland, experience problems of social deprivation in common with others living in the same community. In addition, they often suffer severe social isolation; many either have no close family support or may have alienated partners or relatives through their drug use. Partners themselves may have a drug problem and co-ordinating help for both poses additional difficulties. In addition to the financial problems which they again share with others from the same background, women who use drugs need additional fundings to maintain their habit; such money is most commonly obtained either by shoplifting or by prostitution, both of which in turn lead to legal problems.

Convictions may result in fines, which in turn lead to further illegal activities to raise the necessary money to pay the fines. Where custodial sentences are imposed, these may interrupt the continuity of care and result in loss of contact. Close liaison with prison services is necessary to avoid such problems; simple re-referral by prison authorities on release is inadequate because it takes too long and because correct addresses are often either withheld by the women or are no longer applicable.

Reference has already been made to the effects of deprivation on health and access to health care services. Drug misuse has additional and separate effects on health, and where the life-style is chaotic this further reduces access to services.

Diet and nutritional levels, already often poor in the areas where drug use is most prevalent, are even worse among those using drugs. Nevertheless, in our experience, among pregnant women using drugs, even where levels of use are very high, serious problems of malnutrition, including severe anaemia, are uncommon. Much more common are problems relating to trauma from drug injection and to infection. The former range in severity from thrombosis of peripheral limb veins, significant because of the consequent difficulties in obtaining venous access, to serious problems such as femoral vein thrombosis; arterial injection may cause ischaemic damage resulting in loss of digits or loss of limbs, or even cerebral damage following injection into the carotid vessels. Infections are extremely common, either locally at the site of injection or systemically; important in the latter category are hepatitis B and more recently HIV infection. During pregnancy, breast veins provide an additional site for drug injection and breast abscesses are seen antenatally but more commonly postnatally when maximum breast engorgement occurs; thrombosis as a result of venous damage and infection is no doubt a contributory factor.

Many of the women who use drugs finance their habit with money earned by prostitution; prostitution carries the risk of acquired sexually transmitted diseases, including hepatitis B and HIV infection, and is a worrying health hazard for pregnant women.

Maternal drug use is widely reported to adversely affect fetal health. The already discussed questionable data from self-reporting makes it very difficult to correlate specific harmful effects on the fetus with individual drugs or patterns of use. Difficulties in assessing the risk to the fetus are compounded by the possible effects of the women's social circumstances, other adverse features of life-style such as smoking and drinking, and the tendency for women using drugs not to attend regularly for antenatal care. The most consistently reported effects, however, are increases in perinatal mortality and morbidity, with increased rates of low birthweight due both to preterm delivery and small for gestational age babies (Blinick et al, 1973, 1976; Harper et al, 1974; Perlmutter, 1974; Pelosi et al, 1975; Connaughton et al, 1977; Fricker and Segal, 1978; Stauber et al, 1982; Bolton, 1987).

Management of drug abuse in pregnancy

In considering management of drug abuse in pregnancy, it is necessary to address not only the drug problem itself, but also the need to limit the spread of HIV infection. The point has already been made, however, that drug use is not the most important problem in terms of provision of child care; of greater significance in this context is the effect of drug use on the woman's life-style, and any management plan must aim to stabilize the life-style and involve community agencies to provide ongoing support.

Much of the alleged harmful effect on the fetus of maternal drug use during pregnancy is attributed to fluctuating maternal blood levels due both to variable purity and variable availability of the drugs. This is the basis for the argument in favour of methadone maintenance throughout pregnancy (which eliminates such fluctuations), with the further assertion that maternal detoxification during pregnancy carries a substantial risk to the life of the fetus. A further argument put forward in favour of methadone therapy is that, being oral, it will eliminate the need for i.v. injection and thus reduce the risk of HIV transmission. Detoxification, it is argued on the other hand, may not be completely successful and even occasional intravenous injection carries a risk of HIV transmission.

Pregnancy provides a powerful motivation for modifying life-styles and in our experience most women express a very strong desire to stop using drugs during pregnancy. For such women attending our clinics, therefore, management of i.v. drug abuse has been by immediate or very rapid detoxification; not all were successful, however, so some women went through a process of detoxification or partial detoxification several times during pregnancy. For those women unable or not wishing to stop, methadone maintenance may be appropriate, but only for some drugs of abuse. As already noted, in this group of 113 women, there were no perinatal deaths, 7% of babies were delivered preterm (< 37 weeks' gestation), 10% of babies had birthweights less than 2500 g, and 9% of babies had birthweights less than the 10th centile of weight for gestation. While these numbers are too small to be significant, the favourable pregnancy outcome for these women is gratifying in view of their backgrounds of not only social deprivation but also i.v. drug use; these results also suggest that detoxification during pregnancy may not be as dangerous to the fetus as previously reported. Moreover, while those women successful in controlling their drug use may indeed lapse on occasions, equally methadone maintenance is no guarantee against continued injection of illicit drugs. Thus, while detoxification may not be appropriate for all women in pregnancy, it should certainly be included in the range of treatment options offered. Treatment should be tailored to meet the needs of the individual and, regardless of the chosen method of management, in every case the additional question of risk reduction as regards HIV transmission by drug injection should be addressed.

For those women who opt for detoxification, this is unlikely to prove successful if attempted on an outpatient basis. Initial detoxification should be carried out in the maternity hospital to allow monitoring of fetal well-being during drug withdrawal, but thereafter management is most appropriately provided by a community-based rehabilitation unit. Even for those women unwilling or unable to attempt detoxification or who opt for methadone maintenance, maternity hospital admission may be of value in allowing stabilization of a chaotic life-style or chaotic drug use. While such a period in hospital will delay the start of a comprehensive rehabilitation programme, the time need not be wasted in this respect if there is good liaison with the relevant trained workers who can visit the woman and start working with her while she is in the maternity hospital; this is particularly true in the case of outreach drugs workers based in the woman's own area since such contact may be invaluable once the woman has returned home.

Management of the drug problem must be accompanied by management of all the other medical and social problems which in some cases may be inter-related. For example, dealing with the women's financial problems may be an effective method of risk reduction as regards transmission of HIV infection; it may not eliminate prostitution but for many women it may reduce the frequency with which they are obliged to work, thus benefiting the health of both the woman and her unborn baby. Alleviating social problems, with consequent reduction in stress, will also increase the chances of success in dealing with the problem of drug use.

HIV INFECTION

Information about HIV infection should be offered at the antenatal clinic to allow the woman to make an informed decision about whether she would like HIV screening. Since screening can be carried out in different ways for different reasons, it is essential that the purpose of screening in a particular situation, the issues involved and the arguments for and against screening are clearly understood, not only by the woman to whom screening is being offered, but also by the health care staff involved, and women must feel free to refuse the test if they so wish; only then can genuinely informed consent be given.

Prevalence data for HIV infection is obtained by anonymous screening of a population or group within a population, while named screening of an individual is carried out to allow appropriate management of that individual. Despite the impossibility of matching individual test results to individual people, anonymous screening for prevalence data is a valid exercise; the fact that those people who are HIV-positive cannot be identified and offered appropriate treatment in no way detracts from the value of such testing, which is not carried out for this purpose as this can only be addressed by named screening of individuals. It may be, however, that information obtained by anonymous screening could indicate a group to whom it might be appropriate to offer such individual screening on a named basis. It is important to emphasize, however, that while some basic information can be recorded for those undergoing anonymous screening, it is essential to ensure that any such information will not permit identification of individuals or matching of individuals with their test result.

Named screening of individuals, as already stated, is carried out to allow management of that individual. The view still persists in some quarters, however, that such named screening is carried out to identify those people who are infected so that staff or other patients can be protected from them.

Named screening of an individual can confirm that that person is infected with HIV but conversely, because of the length of time between infection and production of antibodies, seronegativity is no guarantee of non-infection. Named screening is currently offered largely to those who identify themselves as members of 'high-risk' groups. Fear by the women of prejudice among staff may mean that not all those who know themselves to be at risk will choose to disclose this fact; moreover, with increasing heterosexual transmission and spread of HIV infection outside these high-risk groups, increasing numbers of people at risk will be unaware that this is the case. Any risk to staff or patients is therefore most likely to come from those who, for whatever reason, are not identified as being at risk. It is also important to remember that HIV is not the only infection transmitted by blood. The blood and body fluids of all patients should therefore be viewed as potentially hazardous and single tier management, which recognizes this fact and treats all patients in an identical manner, should be applied to all areas of clinical or laboratory practice and to all associated services. With such a management policy, an individual patient's serostatus becomes irrelevant; there is therefore no need for staff to be aware of the result of HIV screening, and named testing of the individual should never be carried out in the mistaken belief that it is in the interests of others but only if there are demonstrable benefits for that individual in knowing their status. If identifiable screening is offered to other than those identifying themselves as high risk, full and relevant pretest counselling should still be provided. It is arguably even more important to provide it for those who consider they are not at risk since a positive result might come as an even greater shock with its implications regarding their partner's behaviour. To argue against such universal counselling on the grounds that the test is unlikely to be positive in 'low-risk' people is illogical; if there were no chance of a positive result there would be no point in carrying out the test.

Given that the test is being carried out only in the individual's own interest, the woman at the antenatal clinic needs to understand precisely what benefits there are for her in knowing her HIV status. For this it is necessary to discuss the risks to mother and baby of maternal HIV infection, but with the recognition that our knowledge is imperfect and consequently the risks are not precisely known.

The general arguments for and against knowledge by an individual of their HIV status will obviously still apply here, but additional issues for the HIV-positive woman who is pregnant relate to the effect of pregnancy on her disease, the effect of her disease on her pregnancy, and the risk of transmission of HIV to the baby.

It appears pregnancy has no adverse effect on the woman's HIV infection (MacCallum et al, 1988) and it appears that the mother's HIV infection has no adverse effect on pregnancy outcome (European Collaborative Study, 1988). The risk of transmission of HIV infection to the baby is not precisely known, but the figures of 24% (European Collaborative Study, 1988) and 33% (Italian Multicentre Trial, 1988) are more optimistic than those prophesied from early experience with mothers already ill with acquired immunodeficiency syndrome (AIDS) (and indeed the baby's prognosis may be worse with more advanced maternal disease) and are better than those for many genetic disorders transmitted from mother to baby for which screening is available; while difficulty in diagnosing HIV infection in babies may mean these figures ultimately prove to be either under- or over-estimates, they are the best available at present.

While pregnancy does not adversely affect the woman's health, there are those who argue that since the woman might die, leaving the child without a mother, to continue with the pregnancy would be irresponsible. While such a possibility undoubtedly exists, this is not an argument which is used to dissuade women with other conditions which reduce life expectancy from having children.

Counselling and advice are not synonymous; although one can speculate on what the ultimate risk to the fetus will be, the risk itself is not a matter of opinion; the acceptability of the risk, however, is entirely a matter of opinion and will vary from one individual to another. No one can make a decision about the acceptability of that risk except the individual woman concerned, and the woman should be *counselled* to allow her to make the decision which she feels is right for her and should not be *advised* to act in the way which health care staff feel is appropriate. It is our experience that for the woman already pregnant, while she may request a termination of pregnancy on grounds relating to social problems, including possible drug use, the decision on whether to continue with the pregnancy is unlikely to be influenced by the discovery that she is HIV positive. It is not the responsibility of those providing her health care to try to influence this decision or give directive advice; moreover, if women feel they are likely to be pressurized into accepting a termination if HIV positive they may feel apprehensive about accepting testing or admitting that they are in a high-risk category, thus preventing them from obtaining help with other problems such as i.v. drug use.

A more appropriate time for many to make decisions involving real choice about the risk of pregnancy might be before they actually become pregnant. Some will feel the risk is unacceptable and decide not to embark on a pregnancy at any time in the future; for others the desire to have children may outweigh the risk of an infected baby and such women should be aware that this risk may be minimized by having their pregnancy sooner rather than later.

Thus the benefits to the pregnant woman of knowing that she is HIV positive are that she can opt for a termination if she so wishes or if she continues with the pregnancy the baby can be followed-up with expert surveillance and treatment. While the opportunity for the woman to decide on her future reproductive plans and the advantages of follow-up for her would apply whether or not she were pregnant, they might have particular relevance at this time. Not all women would consider these benefits sufficient to justify screening. Some might feel unable to cope with a positive result and for those trying to control a drug habit and/or a chaotic life-style this information might jeopardize their chances of success; such women should not be pressurized to accept testing.

For those women who do decide to be tested and are found to be HIV positive there are many issues regarding their reproductive future. For HIV-positive women in general, an integrated well woman/prepregnancy counselling/family planning service is required which can also provide maternity care if she becomes pregnant. The many aspects of care involved for the HIV-positive woman having a baby can take up a lot of her time and lead to involvement of a large number of workers. Many of these women will also need help with drug-related or other social problems. There should therefore be close collaboration among all concerned in providing care for mother and baby, with as many as possible of the necessary services being provided at the same time on the same site. Such rationalization may improve uptake of care as well as considerably improving the quality of life for such women.

SUMMARY

It has long been established that social deprivation adversely affects health, including that of the pregnant woman and her baby; it is therefore justifiable to use medical resources in the treatment of social problems.

Antenatal inpatient care was originally seen as potentially beneficial for women without major medical problems, but such a philosophy is not reflected in current practice. Current antenatal outpatient services do not address the needs of women with social problems who, viewing such services as hostile, may fail to attend. Special services such as help with drugs problems or HIV counselling or screening may be rejected from fear of prejudice and consequent repercussions. Such prejudice often arises because staff do not fully understand the issues involved.

Antenatal care for women with social problems should consider women in the context of their families and social environment and should be provided by a small number of familiar staff forming part of an integrated multidisciplinary team in close and regular contact.

Antenatal admission, if it is the woman's wish, should be viewed as justified in the management of social problems; conversely, women should not be pressurized into admission or made to feel guilty if unable to comply.

Outpatient antenatal services should be conveniently sited in the community close to other relevant services and should be flexible, not only in terms of organization and format, but also in the roles of the participants. They should be comprehensive, but with special services in addition to, not instead of, routine care, and provided by a team of appropriately trained staff.

In the provision of antenatal care for women with social needs, no single format will be universally applicable or desirable, and the precise design and content of the service should be variable according to local requirements and should take account of the women's wishes as well as their needs. Ultimately it will only be if the women perceive the service as being in their interests and as meeting their needs that they will use it; only if they choose to use it, will it have any chance of success.

REFERENCES

Baird D (1945) The influence of social and economic factors in stillbirths and neonatal deaths. *Journal of Obstetrics and Gynaecology of the British Empire* **52**: 217–234.

Baird D (1985) Changing problems and priorities in obstetrics. *British Journal of Obstetrics and Gynaecology* **92**: 115–121.

Baird D & Wyper JFB (1941) High stillbirths and neonatal mortalities. *Lancet* **ii**: 657–659.

Ballantyne JW (1901) Plea for a promaternity hospital. *British Medical Journal* **i**: 813–814.

Blane D (1985) An assessment of the Black Report's explanations of health inequalities. *Sociology of Health and Illness* **7**: 423–445.

Blinick G, Jerez E & Wallach RC (1973) Methadone maintenance, pregnancy and progeny. *Journal of the American Medical Association* **225**: 477–479.

Blinick G, Wallach RC, Jerez E et al (1976) Drug addiction in pregnancy and the neonate. *American Journal of Obstetrics and Gynecology* **125**: 135–142.

Bolton PJ (1987) Drugs of abuse. In Hawkins DF (ed.) *Drugs and Pregnancy. Human Teratogenesis and Related Problems*, pp 180–210. Edinburgh, London, Melbourne and New York: Churchill Livingstone.

Brooke OG, Anderson HR, Bland JM et al (1989) Effects on birth weight of smoking, alcohol, caffeine, socio-economic factors and psychosocial stress. *British Medical Journal* **298**: 795–801.

Browne FJ (1932) Antenatal care and maternal mortality. *Lancet* **ii**: 1–4.

Connaughton JF, Reeser D, Schut J et al (1977) Perinatal addiction: outcome and management. *American Journal of Obstetrics and Gynecology* **129**: 679–686.

Department of Health and Social Security. Central Health Services Council Standing Midwifery and Maternity Advisory Committee (1970) *Domiciliary Midwifery and Maternity Bed Needs*, Chairman Sir JH Peel. London: HMSO.

Department of Health, Scotland (1959) *Maternity Services in Scotland*. Report by a Committee of the Scottish Health Services Council, Chairman Professor GL Montgomery. Edinburgh: HMSO.

Enkin M & Chalmers I (eds) (1982) Effectiveness and satisfaction in antenatal care. In *Effectiveness and Satisfaction in Antenatal Care*, pp 266–290. London: Heinemann.

European Collaborative Study (1988) Mother-to-child transmission of HIV infection. *Lancet* **ii**: 1039–1042.

Fricker HS & Segal S (1978) Narcotic addiction, pregnancy and the newborn. *American Journal of Diseases of Childhood* **123**: 360–366.

Hall MH, Chng PK & MacGillivray I (1980) Is routine antenatal care worthwhile? *Lancet* **ii**: 78–80.

Halmesmaki E, Raivio KO & Ylikorkala AO (1987) Patterns of alcohol consumption during pregnancy. *Obstetrics and Gynecology* **69**: 594–597.

Harper RG, Solish GI, Purow HM et al (1974) The effect of a methadone treatment program upon pregnant heroin addicts and their newborn infants. *Pediatrics* **54**: 300–305.

Heller J, Anderson HR, Bland JM et al (1988) Alcohol in pregnancy: patterns and associations with socio-economic, psychological and behavioural factors. *British Journal of Addiction* **83**: 541–551.

Hepburn M (1987) *The role of antenatal inpatient care in obstetric practice*. MD thesis, University of Edinburgh.

Hill RM & Tennyson LM (1986) Maternal drug therapy: effect on fetal and neonatal growth and neurobehaviour. *Neurotoxicology* **7**: 121–140.

House of Commons Social Services Committee (1980) *Perinatal and Neonatal Mortality: Second Report of the Social Services Committee*, Chairman R Short. London: HMSO.

Ilsley R (1983) Social aspects of pregnancy outcome. In Baron SL & Thomson AM (eds) *Obstetrical Epidemiology*, pp 449–476. London: Academic Press.

Italian Multicentre Trial (1988) Epidemiology, clinical features and prognostic factors of paediatric HIV infection. *Lancet* **ii**: 1043–1045.

Jones KL & Smith DW (1973) Recognition of the fetal alcohol syndrome in early infancy. *Lancet* **ii**: 999–1001.

Kerr JMM (1933) *Maternal Mortality and Morbidity*. Edinburgh: E & S Livingstone.

Little RE (1977) Moderate alcohol use during pregnancy and decreased infant birthweight. *American Journal of Public Health* **67**: 1154–1156.

MacCallum RL, France RJ, Jones ME et al (1988) The effects of pregnancy on the progression of HIV. *Abstract 4032, IVth International Conference on AIDS*, Stockholm.

Marbury MC, Linn S, Moyson R et al (1983) The association of alcohol consumption with outcome of pregnancy. *American Journal of Public Health* **73**: 1165–1168.

McKinlay PK (1929) Some statistical aspects of infant mortality. *Journal of Hygiene* **28(4)**: 394–417.

Mills JL, Graubard BI, Harley EE et al (1984) Maternal alcohol consumption and birthweight. How much drinking during pregnancy is safe? *Journal of the American Medical Association* **252**: 1875–1879.

Ministry of Health (1930) *Memorandum on Antenatal Clinics: Their Conduct and Their Scope*. London: HMSO.

Ministry of Health (1959) *Report to the Maternity Services Committee*, Chairman Earl of Cranbrook. London: HMSO.

Morrison J, Najman JM, Williams GM et al (1989) Socio-economic status and pregnancy outcome. An Australian study. *British Journal of Obstetrics and Gynaecology* **96**: 298–307.

Najman JM, Morrison J, Williams GM et al (1989) Unemployment and reproductive outcome. An Australian study. *British Journal of Obstetrics and Gynaecology* **96**: 308–313.

Newton RW, Webster PAC, Binn PS et al (1979) Psychosocial stress in pregnancy and its relation to the onset of premature labour. *British Medical Journal* **ii**: 411–413.

Oakley A, Chalmers I & MacFarlane JA (1982) Social class, stress and reproduction. In Rees AR & Purcell H (eds) *Disease and the Environment*, 11–50. Chichester: John Wiley.

Office of Population Censuses and Surveys (Social Survey Division) (1984) *General Household Survey*. London: HMSO.

Parboosingh J & Kerr M (1982) Innovations in the role of obstetric hospitals in prenatal care. In Enkin M & Chalmers I (eds) *Effectiveness and Satisfaction in Antenatal Care*, pp 254–265. London: Heinemann.

Pearson K (1913) The Chadwick Lecture. Cited in Lewis J (1980) *The Politics of Motherhood*. London: Croom Helm.

Pelosi MA, Frattarda M, Apuzzio J et al (1975) Pregnancy complicated by heroin addiction. *Obstetrics and Gynecology* **45**: 512–515.

Perlmutter J (1974) Heroin addiction and pregnancy. *Obstetrical and Gynecological Survey* **29**: 439–446.

Reid M, Gutteridge S & McIlwaine G (1983) A *Comparison of the Delivery of Antenatal Care between a Hospital and a Peripheral Clinic*. Edinburgh: Scottish Home and Health Department.

Royal College of Obstetricians and Gynaecologists (1982) *Report of Working Party on Antenatal and Intrapartum Care*, pp 10–13. London: Royal College of Obstetricians and Gynaecologists.

Royal College of Obstetricians and Gynaecologists (1985) *Statement from the Scientific Advisory Committee on Alcohol Consumption in Pregnancy*. London: Royal College of Obstetricians and Gynaecologists.

Standing Committee on Drug Abuse (1985) *Drug Problems in Greater Glasgow: Report of the SCODA Fieldwork Survey in Greater Glasgow Health Board*. London: Chameleon Press.

Stauber M, Schmerdt M & Tylden E (1982) Pregnancy, birth and puerperium in women suffering from heroin addiction. *Journal of Psychosomatic Obstetrics and Gynaecology* **1**: 128–138.

Townsend P & Davidson N (1982) The Black Report. *Inequalities in Health: The Black Report*. Harmondsworth: Penguin Books.

Tudor Hart J (1971) The inverse care law. *Lancet* **i**: 405–412.

Williams SS (1989) *Community antenatal care in the east end of Glasgow*. MSc thesis, University of Glasgow.

Wright JT, Waterson EJ, Barrison IG et al (1983) Alcohol consumption, pregnancy and low birthweight. *Lancet* **i**: 663–665.

Zuckerman BS & Hingson R (1986) Alcohol consumption during pregnancy: a critical review. *Developmental Medicine and Child Neurology* **28**: 649–661.

10

Antenatal care in developing countries

PERCY P. S. NYLANDER
ADEYEMI O. ADEKUNLE

It is now universally accepted that antenatal care is probably the most important factor which determines the outcome of pregnancy. In 'advanced countries' the standard of care in many areas has risen to such an extent that maternal mortality has virtually disappeared and perinatal mortality has reached very low limits. However, in many other parts of the world (the developing countries) the care of the mother during pregnancy, though of a fairly high standard in some areas (e.g. in most teaching hospitals), may still be of low standard or may be non-existent in other areas.

Many factors interfere with satisfactory antenatal care in developing countries:

Inadequate resources. In most developing countries, there is gross shortage of doctors, midwives and maternity units due to financial constraints. In many places, the few medical personnel available congregate in the urban areas, leaving the rural areas with very minimal medical facilities. Many investigators have confirmed these findings (e.g. Mangay-Maglacas and Pizurki, 1981).

Widely dispersed population. In some places, rural areas in particular, the population may be widely dispersed because small groups of people or villages are spread over a wide area, because the people are nomadic in nature, like the Fulanis in the northern parts of West Africa, or because many women spend a great part of the year in vast farms assisting their husbands and so cannot easily reach maternity centres, especially where roads are bad or impassable.

Literacy and financial status. Illiteracy and poverty are important factors which contribute to the poor antenatal care in most developing countries (Editorial, 1983, 1987; Harrison, 1985; Ekwempu, 1988). There is evidence that literacy plays a more important role in determining the standard of antenatal care in such a community than the degree of affluence of the people. Nortman and Hofstatter (1981) in a study in 47 countries in Africa, the Middle East and Asia showed that infant mortality rates were associated far more with literacy rates than with gross national products. Other investigators (Harrison, 1985; Ekwempu, 1988) have shown similar findings.

Baillière's Clinical Obstetrics and Gynaecology—
Vol. 4, No. 1, March 1990
ISBN 0–7020–1476–1

Cultural and traditional practices. The care or lack of care of women during pregnancy is determined to a large extent in most developing countries by the influence of cultural and traditional factors. Most communities in these areas, especially those in non-urban parts, tend to adhere to the old local belief of their forefathers that pregnancy and delivery is the province of traditional birth attendants. No antenatal care is performed in many of such cases. Ekwempu (1988) in his study of the care of pregnant women in Zaria, northern Nigeria, has shown that this influence is so strong in the population that even some educated patients do not go to the maternity centres during their pregnancy, preferring to remain at home and adopt the traditional methods.

The cultural pattern in some developing countries is such that women occupy a subordinate position in the community. The acceptance or not of modern maternity practices may therefore depend on the husbands, who may prefer their pregnant wives to assist in their farms or perform household duties rather than attend maternity clinics.

Some traditional and cultural practices not only prevent a large number of women from utilizing the maternity services but also have harmful effects on the patients, thus detracting from the value of antenatal care:

1. Marriage before menarche leading to teenage pregnancy (Madauci et al, 1968).
2. The gishiri cut—this is a traditional operation practised among the Hausas in northern Nigeria (Harrison, 1985) in which the vagina is cut, usually by old women using razor blades. It is used in the treatment of coital difficulties, menstrual and marital problems, infertility, backache, headache, dysuria, goitre and some other conditions.
3. 'Kunya'—this is a custom which also occurs among the Hausas of northern Nigeria. It prevents a girl during her first pregnancy from discussing her pregnancy or its outcome with anyone (Trevitt, 1973), because young girls having their first babies are expected to be shy and modest.
4. Others are failure to give young children fish because it is believed to produce worms (Malaya), prohibiting eggs, chicken and some types of fish during pregnancy (East Africa), forbidding eggs to children (Lesotho), restricting the diet in an attempt to avoid a large fetus and difficult labour (certain Indian communities in Guatemala) (Cruickshank, 1967).

Religious practices. Certain groups of people (Jehovah's Witnesses) refuse blood infusion on religious principles. This may create problems during the antenatal period in the management of conditions such as severe anaemia. In Muslim communities, the subordinate position of women, many of whom are secluded in purdah, may make acceptance of obstetric care in maternity units difficult, especially where such units are manned by male doctors.

Basic health of the population. In many developing countries the general health of the population is poor. Treatment must therefore be directed towards improving the basic health of the pregnant patient and dealing with any general problems in addition to carrying out antenatal care. Pinatti and Faundes (1983) working in Brazil have also stressed this point. Conditions such as malaria, malnutrition, pulmonary tuberculosis, diarrhoeal diseases and haemoglobinopathy, which are prevalent in many places, not only detract from the value of obstetric care if they are not detected and treated, but may also lead to serious consequences for the mother and baby. The general health of the pregnant mother is therefore not only the responsibility of the general practitioner and the public health authorities but very much that of the obstetrician as well.

Although it is common knowledge that the maternity services in many developing countries are poorly utilized and that some areas have very scanty or no maternity services, it is nevertheless very difficult to assess the degree to which facilities are used. This is because of difficulties in obtaining the relevant data. Whereas in developed countries, accurate data are readily obtained from hospitals, maternity centres or national health statistics and these data are very often representative of the situation in the general population, in most developing countries, especially in the rural areas, national health statistics are either not available or at best are inaccurate and the data from hospitals or maternity centres are heavily biased due to selection factors (Nylander, 1969). This selectivity may be caused by women being unable to use obstetric services for various reasons, including restrictive practices in some hospitals. However, a more important reason is that many women do not utilize hospital facilities because they are frightened, because they cannot afford the expenses or because they prefer to use the traditional methods mentioned earlier.

This bias accounts for the small proportion of pregnant women (particularly those in rural areas) who use hospitals or maternity centres. It also explains why most epidemiological investigations (using hospital data) from developing countries (Harrison, 1985; Ekwempu, 1988) cannot give a true representation of what obtains in the general population.

In a recent publication by the World Health Organization (World Health Organization, 1985) an attempt has been made to estimate the proportion of births attended by trained personnel (doctors, midwives and trained primary health care workers) in different groups of developing countries all over the world. The findings are summarized as follows:

Northern, western, eastern and middle Africa —between 29 and 36%
Middle America and the Caribbean —between 51 and 58%
Tropical and temperate South America —between 69 and 89%
Middle south Asia —20%
Western and eastern south Asia —between 53 and 61%

The report stresses the fact that the estimates should be treated as orders of magnitudes rather than precise figures. This is understandable in view of the difficulties of obtaining accurate data in developing countries as mentioned above. These figures give only an indication of the extent to which maternity institutions or trained personnel are utilized for antenatal care in these groups of developing countries. This is because a number of pregnant women utilize maternity institutions for antenatal care but do not deliver in these centres. There is evidence that such women, while using maternity centres for antenatal care, prefer to be delivered by traditional birth attendants (herbalist, spiritualists, etc.) or to deliver in church institutions.

The figures mentioned above are averages for the various regions. In most countries, there will be, as it were, a spectrum of different levels of antenatal care ranging from those areas where such care is non-existent (e.g. some rural areas) to urban areas where utilization of maternity facilities may be maximal. It is obviously not feasible to discuss every level of antenatal care in these developing areas. Therefore, in the next section, antenatal care as carried out at two levels in an urban area will be described, while antenatal care in a rural area will be discussed in the second section. Lastly, problems of particular importance in developing countries are discussed.

ANTENATAL CARE IN URBAN AREAS

As mentioned earlier, an urban area in a developing country is likely to have many levels of antenatal care available. In Ibadan, Nigeria, for example, the following levels can be identified:

1. Tertiary health centres, i.e. the teaching hospitals and some well-equipped private and government 'specialist hospitals'.
2. Private medical clinics and government hospitals manned by medical practitioners with no specialist training in obstetrics.
3. Health centres and private maternity clinics manned by trained midwives.
4. 'New churches' offering maternity services: some employ the services of trained midwives, while others employ elderly devotees of the religious organizations who have very little training.
5. Traditional birth attendants (TBAs).

In this section, the maternity services available at the first and last levels will be briefly described.

University College Hospital (UCH), Ibadan

The majority of the patients come from Ibadan and the environs and are referred from private clinics, maternity centres or other hospitals. Due to limited facilities, an attempt is made to select only patients who have certain risk factors associated with their pregnancy for antenatal care and delivery. Services provided at the first (booking) and subsequent (routine) clinic visits will be described.

The first visit

A detailed history is obtained on this first visit, which often proves to be a tedious and difficult exercise, especially with illiterate patients who tend to withhold information either as a result of ignorance or for cultural reasons. Common problems encountered include inability to remember the date of the last menstrual period and inability to provide details of past obstetric performance, such as the dates of previous deliveries and the birthweights of the babies.

Patients with previous caesarean sections require careful questioning on the circumstances that led to the operation. Also, in this part of the world, no history is complete without inquiring about bone pains and jaundice in childhood and a history of twinning in the family.

A thorough physical examination is performed at this visit. Special attention is paid to the patient's height, as those who are 5 ft (150 cm) or below in height are subjected to further scrutiny since they are more likely to have small pelves. Discrepancies between the gestational age, as calculated from the menstrual dates, and the uterine fundal height are noted because of the frequency of occurrence of multiple pregnancy in this environment.

A number of investigations are performed:

1. The haematocrit/value; this is preferred to the haemoglobin concentration value as the latter is not appreciably altered in conditions associated with haemolysis such as malaria and yet the oxygen-carrying capacity of the blood is reduced in such circumstances.
2. Blood group and haemoglobin electrophoretic patterns.
3. Serological screening tests for syphilis and tests for other venereal diseases.
4. The mid-stream urine specimen is tested for the presence of albumin, reducing substances and acetone.

Chloroquine sulphate (800 mg) is administered to each patient at the first visit for malarial prophylaxis. For the duration of pregnancy and the puerperium, the patient is given folic acid (5 mg) daily, ferrous sulphate tablets (200 mg) daily and pyrimethamine tablets (25 mg) weekly.

Subsequent visits

Antenatal clinic visits after the initial interview and examination are usually brief. Patients are seen every four weeks up to 28 weeks of gestation, and fortnightly until 36 weeks, after which they are seen weekly until delivery. Patients with complications are seen more frequently and those with abnormal haemoglobins are seen in a special haemoglobinopathy clinic.

Tetanus toxoid (0.5 ml) is administered intramuscularly at 28 and 32 weeks of gestation. Patients who had previously been immunized against tetanus are given only a single booster dose (Maclennan et al, 1965; Suri et al, 1964; Stanfield et al, 1973).

The pelvis is assessed in all patients at 36 weeks of gestation by vaginal examination. Negro women have a steep angle of inclination of the pelvic brim and in multiparae and most primiparae, the head does not usually engage in the pelvic brim until late in labour. Thus, non-engagement of the fetal head at term is only significant if the fetal head cannot be made to engage in the semi-erect position. When inadequacy is suspected, a single lateral radiograph in the erect position is requested. The mode of delivery is then determined by the consultant obstetrician in charge of the patient.

Ultrasonography is now often being used to assist in determining gestational age, estimating fetal weight and locating the placenta. However, it is only available in few of the best centres.

Health educators are an indispensable part of the health team delivering modern obstetric care. At every antenatal clinic session, the health educator talks to the patients on hygiene, diet and nutrition in pregnancy, the course and conduct of normal labour and the care of the newborn infant. In addition, the patient is encouraged to discuss her worries, doubts and problems, and reassurance is given where necessary.

Lowest level of antenatal care available in an urban area

The lowest level of antenatal care is illustrated by the services provided by traditional birth attendants (TBAs).

Many countries in the developing world still depend on traditional systems of care in pregnancy and labour. About 70% of all babies are delivered by TBAs or relatives (Lettenmaier et al, 1988).

Generally speaking, in some developing countries, e.g. Nigeria, TBAs are noted to have contributed a lot to health care delivery (Ademuwagun, 1969; Adebimpe, 1982; Erinosho and Ayorinde, 1984). They have been seen to make use of traditional psychological and medical techniques while treating their patients (Madu and Ohaeri, 1989).

Due to illiteracy, ignorance, poverty and strong belief in the 'supernatural' intervention in pregnancy and childbirth, many women in Nigeria go to the traditional healers, who are usually well known because they reside in the community.

In most cases, the methods employed by the TBA are not known to modern science. The problem is that these methods are unique to their practice and are often hidden from investigators. Even despite Government intervention and encouragement to integrate their services in the national health care delivery, many of them are still ill-disposed to disclose their techniques. These methods are normally handed down from parent to child or from one member of a traditional healing family to another. In general, women who patronize these services believe that a child is a gift from God and that childbirth is a mysterious and supernatural event. They also believe that TBAs are mediators between God and man, and are in a better position to assist during the 'supernatural' event of pregnancy and childbirth. It is not without significance to note that even when modern, trained providers are available, many women prefer traditional care at delivery.

Some women do not get antenatal care because they cannot afford to pay for transportation or, in some places, services. In Nigeria, for instance, attendance at Government antenatal clinics has been dropping since 1985, when medical fees were introduced (Attah, 1986). If TBAs could be trained, they could provide antenatal care for such women and many others who would not use hospitals or a maternity centre because of their confidence in

TBAs. Many developing countries, including Ecuador, Honduras, Philippines, Sierra Leone, Sudan and Thailand, Ghana, Burma and India, have organized programmes for training TBAs (Mangay-Maglacas and Pizurki, 1981; Mangay-Maglacas and Simons, 1986). Many of these countries have realized training TBAs in modern health care may be the quickest way to improve obstetric care, especially for rural women. Many places can boast of more TBAs than doctors or midwives. They are still the most accessible providers of maternal health care in many developing countries. TBAs are trained to provide antenatal care and to recognize complications and refer such women early to the health care unit. They are also trained to practice good hygiene during delivery, including proper care of the umbilical cord, and to recognize and refer women with abnormalities in the puerperium.

ANTENATAL CARE IN A RURAL AREA

Between 1965 and 1971, one of us (PPSN) was responsible for conducting the obstetric and gynaecological teaching in a rural community (Igbo-Ora) in western Nigeria. Although a number of other medical activities were carried out in Igbo-Ora during this period, only the aspect dealing with antenatal care in the community will be discussed.

Igbo-Ora is a small town in western Nigeria with a population of 30 000. It is the centre of the Ibarapa Project of the University of Ibadan, and is situated about 60 miles away from the University. About 1000 deliveries per year take place in this community, approximately 60% of which are conducted in two maternity centres in the town—a local maternity centre run by the local government and the maternity section of the University Health Centre (Nylander, 1969). Close to the Government clinic was a dispensary set up by the Local Government.

There was no electricity supply in the town during the period being discussed. The Health Centre had a radio telephone system for quick communication with UCH, Ibadan. Water was obtained in the town from wells and springs.

Since the University Project began in 1963, a system of identification for all inhabitants in the town and registration of births and deaths has been developed. The town was divided into six districts, each of which had a 'family visitor'. These local literate women who were resident in their respective district visit each household in the district at least once a fortnight to collect obstetric and other medical data.

Medical students resided in Igbo-Ora for about three months during their clinical posting in order to acquaint themselves with conditions in rural areas in Nigeria.

Although the obstetric care which will be discussed in this section relates to what happened in Igbo-Ora between 1965 and 1971, it is representative of the picture which will be seen in many rural areas of Nigeria and other developing countries *today*. The picture in Igbo-Ora then was truly rural, and had not been appreciably modified by its contact with the University or by the introduction of modern innovations. The pattern then is therefore considered as representative of an important level of antenatal care today. Furthermore, this Igbo-Ora experience is unique because it relates to a total population in which practically every member of the community is identified. In this respect, the situation is similar to that described by Thompson in Keneba in 1962 and 1963 (Thompson and Baird, 1967).

Antenatal care in Igbo-Ora (1965–1971)

Antenatal clinics (midwives' clinics) were held once a week by each of the two local maternity centres in Igbo-Ora. A third antenatal clinic (the consultant's clinic) was conducted in the Health Centre, once a week, by a visiting consultant obstetrician from UCH, Ibadan, as mentioned earlier.

Antenatal care could be said to begin with the visits of the 'family visitors' to each household in the community. Their very presence in the household was an incentive to the women to use the antenatal services.

Pregnant patients were seen at the local maternity centres on any day of the week (except Sundays). They were then given appointments to attend the respective antenatal clinics. Arrangements were made between the midwives' clinic and the consultant's clinic whereby all high-risk patients (to be described later) were referred to the consultant's clinic.

The midwives' clinic

The basic routine adopted in the management of antenatal patients in the midwives' clinics during first and subsequent visits was the same as that described earlier for UCH, with the following modifications or omissions:

1. Blood grouping and other haematological tests were not carried out.
2. The packed cell volume was not carried out, but the Talqvist (Lawson, 1967b) method was used for haemoglobin estimation at each visit.
3. In the Government clinic, there was no sterilizer. Therefore, when necessary, instruments were sterilized by boiling them in a container over a kerosene or firewood stove.
4. Sickling tests were not carried out, but where the patient's history suggested she was a sickler, she was referred to the consultant's clinic.
5. There were no facilities for X-ray or ultrasound investigations in Igbo-Ora.
6. The supplies of iron tablets, folic acid tablets and antimalarials were not always adequate in the Government clinic so that patients had to do without on some occasions.

The consultant's clinic

In the consultant's clinic, the visiting consultant saw all the high-risk antenatal patients referred from the midwives' clinic. The high-risk patients were as follows:

1. All patients who were 5 ft (150 cm) or under in height.
2. All primigravid patients who were 36 weeks' pregnant.

3. All patients who were uncertain of their dates or whose fundal heights disagreed with the calculated period of gestation.
4. All patients whose histories suggested potential abnormal pregnancy, e.g. previous postpartum haemorrhage, history of recurrent bone pains. Also all ill, pregnant patients were referred.

The routine antenatal care carried out at the consultant's clinic was the same as described earlier for UCH, with the following modifications or omissions:

1. Haemoglobin estimation of all patients was carried out at each visit using the Talqvist method. However, in cases where the haemoglobin was low or doubtful, the packed cell volume was determined using the private electric generator of the University Health Centre.
2. Blood grouping and other haematological investigations were not routinely carried out, but in cases where the previous or present obstetric history suggested an abnormality, e.g. jaundiced baby in previous pregnancies, the blood group of such patients was performed using the facilities in the University Health Centre.
3. The sickling test was carried out on all patients suspected to be sicklers by their previous history.

One of the problems encountered in the consultant's clinic was that many pregnant patients did not come to book at the clinic until they were already 18 weeks' pregnant. It appeared that the women felt that the doctors and midwives were not interested in pregnant patients until they reached this point. This impression was quickly dispelled and the family visitors were told to correct this wrong impression during their household visits.

The high risk patients were examined and dealt with in different ways. Pelvic examinations were carried out in the short women, and those with deformed pelves or abnormal pelves were referred to UCH, Ibadan, to continue their antenatal care there, while those with normal pelves were advised to continue their antenatal care at the midwives' clinic at Igbo-Ora, but to report to the consultant's clinic at 36 weeks of pregnancy for repeat pelvic assessment. Pelvic examination was also carried out in the primigravid patients. Those with adequate pelves were allowed to carry on their antenatal care at the midwives' clinic in the University Health Centre, while those with inadequate or doubtfully adequate pelves were referred to UCH.

Every effort was made to investigate patients who were uncertain of their dates or those whose fundal heights disagreed with the calculated period of gestation. It was found to be a common practice among the women to calculate the gestation period from the first day of their last missed period or to express the gestation period in lunar months. In many cases, it was found that there was really no discrepancy between the gestation period and the fundal height after recalculating the gestation period in the light of this knowledge, and such patients were sent back to their respective midwives' clinic.

It was the custom in Igbo-Ora and among women belonging to the lower social class in many other parts of the country that husbands bore the responsibility of remembering the date of their wives' last missed period and of making all the necessary or relevant calculations for pregnancy from that date. The responsibility of the wife ended with informing the husbands of the date when she missed her period. In many cases, therefore, consultation with the husband solved the problem of 'uncertain dates'.

All patients who had had abnormal previous pregnancies were booked to continue their antenatal care in the consultant's clinic. Those who had previous histories of recurrent bone pains were referred to UCH for further investigations.

Although diarrhoeal infections were common among the children in Igbo-Ora, it was only occasionally that pregnant patients were found with this condition. In such cases, they were treated with the appropriate sulphonamide drugs or antibiotics and booked to continue their antenatal care in the consultant's clinic, but if amoebiasis was suspected, they were referred to UCH.

Malnutrition was also common among the children, but this condition generally manifested itself in adult women by anaemia in pregnancy or contracted pelves. In any case, advice was always given about the importance of the diet during the talks given by midwives at the beginning of every clinic.

The diastolic blood pressure in women of child-bearing age in the population appeared to be generally lower than those of their counterparts in the UK or other developed countries. It was not considered significant if a patient's diastolic blood pressure rose from 50 to 70 mmHg without proteinuria. The blood pressure of patients in the clinics seldom reached a diastolic of 80 mmHg.

The visits to Igbo-Ora provided an opportunity to study the social and other set-up in homes as a background to obstetric care in these patients. In many cases, the homes were over-crowded, polygamy being the common practice. Women generally helped their husbands in the farm and therefore could not attend clinics on many occasions. They worked hard at home (especially if they were the junior wives) and it was obviously a waste of time asking such patients at the antenatal clinic to rest at home. The diet consisted mainly of carbohydrates, vegetable oils and fruits; there was very little protein.

Patients were sometimes referred as emergencies from the Igbo-Ora Clinic to UCH. For example, a patient with ectopic pregnancy would be referred, and laparotomy with auto-transfusion (Stewart, 1967) may be carried out in UCH if there was scarcity of the appropriate type of blood at the time of operation.

Antenatal care in the Ibarapa District in 1989

The obstetric care described in Igbo-Ora during 1965–1971 had many disadvantages. There was only one outpatient clinic with a weekly obstetrician and a few other maternity centres to serve the Ibarapa District (an area of approximately 1000 square miles). Many pregnant women, therefore, had to trek several miles in order to reach a maternity centre. There was not even a resident obstetrician in the area, nor was there a hospital with facilities to deal with urgent cases, which had to be sent to UCH (a distance which may be up to 100 miles in some cases).

The situation has now altered. There are over 14 maternity centres scattered all over the area, some of them close to the farm settlements. There is a small fully equipped hospital in Eruwa with a resident obstetrician. There are also a few private hospitals in this town with resident medical personnel. Igbo-Ora Health Centre has also been upgraded to a small hospital. There are facilities for blood transfusion and haematological tests in these hospitals. Eruwa hospital also has X-ray facilities.

Eruwa (which is 20 miles from Igbo-Ora) is thus the focal centre and patients from various maternity centres are now referred to Eruwa or Igbo-Ora and not to UCH. The situation is close to that proposed about 20 years ago by Lawson (Stewart and Lawson, 1967) in which, in a scattered population, maternity centres would be built in strategic areas and these centres would refer their cases to a central hospital unit.

This arrangement has brought marked improvement to obstetric care in the Ibarapa District, especially as pipe-borne water and electricity have been installed in most of the district. This venture, although very expensive, has proved very successful in dealing with the problem of antenatal care in an area where the population is widely dispersed. It is hoped that the authorities will be able to maintain this project and introduce similar projects in other parts of the country in time.

Igbo-Ora is no longer rural. Projects which have been designed to find out about health services in rural Nigeria have used other parts of the country. In a recent study of utilization of health facilities in the total population in rural areas of Nigeria (Ayeni et al, 1985) it was shown, among other things, that pregnant women readily utilized the Government health facilities for antenatal care, but only 45% of them delivered in maternity institutions.

Other investigations in *total rural* populations are hard to come by, but recently some workers in a total rural population in Keneba, the Gambia (Prentice et al, 1987) have shown that birthweights may be increased by supplementation of the diet of rural African women during pregnancy.

ABNORMAL ANTENATAL CONDITIONS ASSOCIATED WITH PREGNANCY

Unlike the situation in developed countries, in developing countries greater emphasis is placed on diagnosing and treating conditions such as anaemia in pregnancy, malaria, haemoglobinopathy, pre-eclampsia, chronic hypertension and infections, including sexually transmitted diseases. Malaria remains endemic, while tetanus continues to be a scourge of the newborn and of puerperal mothers (Adadevoh and Akinla, 1970). Epidemics of cholera and meningitis have been annual events in Nigeria (Whittle and Greenwood, 1976; Harrison, 1979).

It is obviously not feasible to discuss every abnormal condition peculiar to developing countries in this chapter. However, the more important ones will be dealt with.

Malaria

Malaria may alter the course of pregnancy both by affecting the health of the mother and by interrupting the pregnancy. Malaria, which is still endemic in some developing countries, may produce haemolysis when parasitized erythrocytes rupture. Other parasitized cells are constantly removed from the circulation by the lymphoid–macrophage system. In many cases, the level of parasitaemia is low and may not be detected in blood films. The severe degree of anaemia which develops is not usually related to the actual paroxysm of malaria. Lawson (1967a) suggested that the parasitized red cells become antigenic, as a result of which auto-antibodies are produced. These auto-antibodies attack the red cells, causing intravascular haemolysis (or filtration of opsonized cells out of the circulation by the lymphoid–macrophage system). This often occurs in pregnancy since the immuno-logical defences to malaria parasitaemia are lowered. The condition is particularly liable to occur between 20 and 28 weeks of pregnancy.

An accelerated rate of haemopoiesis ensues but, since iron from the destroyed red cells is stored in the body, only the demand for folic acid increases. This may not be met during pregnancy owing to insufficient folic acid in the diet and the competing demands of the developing fetus. Anaemia therefore results and in severe cases megaloblastic changes appear in the bone marrow (Lawson, 1967a).

In areas when malaria is endemic, prophylaxis is therefore advised throughout pregnancy. In some patients, usually primigravidae with enlarge-ment of the spleen and liver, antimalarials alone may fail to correct the severe anaemia that may occur. In such cases, repeated transfusion may be required to maintain the haemoglobin at a safe level. In some severe cases, cortico-steroids may even be required to abate the haemolytic process (Lawson, 1967a).

Anaemia

In this section only severe anaemia (packed cell volume below 14%) will be discussed, since this is the type of anaemia usually peculiar to developing countries.

Although heavy hookworm infestation, malnutrition and iron deficiency (Ogunbode and Oluboyede, 1980) may contribute, the usual cause of severe anaemia in most developing countries is malaria and folic acid deficiency.

The role of malaria as a cause of severe anaemia has already been discussed. Congestive cardiac failure is frequently associated with this type of anaemia as a result of oxygen deprivation of cardiac muscle.

Patients with severe anaemia used to be managed in the early years of UCH, Ibadan, by slow blood transfusion with packed cells. This resulted in a high maternal mortality from cardiac failure. The method of treatment in these patients was therefore altered to exchange blood transfusion (Fullerton and Turner, 1962; Phibbs and Sproul, 1966; Lawson, 1967b). In this procedure the patient was transfused with about 1300 ml of packed red cells and at the same time about 1500 ml of blood was removed from the femoral vein. The result of the treatment was very dramatic. Patients who were almost dying (e.g. with a packed cell volume of 6%) recovered promptly within a few hours. The procedure was very successful because the red cell mass was increased without over-loading the circulation. Furthermore, the sudden increase in the oxygen-carrying power of blood caused marked improvement in cardiac function.

Exchange blood transfusion, however, had a number of disadvantages, among which were the number of medical personnel needed for each operation, the inconvenience of assembling bits of instruments, the waste of blood and above all its unsuitability for use in other institutions, especially in rural areas.

An alternative method was therefore commenced in which a fast-acting diuretic, e.g. ethacrynic acid, was given while packed red cells were infused into the patient (Harrison, 1968). This procedure, though not so dramatic, was equally successful. The packed cells supplied the much needed red cells and the fast-acting diuretic given at the same time removed the extra fluid, thus preventing cardiac failure. Blood transfusion with packed red cells and ethacrynic acid is therefore now employed to treat all patients with very severe anaemia in this hospital. The ancillary treatment with iron, folic acid and antimalarials is, of course, continued after the transfusion.

Haemoglobinopathy

The two commonest forms of abnormal haemoglobins that influence reproduction in many developing countries are haemoglobin S and C. This influence is particularly evident in those homozygous for the S gene and in those suffering from sickle cell haemoglobin C disease (HbSC). Maternal morbidity and mortality, as well as perinatal loss, are considerably increased in these patients (Hendrickse and Watson-Williams, 1966). Other abnormal haemoglobins occur, but they are either rare or do not affect pregnancy profoundly.

Haemoglobin S is much less soluble than normal haemoglobin, particularly in the reduced state, and this leads to red cell deformities that result in rapid haemolysis. In homozygous S patients, erythrocyte life span varies from 2 to 15 days with a mean of 9.1 days instead of the normal 120 days (Hendrickse, 1975). In addition to this, the red cell life is further shortened by endemic malaria infestation. There is rapid haemolysis which leads to a perennial state of anaemia. The incidence of anaemia is particularly increased in the third trimester of pregnancy, when fetal demands for haemopoietic factors compete with those of the mother.

The excessive destruction of red cells results in hyperbilirubinaemia which manifests as jaundice and anaemia, and there is an increased frequency of complications such as an increased susceptibility to infections, bone pain and sequestration crises. Not only do bone pain crises cause distressing pain for the patient, the resulting bone infection may trigger off bone marrow embolism. Such embolism is usually preceded by a 'pseudotoxaemia' syndrome in which there is sudden systolic hypertension and albuminuria (Lawson, 1967c).

In order to prevent these complications at UCH, Ibadan, haemoglobinopathy patients are seen more frequently than other antenatal patients and particular attention is paid to regular checking of their packed cell volume and liver and spleen size throughout pregnancy. Prophylaxis against malaria is important. When bone pain crises occur, the patient is admitted and given adequate relief from pain through the use of strong analgesics. If any infection is present, appropriate antibiotic therapy is given. The packed cell volume is monitored 4- to 6-hourly. If the packed cell volume falls below 26%, attempts are made to raise this level using haematinics, mainly folic acid. If the packed cell volume falls below 20%, the patient is transfused with fresh packed cells of haemoglobin A. A fast-acting diuretic–ethacrynic acid 50 mg i.v. or frusemide (furosemide *USP* 20–40 mg) may also be given to prevent over-load of the heart.

It has been found helpful to heparinize many of these patients to keep their clotting time at two and a half times normal. This step, although having no effect on the severity and duration of the crisis, reduces the risk of sudden death from bone marrow embolism (Lawson, 1967c). Immediate marrow embolism is also treated with exchange blood transfusion with fresh haemoglobin A blood.

Acute bone pains can occur at any time in haemoglobinopathy patients, but they are most common during the last month of pregnancy, in labour and during the first few days after delivery. At these times the danger of sudden dyspnoea and finally death is greatest (Hendrickse and Watson-Williams, 1966).

Malnutrition

A woman's health, especially during her growing years, influences her risk during child-bearing. While there may be considerable racial variation in the average stature of women, the growth to optimum genetically determined height is conditioned by factors which influence development in childhood and adolescence (Cruickshank, 1967). Undernourishment during childhood, commonly seen in developing countries, often leads to stunted growth, which affects not only the skeleton, but most other tissues as well. It is also widely accepted that undernourishment and deficiencies of certain nutrients during a woman's reproductive years increases her risk of infection or haemorrhage during pregnancy or delivery, or of pregnancy toxaemia and premature delivery. In a survey of 80 developing countries, Hamilton et al (1984) reported that 20 to 45% of women aged 15 to 44 do not consume enough energy each day.

Since education is crucial to any effort to improve nutrition, health talks are essential ingredients in any antenatal services provided in developing countries.

Teenage pregnancy

Teenage pregnancy occurs mainly in those areas where custom or tradition allows child or early marriage, e.g. among the Hausas in northern Nigeria (Harrison, 1985), in India, and uncommonly in East Asia and Latin America

(Henry and Piotrow, 1979). The custom is more commonly practised among the uneducated, unemployed and low socio-economic classes (Harrison, 1980; Bulley, 1984; Ojengbede et al, 1987).

A small group of teenage pregnancies belonging to single girls, most with unwanted pregnancy has also been identified by some investigators. For example, S. A. Khasiani (unpublished data) estimated that secondary schools in Kenya lose 10% of their female students to pregnancy every year.

Pregnant teenagers are more liable to certain complications during pregnancy, among which are nutritional deficiency (Wallace, 1965), anaemia, threatened abortion, pre-eclampsia and eclampsia (Harrison, 1985). Special efforts have therefore to be taken during the antenatal care of these patients to anticipate and, where possible, prevent these problems.

The greatest problem with teenage pregnancy, however, is that these patients are still growing and this fact has a profound influence on their future pregnancies. In UCH, Ibadan, several years ago, an early teenager had a caesarean section for cephalopelvic disproportion. The X-ray pelvimetry before the operation showed a pelvis which was definitely subnormal and inadequate for the baby. A few years later, the same patient was seen at the clinic, and a repeat X-ray pelvimetry at 36 weeks revealed a capacious pelvis. The patient later had an easy normal delivery. Many investigators have called attention to this important increase which occurs in the pelvic capacity in this group of patients in a short space of time (Scher and Utian, 1970; Moerman, 1982; Harrison, 1985).

In view of the above consideration, the question arises regarding the best way to deliver these patients (a decision which has to be made during the antenatal period). It has already been mentioned that this teenage group of patients belong to the low socio-economic class and are mostly illiterate. This is the very group of patients who will shun hospitals, especially if they have been previously 'insulted' by caesarean section. They become frightened of hospitals, in case a repeat caesarean section will be performed, and will not approach the hospital unless as a last resort. Many of these patients will, therefore, end up with ruptured uteri.

It has therefore been advocated that these patients should routinely be delivered by 'symphysiotomy' unless there is a contraindication. The procedure is quite simple and easily learnt (Lawson, 1967d; Philpott, 1982). Using this method, it is hoped that a large number of ruptured uteri in these patients will be avoided.

SUMMARY

The problem of antenatal care in developing countries may be considered from two aspects: (a) areas where antenatal facilities are absent or are inadequate, and (b) areas where antenatal facilities are adequate but for some reasons are not adequately utilized.

The solution to the first part of the problem would appear to be simple. The governments concerned should provide the required facilities. This obviously is not an easy task in many areas of the world, especially with the present profound economic depression in many developing countries. The people just have to use the facilities available to their best advantage, or do without the facilities.

The second part of the problem presents more difficulties. Where antenatal facilities are available, inadequate utilization has been shown to be due to a number of factors:

1. The facilities are too distant or too expensive. It has been shown how the Nigerian authorities dealt with this problem in the Ibarapa district. However, it is a very expensive solution and few governments will be able to afford this.
2. Illiteracy or ignorance. The obvious solution to this difficulty is to educate the masses and a few governments have already embarked on these commendable programmes. Unfortunately, this procedure is expensive, may take a long time and, as already pointed out, even literate women may not use the antenatal services.
3. Traditional and cultural beliefs and prejudices. It has already been shown that this factor is a very important one in the population in developing countries, even among literate patients. The saying that 'old habits die hard' is probably apt here. Probably, with time, education and closer contact with the developed world, these prejudices will disappear.

From the above observations, it would appear that an inexpensive short-term solution to the two parts of the problem mentioned above is for governments to train and use the TBAs who are already 'in our midst' and who already enjoy the confidence of the masses. The authorities, however, have to be very careful in integrating the TBAs into the health system. It has to be done very judiciously and tactfully, otherwise antagonism and unhealthy rivalry will be created between the TBAs and other members of the health team. They must be made to realize that they are a *part* of the health team.

REFERENCES

Adadevoh BK & Akinla O (1970) Post-abortal and postpartum tetanus. *Journal of Obstetrics and Gynaecology of the British Commonwealth* **77**: 1019–1023.

Adebimpe VR (1982) Ambivalence of 'Westernized' professionals in Africa traditional medicine. In Erinosho OA & Bell NW (eds) *Mental Health in Africa*, pp 215–219. Ibadan: University Press.

Ademuwagun ZA (1969) The relevance of Yoruba medicine men in public health practice in Nigeria. *Public Health Reports* **84(12):** 1085–1091.

Attah EB (1986) *Under-utilization of Public Sector Health Facilities in Imo State, Nigeria: A Study with Focus Groups* (PHN Technical Note 86-1), 17 pp. Washington DC: World Bank.

Ayeni O, Weiss E, Olayinka I, Otolorin EO & Onadeko MO (1985) *The Baseline Survey: Health Status and the Utilization of Health Facilities.* Proceedings of Conference on the Oyo State CBD Project: Community-Based Delivery of Health and Family Planning Services, January 14–16, 1985, Ibadan, Nigeria.

Bulley M (1984) Early childhood marriage and female circumcision in Ghana. In Senegal Ministry of Public Health (SMOH) and the Non-Governmental Organizations (NGO) working Group on traditional practices of affecting the health of women and children in Africa (Dakar), pp 211–214. Senegal and Geneva SMOH and NGO Working Group.

Cruickshank EK (1967) Nutrition in pregnancy and lactation. In Lawson JB & Stewart DB (eds) *Obstetrics and Gynaecology in the Tropics and Developing Countries*, pp 11–24. London: Edward Arnold.

Editorial (1983) Why retain traditional birth attendants? *Lancet* i: 223–224.

Editorial (1987) Maternal health in sub-Saharan Africa. *Lancet* i: 255–257.

Ekwempu CC (1988) The influence of antenatal care on pregnancy outcome. *Tropical Journal of Obstetrics and Gynaecology* 1: 67–71.

Erinosho OA & Ayorinde A (1984) Traditional medicine manpower in Nigeria. A survey of their attitudes and scope of practice. *Nigerian Journal of Economic and Social Studies* 26: 315–331.

Fullerton WT & Turner AG (1962) Exchange transfusion in the treatment of severe anaemia in pregnancy. *Lancet* i: 75.

Hamilton S, Popkin B & Spicer D (1984) *Women and Nutrition in Third World Countries*, 147pp. New York: Praeger.

Harrison KA (1968) Ethacrynic acid in blood transfusion—its effects on plasma volume and urine flow in severe anaemia in pregnancy. *British Medical Journal* iv: 84–86.

Harrison KA (1979) Better perinatal health: Nigeria. *Lancet* ii: 1229–1232.

Harrison KA (1980) Approaches to reducing maternal and perinatal mortality in Africa. In Pilpott RH (ed.) *Maternity Services in the Developing World: What the Community Needs*, pp 52–95. London: Royal College of Obstetricians and Gynaecologists.

Harrison KA (1985) The influence of maternal age and parity on child bearing with special reference to primigravidae aged 15 years and under. *British Journal of Obstetrics and Gynaecology* 92(supplement 5): 23–31.

Hendrickse JP de V (1975) Sickle cell disease in pregnancy in Nigeria. In Isaacs-Sodeye A (ed.) *Sickle Cell Disease—A Handbook for the General Clinician*, pp 34–45. Ibadan: Caxton Press.

Hendrickse JP de V & Watson-Williams EJ (1966) The influence of haemoglobinopathies on reproduction. *American Journal of Obstetrics and Gynecology* 94: 739–749.

Henry A & Piotrow PT (1979) *Age at Marriage and Fertility*. Population Report, Series M, No. 4, 56pp. Baltimore: Johns Hopkins University Population Information Program.

Lawson JB (1967a) Malaria and pregnancy. In Lawson JB & Stewart DB (eds) *Obstetrics and Gynaecology in the Tropics and Developing Countries*, pp 60–72. London: Edward Arnold.

Lawson JB (1967b) Anaemia in pregnancy. In Lawson JB & Stewart DB (eds) *Obstetrics and Gynaecology in the Tropics and Developing Countries*, pp 73–99. London: Edward Arnold.

Lawson JB (1967c) Sickle cell disease in pregnancy. In Lawson JB & Stewart DB (eds) *Obstetrics and Gynaecology in the Tropics and Developing Countries*, pp 100–132. London: Edward Arnold.

Lawson JB (1967d) Obstructed labour. In Lawson JB & Stewart DB (eds) *Obstetrics and Gynaecology in the Tropics and Developing Countries*, pp 173–202. London: Edward Arnold.

Lettenmaier C, Liskin L, Church CA & Harris JA (1988) *Mothers' lives matter: Maternal Health in the Community*. Population Report, Series L, No. 7, 32pp. Baltimore: Johns Hopkins University Population Information Program.

Maclennan R, Schofield FD & Pittman M (1965) Immunization against neonatal tetanus in New Guinea. Antitoxin response of pregnant women to adjuvant and plain toxoids. *Bulletin of the World Health Organization* 32: 683–697.

Madauci I, Isa Y & Daura B (1968) *Hausa Customs*, p 18. Zaria: Northern Nigeria Publishing Company.

Madu SN & Ohaeri JU (1989) The Nigerian traditional healer's approach to the treatment of obsessional neurosis: a case study in Ibadan. *Tropical and Geographical Medicine* (in press).

Mangay-Maglacas A & Pizurki H (eds) (1981) *The Traditional Birth Attendant in Seven Countries: Case Studies in Utilization and Training*, Public Health Papers, No. 75. Geneva: World Health Organization.

Mangay-Maglacas A & Simons J (1986) *The Potential of the Traditional Birth Attendants*, Offset Publication No. 95. Geneva: World Health Organization.

Moerman MI (1982) Growth of the birth canal in adolescent girls. *American Journal of Obstetrics and Gynecology* **143:** 528–532.

Nortman DI & Hofstatter E (1985) *Population and Family Planning Programmes. A Compendium of Data through 1978* 10th edn, pp 4–11. New York: Population Council.

Nylander PPS (1969) The frequency of training in a rural community in Western Nigeria. *Annals of Human Genetics* **33:** 41.

Ogunbode O & Oluboyede O (1980) Treatment of iron deficiency anaemia with a new intramuscular iron preparation. In *Obstetrics and Gynaecology in Developing Countries*. Proceedings of an International Conference held at Ibadan, Nigeria, October 1977, pp 162–167. Broderna. Ekstrands Tryckeri AB Lund.

Ojengbede OA, Otolorin EO & Fabanwo AO (1987) Pregnancy performance of Nigerian women aged 16 years and below as seen in Ibadan, Nigeria. *African Journal of Medicine and Medical Sciences* **16:** 89–95.

Phibbs RH & Sproul A (1966) Exchange transfusion: blood volume, efficiency. *Pediatrics* **38:** 927–929.

Philpott RH (1982) Obstructed labour. *Clinics in Obstetrics and Gynaecology* **9:** 625–640.

Pinatti JA & Faundes A (1983) Obstetric and gynaecological care of the Third World. *International Journal of Gynaecology and Obstetrics* **21:** 361–369.

Prentice AM, Cole TJ, Foord FA, Lamb WH & Whitehead RG (1987) Increased birthweight after prenatal dietary supplementation of rural African women. *American Journal of Clinical Nutrition* **46:** 912–925.

Scher J & Utian WH (1970) Teenage pregnancy—an interracial study. *Journal of Obstetrics and Gynaecology of the British Commonwealth* **77:** 259–262.

Stanfield JP, Gall D & Bracken PM (1973) Single dose antenatal tetanus immunisation. *Lancet* **i:** 215–219.

Stewart DB (1967) Extra-uterine pregnancy. In Lawson JB & Stewart DB (eds) *Obstetrics and Gynaecology in the Tropics and Developing Countries*, pp 371–384. London: Edward Arnold.

Stewart DB & Lawson JB (1967) The organization of obstetric services. In Lawson JB & Stewart DB (eds) *Obstetrics and Gynaecology in the Tropics and Developing Countries*, pp 303–312. London: Edward Arnold.

Suri JC, Dhillon H & Grewal HS (1964) Active immunisation of women in pregnancy for prevention of neonatal tetanus. *Bulletin of the World Health Organization* **31:** 349–357.

Thompson B & Baird D (1967) Some impressions of child bearing in tropical areas Part I. *Journal of Obstetrics and Gynaecology of the British Commonwealth* **74:** 329–338.

Trevitt J (1973) Attitudes and customs in childbirth among Hausa women, Zaria City. *Savannah* **2:** 223.

Wallace H (1965) Teenage pregnancy. *American Journal of Obstetrics and Gynecology* **92:** 1125–1131.

Whittle HC & Greenwood BM (1976) Meningococcal meningitis in the Northern Savannah of Africa. *Tropical Doctor* **6:** 99–104.

World Health Organization (1985) *Coverage of Maternity Care*. Geneva: World Health Organization, Division of Family Health.

11

Variations in provision and uptake of antenatal care

PIERRE BUEKENS

After reviewing the providers who might be involved in antenatal care, we will measure the variations of antenatal care utilization. Methods of measurement will be discussed and geographical and socio-demographic variations will be reported. Potential causes of those variations will be described as 'barriers' to care. Finally, interventions aiming to improve antenatal care will be reviewed.

ANTENATAL CARE PROVIDERS

The respective role of general practitioners, midwives and obstetricians in the delivery of antenatal care varies from one country to another.

Within the European Community, Denmark and the Netherlands give an important role to midwives and, to a lesser degree, to general practitioners (Blondel et al, 1985). Most of the care is provided by obstetricians in Belgium, Luxembourg, and the Federal Republic of Germany (Blondel et al, 1985; Humblet et al, 1989). The sources of care are more diversified in France and in the UK (Blondel et al, 1985). European studies have shown that maternal characteristics may influence the choice of care provider (Buekens, 1986; Humblet et al, 1989). In France, for example, general practitioners are often frequented by women of low educational level (Hubert et al, 1987).

In Canada (Yukon and Northwest Territories not included), antenatal care is provided by family physicians in 55.4% of cases, by obstetricians in 35.5% and by groups of physicians in 3.1% of the cases (MacKenzie et al, 1987). A pilot study recently proposed an increased participation of Canadian midwives in antenatal care (Buhler et al, 1988).

In the US, 34% of the private general/family practitioners and 93% of the private obstetricians/gynaecologists offered obstetrical care in 1983 (Orr and Forrest, 1985), and 92.5% of the practising midwives provided antenatal care in 1982 (Adams, 1984). However, midwives are far less numerous than obstetricians (Little and Houde, 1988). Care is also provided by nurse practitioners, mostly in public clinics. The proportion of women attending the different providers is difficult to determine in the US. Orr and Forrest (1985) estimated that 46% of the private medical providers of obstetric care were general/family practitioners and that 54% were obstetricians/gynaecologists.

Traditional birth attendants can play an important role in antenatal care in areas with limited access to health personnel (Viegas et al, 1987). Traditional birth attendants provide care to 38.2% of the women in Guatemala (INCAP/IRD, 1989) and to 13% of the women in Mexico (Secretaria de Salud, 1988). In Honduras (HMPH/ASHONPLAFA/FHI/MSH, 1989) traditional birth attendants provide care alone in 21.3% of the cases, and they share the care with institutions in another 33.1% of the pregnancies. Nevertheless, beyond those countries from Central and North America, we have been unable to find any reports of other countries involving traditional birth attendants in antenatal care in more than 5% of cases.

ANTENATAL CARE UTILIZATION

Measuring methods

The percentage of women receiving antenatal care

The 'percentage of women receiving antenatal care' has been proposed by the World Health Organization (WHO, 1981) as an indicator for monitoring progress toward Health for All by the year 2000. According to WHO (1981), it is equal to:

$$\frac{\text{Number of first antenatal contacts}}{\text{Number of expected births}} \times 100$$

This WHO definition includes in the numerator all first antenatal visits and it is to be assumed that an early antenatal visit followed by an abortion should not be excluded. The denominator is the number of expected births according to the birth rate of the area to be evaluated.

The statistics published by the US National Center for Health Statistics (NCHS, 1989) concern the antenatal care of live births only. Where still-births rates are low, the use of live births only will probably not distort the results too much. The corresponding percentage of utilization of antenatal care is:

$$\frac{\text{Number of live births to mothers who received antenatal care}}{\text{Number of live births}} \times 100$$

It is to be noted, however, that in the US the indicator used is generally the percentage of live births without antenatal care instead of the percentage with antenatal care. Many other published statistics do not specify the definition used.

A shortcoming of these indicators is that they do not take into account the fact that the shorter the pregnancy, the smaller the probability of having an antenatal visit. Proportions of the population receiving antenatal care are thus difficult to compare if gestational ages at delivery vary from one population to another. Terris and Glasser (1974) took account of this difficulty by using a life-table analysis.

The timing of the first visit

Early attendance is recommended and gestational age at the first visit is thus to be measured. According to WHO (1977), gestational age should be calculated in completed weeks since the first day of the last menstrual period. However, there is no full agreement on what early attendance is. The US National Center for Health Statistics (NCHS, 1989) takes into account the mothers who attend during the three first months of pregnancy. Opinion may vary about the exact equivalent in weeks of those months. It is also important to define the first visit, preferably as the first contact with a health provider during pregnancy. Some statistics only deal with the first visit at a hospital, after having been referred by a general practitioner.

The proportion of babies born to women receiving late or no care

The US statistics use a combination of those with no care with those who began care in the third trimester as an indicator of inadequate care (NCHS, 1989).

The number of antenatal visits

The mean number of antenatal visits made throughout pregnancy can be compared with a recommended frequency. For example, the frequency recommended by the American College of Obstetricians and Gynecologists (ACOG, 1988) is a visit every four weeks for the first 28 weeks of pregnancy, every two to three weeks until 36 weeks of gestation and every week thereafter. This corresponds to 13 visits if the first visit takes place by the eighth week of pregnancy and if the woman delivers at 40 weeks of pregnancy. However, a recent expert committee (Public Health Service, DHHS, 1989) suggested a reduction in this number of visits to eight for healthy women. In Europe (Blondel et al, 1985; Blondel, 1986), recommended or legal numbers of antenatal visits for uncomplicated pregnancies vary from 5 to 15. It has been suggested that the number of antenatal visits 'could be considerably reduced for women without special problems' (Hall et al, 1980). There is thus no universal standard against which the number of antenatal visits can be compared.

Many studies on the number of antenatal visits have not taken the timing of the first visit and the timing of delivery into account (Buekens, 1986). A low number of antenatal visits can be related to late attendance and to preterm delivery. Antenatal care indexes take both biases into account, and are discussed below.

Indexes of adequacy of antenatal care

These indexes pool the results in broad categories such as 'adequate', 'intermediate' or 'inadequate' care, according to local standards. The indexes also take into account the fact that the expected number of antenatal visits is lower if the women attend later and/or deliver early.

The index which has been most widely used in the US is the 'Kessner index' (Kessner et al, 1973). As shown in Table 1, the Kessner index considers that, in order to be adequate, the number of visits has to be high enough and the care has to start at 13 weeks or less. An adapted version has been used in Mexico by Bobadilla Fernandez (1988).

Kotelchuck (1987) showed that the Kessner index has some shortcomings, the main one being that it takes into account a maximum of only nine visits. This means that adequate antenatal care is attributed to any woman who starts before 13 weeks and has nine visits or more, even if more visits would be required to meet the American College of Obstetricians and Gynecologists recommendations (ACOG, 1988). Kotelchuck (1987) proposed a new 'adequacy of prenatal care utilization (APCU) index' and designed a computer program to calculate it (Kotelchuck, 1988).

In France, a minimum antenatal care schedule is defined by law. Accordingly, Blondel et al (1980) have classified the care as 'adequate' if the first visit took place before 16 weeks of pregnancy and the number of visits was equal to or higher than the required number (four for term deliveries, two or three for preterm deliveries).

Indexes are useful, but the definition of what 'adequate' care is is by no means universal. It also needs to be stressed that the indexes measure mainly

Table 1. Index of adequacy of antenatal care.

Antenatal care	Gestational age (weeks)		Number of antenatal visits
Adequate[*]	13 or less	and	1 or more or not stated
	14–17	and	2 or more
	18–21	and	3 or more
	22–25	and	4 or more
	26–29	and	5 or more
	30–31	and	6 or more
	32–33	and	7 or more
	34–35	and	8 or more
	36 or more	and	9 or more
Inadequate[+]	14–21[‡]	and	0 or not stated
	22–29	and	1 or less or not stated
	30–31	and	2 or less or not stated
	32–33	and	3 or less or not stated
	34 or more	and	4 or less or not stated
Intermediate	All combinations other than specified above		

[*] In addition to the specific number of visits indicated for adequate care, the interval to the first visit has to be 13 weeks or less.
[+] In addition to the specific number of visits indicated for inadequate care, all women who start their antenatal care during the third trimester (28 weeks or later) are considered to have had inadequate care.
[‡] For this gestation group, care is considered inadequate if the time of the first visit is not stated.
Adapted from Kessner et al (1973).

the frequency of antenatal care, and that the adequacy of the content of the care should also be studied whenever possible.

Geographical variations

Data on the proportion of women receiving antenatal care have been reviewed by Royston and Ferguson (1985) and by WHO (1986). Blondel et al (1985) and Blondel (1986) reviewed European data. Data from the European Community are shown in Table 2. Other new data are shown in Table 3. The 'health personnel' category includes any provider except traditional birth attendants or 'others'. None of the studies referred to give separate figures for trained and untrained traditional birth attendants. However, it seems unlikely that any study would include trained traditional birth attendants in the health personnel category. In Table 3, total percentages include health personnel and traditional birth attendants only. When information on the cases with missing data was available, these cases have been excluded from the denominators and the percentages have been adjusted accordingly.

Table 2. Percentages of women receiving antenatal care and number of antenatal visits in the European Community. Data in parentheses are estimates.

| Country | Women receiving antenatal care | | | Number of visits | | |
	Year	%	Reference	Year	Average actual number	Reference
Belgium:						
Dutch-speaking part	ND	ND	—	1986	(10)	a
French-speaking part	1982	98.8	b	1982	9.5	b
Denmark	1981	(>99)	c	1981	(8)	c
Federal Republic of Germany (Munich)	1975–1977	98.9	d	1975–1977	8.5	d
France	1981	99.8	e	1981	7	e
Greece (two counties)	1978	70–85	f	ND	ND	—
Ireland	ND	ND	—	1981	(5–10)	c
Italy	1981	(90)	c	ND	ND	—
Luxembourg	1984	(95)	g	1981	(5)	c
Portugal	1979	(70)	h	ND	ND	—
Spain	1983	(96)	g	—	(6)	i
The Netherlands	1981	ND	—	1981	(12–14)	c
UK:						
England and Wales	1981	(>98)	c	1981	ND	—
Scotland	1978	99.9	c	1981	(10–12)	c

ND = no data.

References: a = Renaer and Eggermont, 1987; b = Wollast et al, 1986; c = Blondel, 1986; d = Selbmann et al, 1980; e = Rumeau-Rouquette et al, 1984; f = Kafatos et al, 1978 (quoted by Blondel, 1986); g = WHO, 1986; h = Royston and Ferguson, 1985; i = Miller, 1987. Adapted from Blondel, 1986.

Figure 1 gives an overview of the world utilization of antenatal care. The more recent data were used to prepare the map, and data from before 1979 were excluded. Figure 1 shows that the proportion of women receiving antenatal care is high not only in industrialized countries, but also in some

Table 3. Recent data on percentages of women receiving antenatal care by health personnel or traditional birth attendants (TBAs).

Country	Year	Antenatal care (%) Health personnel	TBAs	Total	Reference
Brazil	1986*	74.0	ND	74.0	Arruda et al, 1987
Bolivia	1989*	43.9	ND	43.9	INE/IRD, 1989
Botswana	1988*	92.3	ND	92.3	CSO/MOH/IRD, 1989
Burundi	1987*	79.9	0.1	80.0	Segamba et al, 1988
Canada (except Yukon and NW Territories)	1986	95.3	0.7	96.1	MacKenzie et al, 1987
Colombia	1986*	73.0	1.0	74.0	CCRP/MSC/IRD, 1988
Cuba	1981	ND	ND	99	INDS, 1981, cited by Bobadilla Fernandez, 1988
Dominican Republic	1986*	94.8	0.6	95.4	CNPF/IRD, 1987
Ecuador	1987*	ND	ND	69	CEPAR/ININMS/IRD, 1987
Egypt	1988*	52.3	ND	52.3	ENPC/IRD, 1989
Ghana	1988*	82.4	3.4	85.8	GSS/IRD, 1988
Guatemala	1987*	34.2	38.2	72.4	INCAP/IRD, 1989
Honduras	1984*	65.2$^+$	45.8$^+$	83.4	HMPH/ASHONPLAFA/ FHI/MSH, 1986
	1987*	64.9$^+$	54.5$^+$	86.2	HMPH/ASHONPLAFA/ FHI/MSH, 1989
Ivory Coast	1988	ND	ND	66	D. Beghin and E. Wollast, unpublished data
Japan	1984	ND	ND	99	WHO, Western Pacific Region, 1986
Kenya	1989*	77.2	1.9	79.1	NCPD/IRD, 1989
Liberia	1986*	82.9	ND	82.9	Chieh-Johnson et al, 1988
Mali	1987*	32.5	2.9	35.4	Traore et al, 1989
Mexico	1987*	71.2	13.0	84.2	Secretaria de Salud, 1988
Morocco	1987*	24.7	0.1	24.8	Azelmat et al, 1989
Nigeria (Ondo State)	1987*	ND	ND	83	DHS, 1989
Panama	1984*	89.4	0	89.4	Monteith et al, 1987
Peru	1986*	ND	ND	60.2	INE/IRD, 1988
Senegal	1986*	63.6	ND	63.6	Ndiaye et al, 1988
Sri Lanka	1987*	96.6	ND	96.6	DCS/IRD, 1987
Thailand	1987*	77.6	0.9	78.5	Chayovan et al, 1988
Togo	1988*	80.9	ND	80.9	URD/IRD, 1989
Trinidad and Tobago	1987*	98.6	ND	98.6	Heath et al, 1988
Tunisia	1988*	56.7	ND	56.7	ONFP/IRD, 1988
Uganda	1989*	86.8	0.6	87.4	MOH/IRD, 1989
United States	1987	ND	ND	98.0	NCHS, 1989
Zimbabwe	1988*	91.3	ND	91.3	DCS/IRD, 1989

ND = no data available to the author.
* Including the births in the five years preceding the survey.
$^+$ Shared care between health personnel and TBAs.

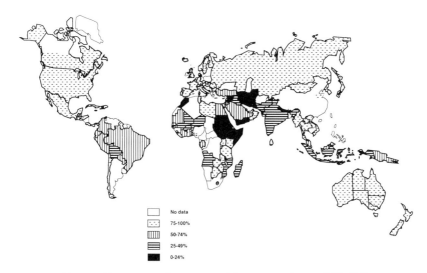

Figure 1. Percentage of women receiving antenatal care, 1979–1989.

developing countries. In Africa, for example, rates of 90% or more have been reported in Botswana and Zimbabwe (Table 3) and in Cape Verde, Gambia, Mauritius, the Seychelles and Tanzania (WHO, 1986); rates lower than 25% are found only in Morocco (Table 3) and in Ethiopia, Somalia and Sudan (WHO, 1986).

In the European Community (Table 2), all countries which reported data had proportions of women receiving antenatal care of 90% or more, except Greece and Portugal. However, we are not aware of any European Community country collecting data on antenatal care on a routine basis, with the exception of Denmark (Knudsen and Borlum Kristensen, 1986). Denmark, however, did not provide results to WHO (1986). It has thus to be assumed that the data published by WHO (1986) are estimates only. In the case of Belgium, the proportion of women receiving antenatal care was estimated by WHO (1986) to be 90%, while an available survey (Wollast et al, 1986) gave a figure of 98.8% for the French-speaking part of the country. When available, data from surveys have been used in Table 2. Two representative surveys give some information about the timing and the number of the visits. The first one has shown that in France in 1981, 97.6% of the women attended before the end of the first trimester (Rumeau-Rouquette et al, 1984). The second survey has shown that the first visit occurred before 13 weeks of pregnancy in 86% of the mothers in the French-speaking part of Belgium in 1982 (Wollast et al, 1986). The average number of visits (Table 2) ranged from 7 in France to 9.5 in Belgium. In Britain, the proportion of women receiving antenatal care has been very high for at least 30 years (Oakley, 1982). Data on gestational age at booking into hospital in Britain have been reviewed by Reid (1986). Between 72 and 89% of women were booked before 20 weeks of gestation, but they presented to their general practitioner well before that.

Table 4. Births to women with early and late or no antenatal care in the United States (Brown, 1989; NCHS, 1989).

Year	Early care (%)	Late or no care (%)
1969	68.0	8.1
1970	67.9	7.9
1971	68.6	7.2
1972	69.4	7.0
1973	70.8	6.7
1974	72.1	6.2
1975	72.3	6.0
1976	73.5	5.7
1977	74.1	5.6
1978	74.9	5.4
1979	75.9	5.1
1980	76.3	5.1
1981	76.3	5.2
1982	76.1	5.5
1983	76.2	5.6
1984	76.5	5.6
1985	76.2	5.7
1986	75.9	6.0
1987	76.0	6.3

In the US, antenatal care attendance is registered on birth certificates. In 1987, 98% of the live births were to mothers with antenatal care (NCHS, 1989). As shown in Table 4, the proportion of live births to women with late (third trimester) or no antenatal care decreased from 8.1% in 1969 to 5.1% in 1979, but then increased from 5.1% in 1980 to 6.3% in 1987 (Brown, 1989; NCHS, 1989). Table 4 also shows that the percentage of babies born to women receiving early care is not improving any more since 1980. The proportion of inadequate care, as measured by the APCU index, was 15.7% in 1984 and 1985, and 15.9% in 1986 (Singh et al, 1989).

Socio-demographic variations

The relation between socio-demographic variables and the utilization of antenatal care is well documented. European data have been reviewed by Buekens (1986) and US data by Brown (1988). Low maternal age, high parity, low socio-economic status, low educational level, immigration, living in a rural area, being unmarried, and having an unplanned or unwanted pregnancy are factors associated with late or no care. Multivariate analysis generally confirms the role of those variables (Brown, 1988). However, late attendance does not necessarily mean irregular care for the rest of the pregnancy. European (Buekens, 1986) and US (Kotelchuck et al, 1988) studies have shown that low socio-economic status populations may have adequate antenatal care utilization after enrolment.

Data on the relation between educational level and antenatal care utilization in developing countries are found in most of the studies listed in Table 3. Those studies always found a strong relationship between low education and absence of antenatal care.

BARRIERS TO ANTENATAL CARE

Financial barriers

Lack of insurance is a major barrier in the US, where 15% of pregnant women have no maternity coverage at all and many have a limited coverage only (Brown, 1988). Most American studies have shown that financial problems were ranked first among barriers perceived by women, and multi-variate analysis of several surveys have confirmed the role of financial barriers (Brown, 1988). The decrease in antenatal care during the economic recession of 1982 (Fisher et al, 1985) is another illustration of the financial barriers existing in the US.

Inadequate system capacity

Early antenatal care may be impaired by long waiting lists, and in some areas care may be completely unavailable. This is the case in various communities in the US in which the capacity of the clinic system relied on by low-income women may be limited (Brown, 1988). Malpractice insurance costs and low reimbursement of the program financing care for low-income women (Medicaid) are also limiting the number of providers available in the US (Brown, 1988). In Europe, a British study (Simpson and Walker, 1980) showed that the median delay by hospitals in giving appointments was more than five weeks in one area.

Distance

Long distance and absence of transportation to reach a provider are barriers to care. In some areas of the US, not having a car can be an insurmountable obstacle (Brown, 1988). American studies of women's perception of barriers to care have shown that transportation was one of the most frequent barriers cited (Brown, 1988). In Ireland, Kaliszer and Kidd (1981) showed that the distance effect existed, but was small in comparison with socio-cultural factors. In Glasgow, Reid and McIlwaine (1980) found that a majority of women would like to have a peripheral clinic in their district, but there was no significant difference in the number of missed visits between peripheral and central clinic attenders (Reid, 1986).

A study from Newfoundland (Girt, 1973) showed that distance may have both a positive and a negative effect on behaviour. Figure 2 shows that in Newfoundland the probability of attending antenatal care increases with distance until at some point it began to decline. A tentative explanation is that the farther women live from a provider they could consult in case of problem, the more worried they are about pregnancy complications, but those living too far away may be discouraged by the additional effort involved in an antenatal visit.

In developing countries, outpatient attendance generally decreases exponentially with distance (Jolly and King, 1966). In a rural area of Kenya, Voorhoeve et al (1982) found a decrease in antenatal care attendance from

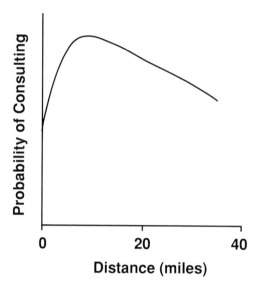

Figure 2. Distance and antenatal care utilization in normal pregnancies. Adapted from Girt (1973).

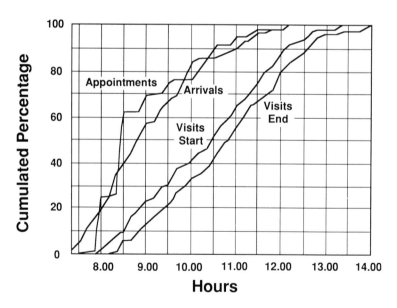

Figure 3. Cumulated percentages of appointments, arrivals, starts and ends of visits according to time of the day in one hospital. Adapted from Llerena and Alvarez (1984).

93% at 8 km to 69% at 24 km from the hospital. In Mexico, a logistic regression analysis taking socio-economic variables into account has shown that a paved road was associated with a 30% increase in antenatal care utilization (Potter, 1988).

Waiting time

Among several factors studied by Flynn (1985), waiting time had the greatest effect on the satisfaction of patients attending for antenatal care. In Britain, during 1975, the average time spent waiting was 62 min in hospitals and 22 min in general practitioners' offices (O'Brien and Smith, 1981). Brown (1988) pointed out that the system of block appointments used by the publicly financed clinics in the US often delays the service routinely. This system schedules only two groups of appointments per day, one early in the morning and another early in the afternoon, with patients seen on a first-come, first-served basis. This can induce long waiting times, as illustrated by Llerena and Alvarez (1984) in a Mexican hospital. Figure 3 shows that women came on time to the antenatal clinic, but that most appointments were given before 8:30 a.m. The consequence is a waiting time increasing to nearly two hours as women accumulate.

Lack of child care

Studies that ask women about reasons for delayed or no antenatal care show that responsibility for other children can be a barrier to care (Reid, 1986; Brown, 1988). Results from two multivariate analyses show that women who had no one to care for their other children had 1.7 to 2.6 more times the probability of having insufficient antenatal care than others (Brown, 1988). Child care is often more easily arranged if clinics open during evenings and weekends.

Culture, attitude and knowledge

Language incompatibility is an important barrier. This is illustrated by a study from France (Stengel et al, 1986), which showed a strong relationship between knowledge of the French language and the probability of having more than six visits.

The failure of providers to appreciate the cultural preferences of some patients may also be a strong barrier. For example, among some populations it is unacceptable to have an examination done by a man (Reid, 1986; Brown, 1988).

Numerous attitudes may act as barriers (Brown, 1988). They include, among others, fear of parental discovery, fear of problems with the Immigration Service, and fear that certain habits will be discovered and criticized (e.g. smoking, drug or alcohol use, eating disorders).

Existing social networks might be influential. McKinlay (1973) has shown that underutilizers of antenatal care frequently rely on readily available relatives and friends as lay consultants before using the service.

Whether or not women work may affect their attitude toward antenatal care. Data from Belgium, France and the UK (Buekens, 1986) show that working women attend earlier than others.

As mentioned before, low education is one of the socio-demographic variables repeatedly found to be associated with poor utilization of antenatal care. Few studies, however, tell us what women with low education know and believe. Studies of working class women showed that their beliefs agree more with the medical doctors' standards than the beliefs of middle class women do (Reid, 1986).

IMPROVING THE UTILIZATION OF ANTENATAL CARE

Improving services

Reducing financial barriers to care, expanding the capacity of the system, decreasing the obstacles due to distance and improving institutional practices are four possible means of action.

The first three points are probably not crucial issues in Europe, but many studies (Reid, 1986) on patient dissatisfaction suggest that improvement of institutional practices is necessary. Successful attempts to increase continuity of care have been reported by Reid (1986). The need for better co-ordination of shared care has also been pointed out (Thomas et al, 1983; Humblet et al, 1989).

A review of American programmes (Brown, 1989) showed a great reluctance to change institutional practices. Many programmes in the US have tried to reduce financial obstacles or improve the capacity of the system. Nonetheless, Brown (1989) concluded that they 'meet with only modest success, primarily because they are anomalies in a complicated, fragmented "non-system" of maternity services characterized by pervasive financial and institutional obstacles'.

In developing countries, financial barriers, inadequate system capacity and distance are often crucial, but the improvement of institutional practices may still be important. In some communities, fixed days and times may not be understood by many women, and the provision of flexible hours for antenatal care could increase its use (Favin et al, 1984). Favin et al (1984) reported a study from Kenya showing a 50% increase in utilization when maternal and child health services were integrated with other clinic services and provided daily.

Outreaching women

Two frequently used approaches are attracting women through a wide variety of case-finding methods and providing social support to encourage continuation in antenatal care (Brown, 1989).

Routine outreach activities exist in Europe, but few have been evaluated. Public advertising has been performed in Belgium among other countries.

Agency networking is extensively used, and women are being referred from agencies such as social assistance. Explicit financial incentives exist only in France and in Luxembourg (Blondel et al, 1982; Blondel, 1986; Miller, 1987). Nevertheless, Miller (1987) pointed out that many benefits are linked to antenatal care attendance in Europe, including, for example, transportation privileges, birthing bonuses and paid leave. Home visiting systems exist in many European countries (Blondel, 1986; Miller, 1987) and may contribute to the good continuation of care (Wollast et al, 1986). A French study (Zmirou et al, 1988) has shown that the number of antenatal visits may be increased by a health education and home visiting programme. Hall et al (1985) have suggested that women who miss their appointments should be visited at home by midwives who could perform examinations as well as recommending clinic attendance. In our opinion, such integration of interventions should be encouraged in the future.

US programmes have been reviewed by Brown (1988). Case-findings have been performed by 'outreach workers' looking for unattended pregnant women in their neighbourhoods. They are on the street, in housing projects, schools and welfare offices. The number of women recruited is often low, and the cost is high. Nevertheless, the results of outreach workers may be comparable to those of private sector salespeople (Brooks-Gun et al, 1989). Intervention of lay health advisors have also been used and have increased antenatal care utilization in migrant populations (Watkins et al, 1990). Hotlines also appeared to be helpful. Referrals or agency networking are another form of case-finding that was felt useful. Use of incentives is under experimentation in the US and has not been extensively evaluated yet. Programmes emphasizing social support have been found to result in an increased number of antenatal visits.

In developing countries, community health leaders have been used by many projects (Favin et al, 1984). These are members of the community trained for a week or less and are normally not paid. One of their tasks is to promote the use of maternal and child care.

Avoiding overutilization

Overutilization of antenatal care is a potential problem. It could induce undue costs, reduce the duration and quality of visits and could lead to iatrogenic problems. Each screening test performed carries a risk of false-positive results. False-positive results might induce unnecessary interventions, which in turn carry their own risks of secondary effects. Unnecessary screenings should thus be avoided, and the number of antenatal visits should not be increased without reason.

As previously discussed, there is no consensus about the ideal number of antenatal visits. However, recommendations to decrease the actual standard number of visits for healthy women have been published in the UK (RCOG, 1982) and in the US (Public Health Service DHHS, 1989). A study from Aberdeen, Scotland, has shown that it is possible to decrease the number of antenatal visits without having a detrimental effect on the health of mother or baby (Hall et al, 1985).

The method of financing could have an impact on the utilization of antenatal care. Whether or not payment of part of the costs by users might
reduce overutilization is an issue which has been addressed by US studies. A
randomized control trial (Lohr et al, 1986) has shown that copayment
decreases the use of ante- and postnatal care in poor populations but not in
non-poor ones, suggesting that copayment increases social inequalities.
Another study (Cherkin et al, 1989) has shown that, in a prepaid group
practice, a 5$ copayment on office visit rates slightly increased the utilization
of obstetric/gynaecological care by women in the child-bearing age group.
This contrasted with a reduction in the utilization of other primary or
speciality care visits. The results of those studies on copayment are not
encouraging. Another important but less well-documented issue is the
impact of the providers' payment system on antenatal care utilization. A
review of studies about financing general medical practice (Shimmura, 1988)
concluded that fee-for-service payment encourages more consultations,
medical doctors of fee-for-service payment systems having an incentive to
see patients more often than doctors of capitation systems. In the US,
prepaid care is provided by Health Maintenance Organizations. Quick et al
(1981) have shown that members of Health Maintenance Organizations had
fewer visits than the general population, but this could be due to late
initiation of antenatal care. Further studies are needed to clarify the
influence of financing methods on the utilization of antenatal care.

CONCLUSION

Poor attendance of antenatal care in some areas of the world and the
decreasing attendance in the US are matters of concern. Nevertheless,
utilization of antenatal care is very high in many countries, including some
developing countries. Where attendance is very high, specific programmes
might still be advisable to reach the last non-attenders, but most of the
efforts should be focused on the improvement of services. Reducing waiting
times, providing child care and improving communication could both
increase attendance and satisfaction. Where attendance is not adequate,
financial barriers seem to be the main obstacle. When financial barriers are
reduced, additional programmes might tackle the remaining barriers.
Overutilization of antenatal care could also be a problem and could be better
addressed by decreasing the recommended number of visits than by requesting payment of a part of the costs by the users.

SUMMARY

Antenatal care providers vary from one country to another. In Europe, most
of the care is provided by obstetricians in some countries, while the role of
midwives is important in other countries. Many women are attended by
general practitioners in Canada and, to a lesser extent, in the US. Involvement of traditional birth attendants in antenatal care in more than 5% of the

pregnancies has been reported in Guatemala, Honduras and Mexico only. Several indicators may be used to measure the utilization of antenatal care: the percentage of women receiving care, timing of the first visit, proportion of women receiving late or no care, number of visits and indexes of adequacy of antenatal care. Recent world data are provided. The percentage of women receiving antenatal care is higher than 90% in many countries, including some developing countries. However, the proportion of women with late or no care is increasing in the US. Women of low socio-demographic status are at high risk of having inadequate care. Financial barriers play a major role. Inadequate system capacity, distance, long waiting time, lack of child care and differences in culture, attitude and knowledge are other important barriers. Improving the services and out-reach of non-participating women may both increase the utilization of antenatal care. Overutilization should also be a matter of concern. It could be better addressed by decreasing the recommended number of visits than by requesting payment of a part of the costs by the users.

Acknowledgements

This paper has been prepared while the author was Visiting Associate Professor at the Department of Maternal and Child Health, School of Public Health, The University of North Carolina at Chapel Hill, US. The author is Research Associate of the Belgian National Research Fund. We thank D. Bender, B. Blondel, C. Infante Castaneda, M. Kotelchuck, C. A. Miller and M. Peoples-Sheps for their comments and suggestions. We thank P. Bailey, D. Beghin, J. L. Bobadilla Fernandez, P. Hernandez, L. Schlaepfer, F. Simini, N. Tremblay, E. Wollast and the Institute for Resource Development Inc. for the data provided.

REFERENCES

ACOG (1988) *Guidelines for Perinatal Care*, pp 54–55. Elk Grove Village, Illinois and Washington DC: American Academy of Pediatrics and American College of Obstetricians and Gynecologists.

Adams C (1984) *Nurse-midwifery in the United States 1982*, p 28. Washington, DC: American College of Nurse-Midwives.

Arruda JM, Rutenberg N, Morris L & Anhel Ferraz E (1987) *Pesquisa Nacional Sobre Saude Materno-infantil e Planejamento Familiar, Brasil 1986*, pp 149–150. Rio de Janeiro: Sociedade Civil Bem-Estar Familiar no Brasil and Institute for Resource Development.

Azelmat M, Ayad M & Belhachmi H (1989) *Enquête Nationale sur la Planification Familiale, la Fécondité et la Santé de la Population au Maroc, 1987*, pp 87–89. Rabat, Maroc and Columbia, Maryland: Ministère de la Santé Publique and Institute for Resource Development.

Blondel B (1986) Antenatal care in the countries of the European Community over the last twenty years. In Kaminski M, Breart G, Buekens P et al (eds) *Perinatal Care Delivery Systems: Description and Evaluation in European Community Countries*, pp 3–15. Oxford: Oxford Medical Publications.

Blondel B, Kaminski M & Breart G (1980) Antenatal care and maternal demographic and social characteristics: evolution in France between 1972 and 1976. *Journal of Epidemiology and Community Health* **34**: 157–163.

Blondel B, Saurel-Cubizolles MJ & Kaminski M (1982) Impact of the French system of statutory visits on antenatal care. *Journal of Epidemiology and Community Health* **36**: 183–186.

Blondel B, Pusch D & Schmidt E (1985) Some characteristics of antenatal care in 13 European countries. *British Journal of Obstetrics and Gynaecology* **92:** 565–568.

Bobadilla Fernandez JL (1988) *Quality of Perinatal Medical Care in Mexico City*, p 138. Mexico: Instituto Nacional de Salud Publica.

Brooks-Gunn J, McCormick MC, Gunn RW et al (1989) Outreach as case finding, the process of locating low-income pregnant women. *Medical Care* **27:** 95–102.

Brown S (ed.) (1988) *Prenatal Care: Reaching Mothers, Reaching Infants*. Washington, DC: Institute of Medicine/National Academy Press.

Brown S (1989) Drawing women into prenatal care. *Family Planning Perspectives* **21:** 73–80.

Buekens P (1986) Determinants of prenatal care. In Kaminski M, Breart G, Buekens P et al (eds) *Perinatal Care Delivery Systems: Description and Evaluation in European Community Countries*, pp 16–25. Oxford: Oxford Medical Publications.

Buhler L, Glick N & Sheps SB (1988) Prenatal care: a comparative evaluation of nurse-midwives and family physicians. *Canadian Medical Association Journal* **139:** 397–403.

CCRP/MSC/IRD (1988) *Colombia: Tercera Encuesta Nacional de Prevalencia del Uso de Anticonceptivos y Primera de Demografia y Salud*, pp 92–95. Corporacion Centro Regional de Poblacion, Ministerio de Salud de Colombia and Institute for Resource Development.

CEPAR/ININMS/IRD (1987) *Ecuador, Encuesta Nacional de Demografia y Salud Familiar 1987: Informe Preliminar*, p 19. Centro de Estudios de Poblacion y Paternidad Responsable, Instituto Nacional de Investigaciones Nutricionales y Medico Sociales, and Demographic and Health Surveys, Institute for Resource Development.

Chayovan N, Kamnuansilpa P & Knodel J (1988) *Thailand Demographic and Health Survey 1987*, pp 94–96. Bangkok, Thailand and Columbia, Maryland: Institute of Population Studies, Chulalongkorn University and Institute for Resource Development.

Cherkin DC, Grothaus L & Wagner EH (1989) The effect of visit copayments on utilization in a Health Maintenance Organization. *Medical Care* **27:** 1036–1045.

Chieh-Johnson D, Cross AR, Way AA & Sullivan JM (1988) *Liberia Demographic and Health Survey 1986*, pp 71–72. Monrovia, Liberia and Columbia, Maryland: Bureau of Statistics, Ministry of Planning and Economic Affairs, and Institute for Resource Development.

CNPF/IRD (1987) *Republica Dominicana, Encuesta Demografica y de Salud, DHS—1986*, p 70. Consejo Nacional de Poblacion y Familia and Institute for Resource Development.

CSO/MOH/IRD (1989) *Botswana Family Health Survey II 1988: Preliminary Report*, pp 12–13. Central Statistics Office, Ministry of Finance and Development Planning, Family Health Division, Ministry of Health and Demographic Health Surveys, Institute for Resource Development.

DCS/IRD (1987) *Sri Lanka Demographic and Health Survey 1987: Preliminary Report*, p 21. Department of Census and Statistics, Ministry of Plan Implementation and Demographic and Health Surveys, Institute for Resource Development.

DCS/IRD (1989) *Zimbabwe Demographic and Health Survey 1988: Preliminary Report*, pp 18–20. Department of Census and Statistics, Government of Zimbabwe and Demographic and Health Surveys, Institute for Resource Development.

DHS (1989) Selected statistics from DHS surveys. *Demographic and Health Surveys Newsletter* **2.2:** 10.

ENPC/IRD (1989) *Egypt, Demographic and Health Survey 1988: Preliminary Report*, p 34. Egypt National Population Council and Demographic and Health Surveys, Institute for Resource Development.

Favin M, Bradford B & Cebula D (1984) Access to maternal health services. In *Information for Action Issue Paper: Improving Maternal and Child Health in Developing Countries*, pp 22–35. Geneva, Switzerland and Washington, DC: World Federation of Public Health Associations.

Fisher ES, LoGerfo JP & Daling JR (1985) Prenatal care and pregnancy outcomes during the recession: the Washington State experience. *American Journal of Public Health* **75:** 866–869.

Flynn SP (1985) Continuity of care during pregnancy: the effect of provider continuity on outcome. *Journal of Family Practice* **21:** 375–380.

Girt JL (1973) Distance to general medical practice and its effect on revealed ill-health in a rural environment. *The Canadian Geographer* **17:** 154–166.

GSS/IRD (1988) *Ghana Demographic and Health Survey 1988: Preliminary Report*, p 16.

Ghana Statistical Service and Demographic and Health Surveys, Institute for Resource Development.

Hall MH, Chng PK & McGillivray I (1980) Is routine antenatal care worthwhile? *Lancet* **ii**: 78–80.

Hall M, Macintyre S & Porter M (1985) *Antenatal Care Assessed: A Case Study of an Innovation in Aberdeen.* Aberdeen: Aberdeen University Press.

Heath K, Da Costa-Martinez D & Sheon AR (1988) *Trinidad and Tobago Demographic and Health Survey 1987*, pp 60–61. Port-of-Spain, Trinidad and Columbia, Maryland: Family Planning Association of Trinidad and Tobago and Institute for Resource Development.

HMPH-ASHONPLAFA/FHI/MSH (1986) *Maternal-Child Health and Family Planning Survey Honduras, 1984*, pp 32–33. Honduran Ministry of Public Health, Association for Family Planning in Honduras, Family Health International, Management Sciences for Health.

HMPH/ASHONPLAFA/FHI/MSH (1989) *Epidemiology and Family Health Survey Honduras, 1987*, pp 81–84. Honduran Ministry of Public Health, Association for Family Planning in Honduras, Family Health International, Management Sciences for Health.

Hubert B, Blondel B & Kaminski M (1987) Contribution of specialists to antenatal care in France: impact on level of care during pregnancy and delivery. *Journal of Epidemiology and Community Health* **41**: 321–328.

Humblet PC, Wollast E, Vandenbussche P, Leleux P & Buekens P (1989) Organization of prenatal care in Belgium. *Biology of the Neonate* **55**: 55–62.

INCAP/IRD (1989) *Encuesta Nacional de Salud Materno Infantil 1987*, pp 12–13. Guatemala, Central America and Columbia, Maryland: Instituto de Nutricion de Centro America y Panama and Institute for Resource Development.

INDS (Instituto de Desarollo de la Salud) (1981) *Investigacion Perinatal.* La Habana, Cuba: Editorial Cientifico-Tecnica.

INE/IRD (1988) *Encuesta Demografica y de Salud Familiar 1986*, pp 102–104. Lima, Peru: Instituto Nacional de Estatistica, Direccion General de Demografia, Consejo Nacional de Poblacion and Institute for Resource Development.

INE/IRD (1989) *Bolivia Encuesta Nacional de Demografia y Salud 1989: Informe Preliminar*, p 18. Instituto Nacional de Estatistica and Demographic and Health Surveys, Institute for Resource Development/Macro Systems.

Jolly R & King M (1966) The organization of health services. In King M (ed.) *Medical Care in Developing Countries: A Symposium from Makerere*, pp 2.1–2.15. Nairobi: Oxford University Press.

Kafatos A, Pantelakis S & Doxiadis S (1978) Prenatal care in two counties of Greece with different infant mortality rates. *Iatriki* **33**: 514.

Kaliszer M & Kidd M (1981) Some factors affecting attendance at ante-natal clinics. *Social Science and Medicine* **15D**: 421–424.

Kessner DM, Singer J, Kalk CE & Schlesinger ER (1973) *Infant Death: An Analysis by Maternal Risk and Health Care*, p 59. Washington DC: Institute of Medicine, National Academy of Sciences.

Knudsen LB & Borlum Kristensen F (1986) Monitoring perinatal mortality and perinatal care with a national register: content and usage of the Danish medical birth register. *Community Medicine* **8**: 29–36.

Kotelchuck M (1987) *The mismeasurement of prenatal care adequacy in the US and a proposed alternative two-part index.* Paper presented at American Public Health Association Annual Meeting, New Orleans, Louisiana.

Kotelchuck M (1988) *Adequacy of Prenatal Care Utilization Index, SAS Computational Program.* Chapel Hill NC 27599-7400: School of Public Health.

Kotelchuck M, Wise PH & Costello CA (1988) *Prenatal care utilization after enrollment.* Paper presented to American Public Health Association, Boston, Massachusetts.

Little GA & Houde CT (1988) Changing professionals in maternal and child health. In Wallace HM, Ryan G & Oglesby AC (eds) *Maternal and Child Health Practices*, pp 149–159. Oakland, California: Third Party Publishing Company.

Llerena CM & Alvarez GA (1984) En espera de atencion medica. *Salud Publica de Mexico* **26**: 50–59.

Lohr KN, Brook RH, Kamberg CJ et al (1986) Use of medical care in the Rand Health Insurance Experiment: Diagnosis- and service-specific analyses in a randomized controlled trial. *Medical Care* **24(supplement S22)**.

MacKenzie T, Lees REM, Roberts JH, Willan AR & Thompson HM (1987) *Satisfaction with Obstetrical Care among Canadian Women*. Canadian Medical Association.

McKinlay J (1973) Social networks, lay consultation and help-seeking behavior. *Social Forces* **51**: 275–292.

Miller CA (1987) *Maternal and Infant Survival*. Washington, DC: National Center for Clinical Infant Programs.

MOH/IRD (1989) *Uganda Demographic and Health Survey 1988/1989: Preliminary Report*, p 14. Ministry of Health and Demographic and Health Surveys, Institute for Resource Development.

Monteith RS, Warren CW, Stanziola E, Lopez Urzua R & Oberle MW (1987) Servicios de salud maternoinfantil y vacunacion en Panama y Guatemala. *Boletin de la Oficina Sanitaria Panamericana* **103**: 210–226.

NCHS (1989) Advance report of final natality statistics, 1987. *Monthly Vital Statistics Report, National Center for Health Statistics* **38(supplement)**.

NCPD/IRD (1989) *Kenya Demographic and Health Survey 1989: Preliminary Report*, p 14. National Council for Population and Development, Ministry of Home Affairs and National Heritage and Demographic and Health Surveys, Institute for Resource Development/Macro Systems.

Ndiaye S, Sarr I & Ayad M (1988) *Enquête Démographique et de Santé au Sénégal, 1986*, pp 87–89. Ministère de l'Economie et des Finances, Direction de la Statistique, Division des Enquêtes et de la Démographie and Institute for Resource Development.

Oakley A (1982) The relevance of the history of medicine to an understanding of current change: some comments from the domain of antenatal care. *Social Science and Medicine* **16**: 667–674.

O'Brien M & Smith C (1981) Women's views and experiences of ante-natal care. *Practitioner* **225**: 123–125.

ONFP/IRD (1988) *Enquête Démographique et de Santé en Tunisie: Rapport Préliminaire*, p 16. Office National de la Famille et de la Population and Demographic and Health Surveys, Institute for Resource Development.

Orr MT & Forrest DJ (1985) The availability of reproductive health services from US private physicians. *Family Planning Perspectives* **17**: 63–69.

Potter JE (1988) Utilizacion de los servicios de salud materna en el Mexico rural. *Salud Publica de Mexico* **30**: 387–402.

Public Health Service DHHS (1989) *Caring for our Future: the Content of Prenatal Care:* A report of the Public Health Service Expert Panel on the content of prenatal care. Washington, DC: Department of Health and Human Service.

Quick JD, Greenlick MR & Roghmann KJ (1981) Prenatal care and pregnancy outcome in an HMO and general population: a multivariate cohort analysis. *American Journal of Public Health* **71**: 381–390.

RCOG (1982) *Report of the RCOG Working Party on Antenatal and Intrapartum Care*, p 39. London: Royal College of Obstetricians and Gynaecologists.

Reid M (1986) Non-medical aspects in the evaluation of prenatal care for women at low risk. In Kaminski M, Breart G, Buekens P et al (eds) *Perinatal Care Delivery Systems: Description and Evaluation in European Community Countries*, pp 59–76. Oxford: Oxford Medical Publications.

Reid ME & McIlwaine GM (1980) Consumer opinion of a hospital antenatal clinic. *Social Science and Medicine* **14A**: 363–368.

Renaer M & Eggermont E (1987) Bijdragen tot de sociale verloskunde. XI. De organisatie van de pre en perinatale zorgen. *Tijdschrift voor Sociale Geneeskunde* **43**: 1025–1034.

Royston E & Ferguson J (1985) The coverage of maternity care: a critical review of available information. *World Health Statistics Quarterly* **38**: 267–288.

Rumeau-Rouquette C, du Mazaubrum C & Rabarison Y (1984) *Naître en France, 10 Ans d'Évolution 1972–1981*, pp 57–73. Paris: Doin and Les Editions INSERM.

Secretaria de Salud (1988) *Encuesta Nacional Sobre Fecundidad y Salud, 1987*, p 207. Mexico: Subsecretaria De Servicios De Salud, Direccion General De Planificacion Familiar.

Segamba L, Ndikumasabo V, Makinson C & Ayad M (1988) *Enquête Démographique et de Santé au Burundi, 1987*, pp 66–68. Gitega, Burundi and Columbia, Maryland: Ministère de l'Interieur, Département de la Population and Institute for Resource Development.

Selbmann H, Brach M, Elser H et al (1980) *Munchner Perinatal-Studie 1975–1977*. Koln-Lovenich: Deutscher Arzte-Verlag.

Shimmura K (1988) Effects of different remuneration methods on general medical practice: a comparison of capitation and fee-for-service payment. *International Journal of Health Planning and Management* **3**: 245–258.

Simpson H & Walker G (1980) When do pregnant women attend for antenatal care? *British Medical Journal* **ii**: 104–107.

Singh S, Darroch Forrest J & Torres A (1989) *Prenatal Care in the United States: A State and County Inventory*, vol. 1, p 19. New York and Washington, DC: The Alan Guttmacher Institute.

Stengel B, Saurel-Cubizolles MJ & Kaminski M (1986) Pregnant immigrant women: occupational activity, antenatal care and outcome. *International Journal of Epidemiology* **15**: 533–539.

Terris M & Glasser M (1974) A life table analysis of the relation of prenatal care to prematurity. *American Journal of Public Health* **64**: 869–875.

Thomas H, Draper J & Field S (1983) An evaluation of the practice of shared antenatal care. *Journal of Obstetrics and Gynaecology* **3**: 157–160.

Traore B, Konate M & Stanton C (1989) *Enquête Démographique et de Santé au Mali*, pp 80–81. Bamako, Mali and Columbia, Maryland: Centre d'Etudes et de Recherches sur la Population pour le Développement, Institut de Sahel and Institute for Resource Development.

URD/IRD (1989) *Enquête Démographique et de Santé au Togo 1988: Rapport Préliminaire*, p 13. Unité de Recherche Demographique, Université du Benin, Demographic and Health Surveys, Institute for Resource Development.

Viegas OAC, Singh K & Ratnam SS (1987) Antenatal care: when, where, how and how much. In Omran AR, Martin J & Hamza B (eds) *High Risk Mothers and Newborns*, pp 287–302. Thun, Switzerland: Ott Publishers.

Voorhoeve AM, Kars C & Van Ginneken JK (1982) Machakos project studies: agents affecting health of mother and child in a rural area of Kenya. *Tropical and Geographical Medicine* **34**: 91–101.

Watkins E, Larson K, Harlan C & Young S (1990) A public health model for maternal and child health at a migrant health center. *Public Health Reports* (in press).

WHO (1977) *Manual of the International Statistical Classification of Diseases, Injuries, and Causes of Death*, p 764. Geneva: World Health Organization.

WHO (1981) *Development of Indicator for Monitoring Progress Towards Health for All by the Year 2000*, pp 57–61. Geneva: World Health Organization.

WHO (1986) *World Health Statistics Annual*. Geneva: World Health Organization.

WHO, Western Pacific Region (1986) *Evaluation of the Strategy for Health for All by the Year 2000: Seventh Report on the World Health Situation*, p 146. Manila: World Health Organization.

Wollast E, Vandenbussche P & Buekens P (1986) Evaluation de la surveillance prénatale en Belgique et comparaison entre les secteurs médicaux publics et privés. *Revue d'Epidémiologie et de Santé Publique* **34**: 52–58.

Zmirou D, Charrel M & Veyre C (1988) Bien naître en milieu rural: une évaluation de la prévention éducative du risque périnatal en milieu rural. *Pediatrie* **43**: 143–148.

12

Information systems and audit in antenatal care

K. A. GUTHRIE
M. KELLY
R. J. LILFORD

RECORD CONTENT

Obstetric records vary widely in the amount, content and relevance of the information held (Lilford et al, 1985). Information is collected for four main purposes—administration, the identification of maternal and fetal risk, and the identification of special requirements.

Administration

A basic data set is required for patient identification, recall, communication with the primary care team and unit statistics. Also required is pertinent social data, such as religion, next of kin and home telephone number (Table 1). This sort of information is required for all hospital inpatients.

Table 1. Basic data set for patient identification and administration.

Marital surname	Date of birth
(current and previous)	NHS number
Maiden name	Casefile number
Forenames	Ethnic origin
Title	Country of birth
Address	Occupation of self
Home telephone number	Occupation of partner
Next of kin:	Religion
Name	
Address	
Telephone number	
General practitioner:	
Name	
Address	
Telephone number	
Hospital consultant	

Fetal risk factor identification

One of the major objectives of antenatal care is the detection of asymptomatic women whose fetuses have a greater than average risk of significant pregnancy-related problems. The booking history is part of a screening process aimed at early identification of conditions which might require specific intervention, e.g. utero-placental failure, cervical incompetence, serious fetal anomalies. It also records an accurate menstrual history, correct gestational age being essential to the appropriate management if serious complications occur.

Maternal disease identification

Patients who present with symptoms and those with an established disease which is known to affect pregnancy require a specific care-plan, e.g. diabetics, low-income single parents, mothers with no social support.

Special requirements

Identification of factors which, although not relevant to the usual mortality and morbidity statistics, nevertheless affect the quality of the patient's pregnancy experience and her satisfaction with care, e.g. backache, desire for non-interventionist confinement (Chalmers et al, 1989).

The latter three groups are what clinicians require to give their patients well-rounded and appropriately tailored care. There is, however, a wide variance in information collected, both in amount and in content. A distinction must be made between retrospective systems, where a 'minimal database' is required for administrative and epidemiological research (Van Hemel, 1977), and antenatal questionnaires, which are used primarily for patient management (Lilford et al, 1983). The latter must come as close as possible to fulfilling Baird's maxim 'A medical history (at booking) should be sought down to the most intricate detail; any condition may be significant' (Baird, 1976). The primary function of antenatal history-taking is the identification of the fetal and maternal risk factors.

Thus, while the recommendations of the Standard Maternity Information System (Thomson and Barron, 1980) and the Steering Group for Health Service Information (Körner report, 1982) contribute towards standardizing the minimal database, the information required for optimal clinical care is less tightly defined. High-quality information enables formal or informal risk scoring whereby patients requiring special care are accurately pre-selected whilst low-risk cases can be managed, with minimal intervention, by their primary health care team. An analysis of the obstetric case notes from 41 different UK teaching hospitals (Lilford et al, 1983) showed them to contain a mean of 80 items concerned with the booking history; the minimum number was 29 and the maximum 136. Fifteen hospitals had very detailed case notes containing over 100 items, yet many totally omitted contraception, specific gynaecological history or history of the present pregnancy. In addition, several of the departments gave only open headings to sections on family or social and personal history and, although 71% included a history of tobacco-smoking, there was little emphasis on alcohol intake (15%), diet (2.5%) or domestic support (12%). Such poor standardization, however, is not unique to the UK (Van Hemel, 1977).

How detailed should a booking history be? The *quantity* of information collected has no intrinsic value; *relevance* is the most important factor. The clinical checklist developed at Sighthill, Edinburgh, and recommended by the Royal College of Obstetricians and Gynaecologists Working Party on Antenatal Care attempts to identify clinically relevant information (RCOG, 1982). However, this list contains only 30 items. Lilford and Chard (1984) isolated 82 items which may be identified at booking and which, if present, require specific action. We have now extended this list to 98 items. A list of these items is given in Table 2.

Table 2. Risk factors identified at booking with generated action suggestions.

MEDICAL HISTORY

1. **Cardiac system**
   History of cardiac disease
   —*Cardiac status*
   —*Consider specialist referral*
   —*?Necessity of antibiotic cover in labour*

2. **Hypertension**
   —*Renal function tests*
   —*Fetal assessment*

3. **Epilepsy**
   On treatment
   —*Monitor treatment*
   —*Implications for breast-feeding*

4. **Epilepsy**
   On treatment, but not attending specialist clinic
   —*Review medication*
   —*Consider specialist referral*

Surgical

5. Cone biopsy in primigravida or with subsequent caesarean section or preterm delivery in multigravida
   —*Consider cervical stenosis/incompetence*

6. Previous myomectomy
   —*?Mode of delivery*

7. Previous vaginal surgery
   —*?Mode of delivery*

8. Previous tubal surgery
   —*?Ectopic pregnancy*
   —*Early scan*

9. Previous atypical cervical smear
   Never had smear performed
   No smear for 3 years
   —*Suggest smear*

10. **Anaesthetics**
    Problems with anaesthetics in the past
    —*Discuss case with anaesthetist*

Brain and nervous system

11. Myasthenia gravis
    —*Alert paediatrician re transplacental passage of antibodies*

12. Multiple sclerosis
    —*Alert anaesthetist re epidural*

13. Paralysis
    —*?Mode of delivery*

14. **Psychiatric illnesses**
    —*Suggest case notes review*

Eyes, ears, nose, throat, lungs and air passages

15. Asthma
    —*Drug information on prostaglandins re use of Prostin as ripening agent*

16. Cystic fibrosis
    —*Check for liver disease and diabetes*
    —*Monitor fluid and electrolyte balance during delivery*

17. istory of tuberculosis
    —*Alert paediatrician re BCG to infant*

18. Tuberculosis on current treatment
    —*Review chest X-ray*
    —*?BCG to infant*

19. Pneumothorax
    —*Passive 2nd stage*

Table 2.—*(cont).*

Intestines, liver and gall bladder

20. History of hepatitis (either hepatitis B
or of unknown origin)

—*Check hepatitis antibodies*
—*Counsel re HIV testing*
—*Check liver function tests*
—*Alert paediatrician re infant*

21. Hepatitis (active) carrier of hepatitis B

immunization
—*Check antibodies*
—*Counsel re HIV testing*

Blood disorders

22. Thalassaemia

—*?Necessity of counselling and antenatal
diagnosis*
—*Folic acid supplement with or without iron*

23. Sickle cell disease

—*Avoid anaemia, infection, hypoxia,
dehydration and cooling, especially in
labour*
—*Review mode of delivery*

24. Idiopathic thrombocytopenia

—*Alert paediatrician*

25. Von Willebrand's disease

—*Alert paediatrician*

26. Haemophilia

—*Antenatal counselling*
—*Alert paediatrician*
—*?Diagnosis*

27. **Diabetes**

Gestational or otherwise

—*Referral to specialist clinic*

28. **Diabetes**

Treated by tablets

—*Change to insulin therapy*

Thyroid

29. History of thyroid disease

—*Review thyroid function*

30. Hyperthyroidism

—*Alert paediatrician re transplacental
passage of antibodies in Graves' disease*

31. Hypothyroidism

—*Alert paediatrician re transplacental
passage of antibodies in autoimmune
thyroiditis*

32. Hypothyroid (Previously hyperthyroid)
(due to therapy)

—*Transplacental passage of antibodies in
Graves' disease*
—*Alert paediatrician re neonatal
thyrotoxicosis*

33. History of radio-iodine therapy

—*Check for secondary hypothyroidism*

34. Drug therapy for thyroid problem

—*Check thyroid function*
—*Note possible effect on fetus*
—*Implications for breast-feeding*

Pituitary tumour

35. Prolactinoma

—*Monitor thyroid function*
—*Serial checks on visual fields*
—*Not a contraindication to breast-feeding*

36. ?Prolactinoma

—*Case note review*
—*Serial checks on visual fields*
—*Monitor thyroid function*
—*Not a contraindication to breast-feeding*

Urinary tract

37. Recurrent urinary tract infection (×3)
involving kidney

—*Renal function tests*
—*Fetal assessment*
—*Mid-stream specimen of urine each visit,
including general practitioner visit*
—*Kidney ultrasound scan*

Table 2.—(cont).

38. Recurrent urinary tract infection (× 3) involving kidney, never having had an intravenous urogram	*—Intravenous urogram 9 months post-delivery*
Venous thrombosis and pulmonary embolus	
39. History of deep vein thrombosis/ pulmonary embolus (confirmed)	*—?Prophylactic anticoagulants*
40. Deep vein thrombosis/pulmonary embolus on clinical grounds alone	*—Review case notes*
41. **Medical allergies**	*—Suggest review signs and symptoms*
Musculo-skeletal	
42. Systemic lupus erythematosus	*—Alert paediatrician re association with congenital fetal heart block*
	—Review immunological status and therapy
43. Rheumatoid arthritis	*—Note risk of fetal heart block*
	—Risk to joints during delivery (neck and hip hyperextension/abduction)
44. Congenital abnormality/bony injury to spine/hips/pelvis	*—Implications for epidural/spinal analgesia*
	—Implications for mode of delivery
PERSONAL AND FAMILY HISTORY	
45. Smokes > 10 cigarettes per day	
46. Drinks > 4 units alcohol per day	*—Fetal assessment*
47. Uses illegal drugs	
48. Intravenous drug abuse	*—Suggest Counsel re HIV testing/hepatitis surface antigen*
49. Vegetarian diet	*—Check iron/folate status*
50. Vegan diet	*—Check iron/vitamin B$_{12}$/folate status*
51. Poor grasp of English language	*—Arrange for interpreter*
52. Poor social circumstances/problems	*—?Medical social worker*
53. Ethnic origin:	
European/Asian	*—Consider thalassaemia risk (should be checked routinely by antenatal clinic booking staff)*
African Asian	
Arabic/Part Asian	
African	
Afro-Caribbean	*—Consider risk of sickle cell disease*
Part Black	
Ethnic Chinese	*—Check hepatitis B status*
54. Diabetes in 1st-degree relative	*—Consider glucose tolerance test at 30 weeks*
55. Tuberculosis: contact within last year or living with someone with tuberculosis	*—Check chest X-ray*
PREVIOUS PREGNANCIES	
Antenatal	
56. Self or child with neural tube defect	*—Counsel*
	—Check α-fetoprotein/ultrasound screening
57. History of cervical suture	*—?Necessity this pregnancy*
58. History of ectopic	*—Early scan to exclude another*
59. Previous mid-trimester abortion (> 16 wks with < 4 h contracting)	*—?Incompetent cervix*
	—?Necessity for cervical suture
60. Molar pregnancy	*—Early scan*
61. Pregnancy termination due to medical/ genetic/neural tube lesions	*—Counsel*
	—?Antenatal diagnosis
62. Previous pre-eclamptic toxaemia with proteinuria	*—Consider CLASP trial/aspirin*
63. Rhesus/antibody sensitization	*—Alert paediatrician*
	—Serial antibody checks

Table 2.—*(cont).*

Labour

64. Delivered at < 37 completed weeks with spontaneous rupture of membranes prior to contractions or contractions lasting < 4 h prior to delivery
—*Consider incompetent cervix*
—*?Cervical suture*

65. Previous caesarean section
—*Discuss mode of delivery this time*
—*Send for old notes*

66. Previous baby breech/oblique/transverse lie at time of delivery
—*Consider uterine anomaly*

67. Previous 3rd-degree tear
—*Registrar present at subsequent delivery*

68. Delivery by caesarean section for failed forceps/ventouse or cephalopelvic disproportion
—*?Pelvimetry considered*

Puerperium

69. History of puerperal depression
—*Consider psychiatric referral antenatally*

70. Severe puerperal depression requiring psychiatric care
—*Consider psychiatric re-referral antenatally*

71. Infant weighing > 4500 g
—*Glucose tolerance test at 30 weeks*

72. Infant < 2500 g, taking into account sex/birth order/gestation
—*Fetal assessment and CLASP trial if genuine intrauterine growth retardation*

73. Previous stillbirth
—*Glucose tolerance test at 30 weeks*
—*Antenatal fetal assessment*

74. Previous fetal anomaly
—*Consider counselling*
—*Consider anatomy scan*

75. Previous child live at birth but now dead
—*Alert paediatrician*

CONTRACEPTION AND MENSTRUAL HISTORY

76. Age less than 18 or greater than 37
—*Antenatal fetal assessment*

77. Age greater than 37
—*Trisomy counselling*

78. Age less than 37 and greater than 29
—*Consider α-fetoprotein/trisomy trial*

79. Intrauterine contraceptive device removed during pregnancy
—*Consider ectopic pregnancy*

80. Intrauterine contraceptive device in situ
—*Counsel*
—*Consider removal*

81. Bromocriptine treatment for infertility
—*Review notes for hyperprolactinaemia*

82. Abnormal last period/light
—*?Ectopic*

PRESENT PREGNANCY

83. Rubella contact since becoming pregnant
—*Check IgM/IgG titres*

84. Rubella non-immune or ?non-immune
—*Check antibody status re postnatal immunization*

Medications

85. Steroids within last 6 months
—*Consider steroid cover in labour*

86. Anticoagulants during this pregnancy other than heparin
—*Assess for fetal anomaly*
—*Change to heparin 1st and 3rd trimesters*
—*Breast-feeding implications*

87. Phenytoin during pregnancy
—*Fetal anatomy scan*
—*Monitor levels*
—*Folate supplements*
—*No contraindication to breast-feeding*

88. Valproate in pregnancy
—*Fetal anatomy scan*
—*Folate supplements*
—*No contraindication to breast-feeding*

89. Phenobarbitone in pregnancy
—*Monitor serum levels*
—*Folate supplements*
—*No contraindication to breast-feeding*

Table 2.—*(cont).*

90. Carbamazepine in pregnancy	—*Monitor serum levels*
	—*No contraindication to breast-feeding*
91. Lithium in pregnancy	—*Monitor serum levels*
	—*Implications for breast-feeding*
	—*Cardiac scan*
Problems in current pregnancy	
92. Constipation	—*Prescribe diet and laxatives*
93. Varicose veins	—*Prescribe support tights/advise*
94. Dysuria/frequency/haematuria	—*Check mid-stream specimen of urine*
95. Irritant vaginal discharge	—*Swabs*
96. Severe vomiting	—*Scan for multiple/molar pregnancy*
97. Vaginal bleeding	—*Viability scan*
98. Headaches, other than usually experienced	—*Check fundi*
99. **Extras**	

RECORD STORAGE—BY HOSPITAL OR PATIENT?

The attitude of the medical profession to personal access to medical records is changing, no doubt influenced by pressure from the public culminating in the Data Protection Act (1984) and a general disenchantment with paternalistic practice.

The shared-care card allows the patient record to be updated whenever the patient is seen, but laboratory results will often have to be stored elsewhere, at least in the short term, until they can catch up with the card.

Two experimental programmes in which women holding their own case notes have been compared with conventional systems showed that fewer records were lost or unavailable in the experimental (patient-carried) group (Elbourne et al, 1987; Lovell et al, 1987). Certainly in Bradford, with an annual delivery rate of 6000 in two sites, less than ten sets of patient-carried case notes were lost in 12 years. Studies have also shown that women carrying their own notes felt more in control of their antenatal care, more able to communicate effectively with the caregivers and would want to carry their own notes again in a subsequent pregnancy (Elbourne et al, 1987; Lovell et al, 1987). Until the next generation of information storage, which may include electronic transmission of clinical findings and investigation results between sites with spin-off hard copy, patient-carried data has much to recommend it. Doctors and midwives should, however, record information which can be read by the patient in a form that she can understand.

COMPUTERIZED SYSTEMS OF ANTENATAL RECORDS

There are two methods of collecting clinical information by computer: prospective and retrospective. In the former, data is entered 'on-line', i.e. 'live' as it is collected; in the latter, data is collected *after* the event from paperwork generated *during* the event.

Retrospective data collection

This can be done after discharge, after delivery or after each patient encounter.

Systems for data entry after discharge have existed for many years for collecting medical (Gledhill et al, 1970) and obstetric (Jelovsek and Hammond, 1978) histories after discharge. Typically, information is transferred from the handwritten notes to the computer by way of coding forms which may be completed by medical or secretarial staff. In Britain, for example, the Hospital Activity Analysis (HAA) and Körner statistics use the International Classification of Diseases (ICD) and the Office for Population and Census Surveys (OPCS 4) codes. The main purpose of these systems is to provide a large and rapidly accessible database for routine clinical and epidemiological studies. This form of data collection is removed in time and place from the critical events in patient care. The most important drawback of these retrospective systems of data entry after discharge is failure to obtain complete and correct information as a result of omissions or illegibility in the core manual records and inadequate training of the clerical staff; the HAA is notorious in this regard. The accuracy of the computerized record is, therefore, limited by the quality of the handwritten case notes, by errors in transferring information to the coding forms and by errors in entering information on the computer. Data entered in this retrospective, labour-intensive and inaccurate way has no value in the clinical management of patients.

Data collection after labour has been facilitated by the introduction of microcomputer systems which can be used by the staff responsible for the delivery and which should incorporate error-checking within an interactive programme (Maresh et al, 1982). On-line vetting has been shown to enhance the accuracy of data. Introducing error trapping into the programme

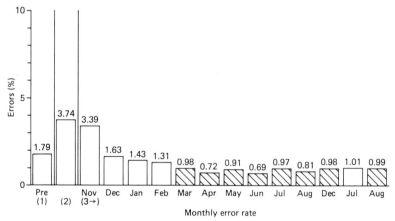

Figure 1. Labour ward data: error rates for six months pre-computerization vs monthly computer error rates before and after introduction of error trapping. 1 = pre-computer (manual records); 2 = computerized records pre-error trapping (three months' data); 3 = computerized records with error trapping. Monthly error rates during 1987–1989; those below 1% are highlighted by hatching.

designed for in-house use in St James's labour ward rapidly reduced the error rate from 3.74% to less than 1%, which is well below the precomputer level of 1.79% (Figure 1).

Computerization after each patient encounter extends this principle to other events in a patient's progress through a maternity department. These systems rely on information collected manually by professional staff. Data is then entered by them or other staff. If the entire antenatal history is included on the computer record, then a large number of coded questionnaire forms must be completed after the booking encounter with the expense of subsequent data entry. Systems of this type are widely used in North America (Sokol and Chik, 1982).

On-line data collection

On-line data is entered directly onto the computer without first being recorded on paper. 'Hard copy' is subsequently produced by the computer. This method may be used to collect the booking history and has many advantages (Table 3); it offers unlimited branching capacity, gives a comprehensive history for clinical management and obviates coding errors without the expense of employing extra personnel. Simply altering the programme to change the database is far cheaper than reprinting questionnaires and more reliable than human memory.

Table 3. Comparison of the advantages and uses of the three basic methods of computerized data collection.

	Retrospective code forms	Clinical questionnaires	On-line
Database for retrospective research	+	+	+
Automatic discharge summary	+	+	+
Database for clinical use	−	+	+
Clinical advice and reminders	−	+	+
Unlimited branching capacity to produce comprehensive records	−	−	+
Does not require extra personnel	−	−	+
Questionnaire can be easily and inexpensively altered	−	−	+

COMPUTERIZED HISTORY-TAKING SYSTEMS

Information recording

The reduction in size of computer processors over the last 20 years has bred the microcomputer—no different in principle from its larger mainframe predecessors, but much less expensive. Microcomputers lend themselves to clinical application, either free-standing or as part of a microcomputer network linked to a hard disc, in which terminals give input to preselected microcomputers linked to printers which provide 'hard copy' for case notes, discharge summaries, etc. Terminals can be placed in various geographical

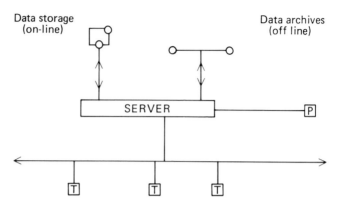

Figure 2. A microcomputer network or clinical information service (CIS). T = terminals; P = printer.

sites, e.g. the antenatal clinic, radiology and pathology departments, and the general practitioner's surgery, building the network up to a clinical information system (CIS) (Figure 2). These systems can be extended to other disciplines as medical information systems or to a hospital information support system (HISS) (Figure 3).

A number of systems have been developed for on-line data collection, but the archetypal method uses a visual display unit (VDU) and keyboard. The

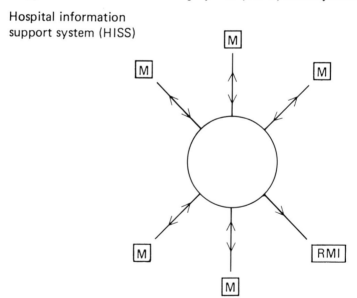

Figure 3. An obstetric network, as a major service provider, could link into a hospital information support system (HISS). Data from other major service providers comes back into the obstetric network via HISS. RMI = resource management initiative; M = clinical support systems, e.g. clerical, pathology, haematology, nursing support services, cytogenetics, anaesthetics.

questions are displayed in sequence on the screen of a computer terminal and answered on a keyboard, either by the patient or an accompanying medical attendant. 'Yes' or 'no' answers are required most often, and keyboards can be correspondingly simplified with a reduction in the number of keys. The computer actively selects the next question on the basis of the previous answer, thereby offering unlimited branching capacity without the need for a specific intervention by the user.

New data entry systems are also available such as light- and touch-sensitive screens. Computers can also 'ask' questions verbally using voice technology (Marg et al, 1972; Stead et al, 1977; Friedman et al, 1978). Systems also exist where questions are posed both verbally and on the VDU (Simmons and Miller, 1971). The next generation of computers currently being designed by the armed forces will respond to the spoken command.

To simplify keyboard entry, systems have been developed which rely on a special questionnaire with bar codes which are read by drawing a light pen over the question, transmitting the bar code to the computer. It is essentially the same system as used at supermarket checkouts. Such a system was developed in the antenatal clinic at Kings College Hospital in London (Saunders et al, 1982).

Information storage and retrieval

Clinical information is usually stored on disc as well as on tape as a back-up for archive and security. Information can be returned for display on a VDU; alternatively 'hard copy' can be transcribed by printer for the case notes or for letters. Programmes can be designed to reproduce all clinical data as 'pages' on the VDU and summarize key findings. The great strength of computer data-handling systems is that as much or as little as is required can be retrieved from the system; for example, you could review one patient's single haemoglobin, all of one patient's haemoglobins or all of all patients' haemoglobins, as required, maintaining confidentiality if required by way of a password.

Many of the earlier information systems were based on in-house software development (e.g. Gibbons et al, 1982). Much of this development was very hardware- and environment-specific. This made it difficult, if not impossible, to install one of these information systems into another hospital with a different information technology/medical environment. The last five years have seen the rapid development of standard 'computing platforms', platform-independent computing environments and international standards for inter-platform communication. A 'computer platform' is essentially a standard combination of computer hardware and software in terms of an operating system/environment. An example of this would be a personal computer running the MS-DOS operating system. For information handling, relational database management systems have become the *de facto* standard, and structured query language is fast becoming the standard relational database interface across the whole range of computing platforms. Utilizing modern fourth-generation languages, basic clinical data entry, storage and retrieval systems using a relational database management system backend can be rapidly built and ported across a wide range of computer platforms (e.g. MS-DOS local area network, UNIX minicomputer and IBM mainframe). With open systems interconnection, both distributed and server-based database systems will play an increasingly important role in the near future. They will allow the true integration of clinical data into a HISS (Figure 3).

However, the majority of present commercial and in-house developed information systems still do not offer a fully open architecture in terms of standards or communication. Growing pressure from information technology literate clinicians, resource management initiatives and HISS will force vendors and developers to change this situation in the near future.

Questionnaire design

The overriding principle in questionnaire design is to make use as easy as possible. A password allows entry to the system and the simplest format thereafter is based on a 'menu' from which the user may simply select a function (Figure 4). After the function is complete, the system will revert to the menu, allowing the operator to concentrate on the patient and the questions as they appear on the VDU, effectively ignoring the operation of the computer.

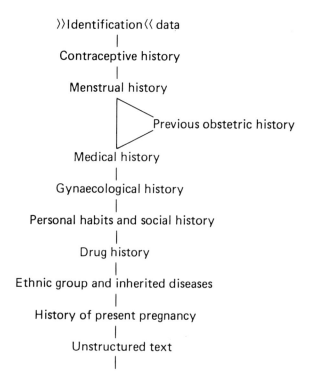

Figure 4. Overall scheme ('menu') for booking questionnaire.

The history ideally follows a highly branching pattern, simulating an idealized manual history. Thus, if the response to 'Has Ms Roberts used contraception prior to this pregnancy?' is 'Yes', the programme automatically branches out into an appropriate series of questions about contraception. Similarly, in a primigravida, questions about past obstetric history are omitted.

There are five basic types of questions: yes/no, yes/no/don't know, mutually exclusive multiple choice questions, multiple choice questions where more than one answer may apply, and free text entry. A 'protected field' is displayed for entry of dates and text. The questionnaire should be exhaustive and seek to include any feature and combination of features which may arise. As this cannot be guaranteed in all cases, some multiple choice questions must include 'don't know' and 'other' categories, the latter leading to a limited free text field. Free text fields are required for proper nouns, such as the previous place of confinement, and for recording rare disease or drug therapy. Free text is also required at the end of each section of the programme for entry of other relevant information that may have arisen. Errors typed during entry should be erasable using the 'delete' button.

The accuracy of information recorded can be enhanced by various manoeuvres:

1. The computer will not accept an answer not listed as an optional answer for that question.
2. Branching eradicates the inconsistencies of a non-branching programme—data collecting is therefore very 'tight'. Data insertion in the wrong place should not occur in the on-line interactive systems where the programme branches round irrelevant or non-applicable portions of history.
3. Missing values—the interactive programme will not proceed until data is entered.
4. Protected fields for numeric information will not accept text and vice versa.
5. After each section, the summary of answers may be displayed so that the user can correct any errors or to permit the patient to change her mind. A 'go back' facility with the return button makes this quick and easy, without having to retype all the information.
6. 'Help boxes' may be available on request for detailed explanation, e.g. to define parity vs gravidity, give a list of oral contraceptives or explain why a question on ethnic origin is asked. Routine display would slow down the programme and is not required anyway in the majority of cases.
7. Facts, rather than diagnoses, are requested for accuracy, e.g. to enquire about hypertension and proteinuria rather than pre-eclampsia.
8. Error (plausibility) checks can be included. Unlikely values can be accepted only after verification (value questioned on the screen and re-entry invited) and impossible answers rejected. For example, a maternal age of 14 is possible but not probable, so would require

verification. A maternal age of 64 is not possible in the post-biblical era, and simply would not be accepted. An alternative value would be requested.

9. Unlikely combination of answers—the programme will pick up and reject impossible combinations of independently plausible data, e.g. time of delivery prior to the time of commencement of second stage.

Detection of informal errors by 'trapping' has been shown to considerably increase the accuracy of records, as shown by our own labour ward audit (Figure 1).

A good interactive programme will provide an opportunity for patients to change their minds, contain carefully worded questions for clarity, use non-interpreted data and keep the tone of the interview friendly. The last, however, should not be achieved at the expense of irritating the medical/ nursing staff (Malone-Lee, 1987). It could also present the questions multi-lingually if required.

Antenatal database content

As said before, there is extremely poor standardization of obstetric data collection and the performance of any obstetric database depends on the questions included. Lilford et al (1983) describe the genesis of an antenatal database from the current hospital manual system, an analysis of the British teaching hospitals case records, the Royal College of Obstetricians and Gynaecologists recommended antenatal booking record and medical text-books on history-taking. They used the computer to calculate gestational age, taking into account possibility of pregnancy after prolonged amenor-rhoea, pregnancy following confinement amenorrhoea, and even pregnancy prior to the first menstruation. Protected fields for free text were provided to cover rare conditions not covered in multichoice questions.

A complete history with no omissions, computer-based, eliminates memory lapse by the operator. The computer provides a larger amount of practically useful information (Schuman et al, 1975; Bulpitt et al, 1976), although probably at the expense of over-reporting trivia (Robinson et al, 1975). A cross-over trial of manual and computerized data systems in antenatal care showed that the computer provided a qualitative and quanti-tative improvement (Lilford et al, 1983). Certainly the patient is reminded of symptoms which would have been ignored in a conventional interview (Simmons and Miller, 1971).

A further requirement is risk scoring and action suggestions. Risk scoring has been widely tried in obstetrics (Edwards et al, 1979). Computerized data gathering lends itself to formal risk scoring as this can be done automatically with no loss of efficiency (Rosen et al, 1978). However, a clinical data retrieval system can easily be designed to alert the obstetrician to a high risk by identifying the specific factors involved rather than simply providing an overall summarized assessment. These can be printed in a different colour or type face, and can be associated with specific clinical advice (Lilford and Chard, 1984; Lilford et al, 1985). More complex medical information systems can also alert the physician to abnormal or missing results.

Transcript

The acceptability of a system in clinical practice depends largely on the quality of the computer print-out ('hard copy'), which must be laid out clearly and compartmented, with important positive and negative features and action suggestions heightened by type face or colour. To avoid information over-load, negative responses may have to be omitted or typed in very small print. Such transcripts are incorporated into case notes. An alternative would be display of information on a VDU, an essential in a paperless and completely on-line obstetric record such as has been developed in the Columbian Presbyterian Medical Centre (Gonzalez and Fox, 1989).

In summary, the advantages of computerized data collection include standardization, high-quality presentation, time-saving for trained staff (with poorly trained or junior staff, the loss of time should be compensated for by the quality of the history), rapid availability of records and reminders of risk factors, action suggestions, omissions, reports and actions. The disadvantages are its inability to accept unlimited discursive information, the lack of confidentiality and mechanical breakdown:

1. Limited discursive information—the computer cannot gauge a patient's reaction to a given question; it cannot register non-verbal communication, although one imaginative system attempted to do this by recording the patient's pulse rate (Slack, 1971). It could be argued impartiality is a benefit, as the computer has no preconceived ideas and cannot influence a patient to modify her response to please the questioner.

2. Lack of confidentiality—this may be the case with centralized data-banks (Newcombe and Trimble, 1975), but in the context of clinical departments computer files are, perhaps, better protected than case notes stored in a standard file. Specific security measures such as passwords limit access to relevant sections of data; for example, a research worker would have access to results but not to patient identification data. In the future, access may be limited by fingerprint identification.

3. Computer breakdown—as a result of hardware failure, this is rare. Power surge and loss can be dealt with by appropriate 'power-smoothing' devices. Most problems lie in software design, an area essential for improvement if computers are to be widely accepted for clinical use.

THE PSYCHOLOGICAL EFFECT OF CLINICAL COMPUTING

Arguments that computers depersonalize the doctor–patient relationship have not been supported by practical experience. Computer histories do not diminish the time spent with the patient. Use of the computer as an intermediary makes 'personal' questioning, e.g. drug abuse or alcohol consumption, less pejorative (Lucas, 1977). Ninety-seven per cent of women in a pregnancy termination clinic (Lilford et al, 1985) and 99% of women in an antenatal clinic (Brownbridge et al, 1988) did not object to the use of a computer, which agrees with other surveys of patients' views on history-taking by computer (Cruikshank, 1984; Brownbridge et al, 1985).

Nursing staff did not object to using a computer but found it a constraint on time (Lilford et al, 1985; Brownbridge et al, 1988). An activity analysis of videotapes showing midwives performing computer versus manual bookings showed that automation did not distract the midwife from the patient once she had become proficient with the keyboard. Midwives did, however, tend to use more leading questions (Brownbridge et al, 1988) when the computer was used.

OPERATIONAL EFFECTS OF THE ANTENATAL CLINIC COMPUTER

This question is, as yet, unanswered. It has been shown that a larger, more structured, relevant booking history not confounded by the human error of omission is superior in quality to manual methods (see above). However, it has not yet been shown that increasing the level of relevant data and providing action suggestions leads to an improved standard of care as judged against a bench-mark standard. We are currently investigating the quality of the process of care with and without computer histories in an antenatal clinic; 2400 referrals to the clinic have been randomized to have their booking history taken by computer, highly structured manual or relatively unstructured manual questionnaire. The same pool of midwives are being used throughout. The effect of these methods on subsequent care are being assessed.

AUDIT—THE STUDY OF PROCESS

Audit means different things to different people and one's view on the subject depends on which definition is selected. Obstetricians are quick to take credit for instituting audit in the form of local and national data collection exercises, such as statistics on perinatal mortality, birthweight, etc. While these exercises certainly constitute observational studies, they cannot be used to make conclusions about the quality of care. In particular, birthweight is probably one of the less important variables affecting out-comes such as perinatal mortality and neurological morbidity. Thus, any argument for a change in resourcing or patterns of care, predicated on these statistics, is likely to be specious. It is often claimed that the proliferation of computer systems, such as those used to collect the Körner maternity data set, contribute to audit. This argument is based on the notion that these more detailed data sets contain sufficient information to allow researchers to control for other variables such as social class. This idea is fallacious for two reasons. Firstly, these data sets are often inadequately detailed 'minimal data sets' and this rationalization appears necessary in order to ensure the quality of retrospective data at a national level. Secondly, and far more important, statistical techniques, such as multivariate analysis and logistic regression, can only control for known sources of bias, yet unknown factors are likely to be more important, especially in a socially and economically sensitive subject such as perinatology. There is, therefore, no sound inference that can be made from a review of information contained in amalgamated databases of hospital statistics. Audit, as properly defined, hinges on inference: the inference that the quality of care was or was not of a high standard. Descriptive statistics, therefore, can be used to generate hypotheses but should not be used as a form of audit.

Rather different to the anonymous data collections mentioned above are national surveys which not only measure overall mortality and morbidity, but which also examine each case with a bad outcome in detail. Here, experts make an informed, albeit subjective, judgement as to whether the bad outcome could have been prevented by a higher standard of care. This process, therefore, is similar to cases of civil tort, where the Court must decide about negligence and causality on the balance of probability. However, unlike a court of law, this form of audit is *designed* to warn other doctors about problems and pitfalls (e.g. be careful to count your swabs during episiotomy repair). Such reports make compelling reading for doctors and are much like the yearly reports published by the defence societies. While thoroughly supporting these activities and finding them very informative in warning about pitfalls which lie ahead, a minor note of caution must be sounded. These are one-sided audits, in which only those cases with a bad outcome are examined. This, by its very nature, is likely to bias an assessor in the direction of criticizing clinical care. An assessor or reader must therefore avoid the superficially plausible question—would the bad outcome have been avoided by a different form of care? The answer will often be 'In all probability—yes', but it does not follow from this that care was of a poor quality. The fact that a *particular* patient would have most likely been spared a bad outcome by a different form of care does not mean that other such patients should receive this treatment. One of us (RJL) recently attended a coroner's inquest into a maternal death from septicaemia and liver failure following prolonged labour and caesarean section. The coroner asked 'Would this patient have survived if an earlier caesarean section had been carried out?' The answer was 'More probably'. However, the question was not well put. The more appropriate question was 'Should all such women have earlier caesarean sections?' or 'Would earlier caesarean section have had an higher expected utility?' In this case the answer was 'No', but in more ambiguous cases experts are likely to subconsciously bias assessment against the form of treatment associated with the poor outcome.

A method to avoid such subtle biases that can be introduced by non-blinded one-sided audit is to take random controls with similar presenting features and examine the methods of care in these patients. Of course, if no difference is found, this leaves open the question of whether care was generally poor, as opposed to poor only in those patients with a bad outcome.

The above consideration takes us straight into discussion of how we decide on the appropriate standards of care. These standards must be those which maximize the chances of a good outcome (we will deal here with the simple case where there are no trade-offs between various outcomes). The first point to make is that auditing the quality of care involves a study of *process*. It therefore depends on the assumption that we know which practices maximize beneficial outcomes. This exercise is therefore only relevant when we have good evidence linking the process of care with these outcomes. Judgement about whether particular clinical or management policies are more likely to do good than harm will be based on different forms of evidence. At one extreme, the effects of policies may be obvious, e.g. the beneficial effect of blood transfusion after massive haemorrhage, the drainage of wound abscesses or the prescription of antibiotics for life-threatening infection. The trouble is that, the more obvious the benefit of the medical intervention, the less likely are doctors to ignore it. Thus, assessment of the quality of medical care in deaths from massive postpartum haemorrhage usually hinges on whether blood transfusion was adequate or excessive, a somewhat more subtle and contentious point than failure to establish an intravenous line!

There is, however, one area where clear guidelines can be laid down as to the process of care and where, in our view, audit has its greatest role. This is in the quality of administrative arrangements. Many of the appropriate processes are simply good manners but these can be effectively audited. Thus audit can include such factors as 'Was the general practitioner and midwife informed of a perinatal death before the patient's discharge?' or 'Have doctors recognized and acted upon an abnormal smear result?' It is our view that it is in these organizational matters that the National Health Service most often falls down and where audit has the most to offer. The on-line action suggestions which we have discussed act as a form of automated audit, with the advantage that they identify deficiencies or potential errors *before* any harm can come to a patient.

In the above examples the accepted standard against which the process of care can be compared is very obvious. In other cases, however, the accepted standard should itself be audited to ensure that it is based on sound evidence. I. Chalmers (personal communication) pointed out the fundamental flaw in any form of audit that was restricted to an examination of the process of health care by citing the first known example of medical audit; this involved censure of a Boston physician who had not prescribed the then standard treatment for pneumonia—blood letting. It is important that audit does not become an authoritarian tool to restrict the advance of medical knowledge. Thus, any requirement of particular policies for care or management within the health services should be based on good evidence that these policies are more likely to do good than harm.

Evidence about the effects of care may take a variety of forms, including seeking the views of people who have used the health service. Here again, however, caution is needed, since we do not know how prior expectations among different groups of people influence their reactions to the health service. Other methods of care have been evaluated in properly controlled studies, thus generating evidence required for informed audit of practice. There is now good evidence that certain forms of care are more effective than others (e.g. catgut sutures cause more pain following perineal wound repair, steroids promote fetal lung maturity, prophylactic antibiotics reduce the morbidity and financial costs of caesarean section, and oxytocic agents reduce the incidence of postpartum haemorrhage) (Chalmers et al, 1989). However, many practices which are enshrined in obstetric dogma are of completely unproven value and may even be harmful; the best example of this is the glucose tolerance test. Therefore we have some good evidence on which to base certain policies and these can be used as a 'gold standard' against which the process of care can be judged. Other examples are much more tenuous and before resorting to audit, more properly controlled randomized experiments should be carried out. In a rather more parochial British sense, audit forms an important component of the proposed National Health Service reforms. The essence of these is the separation of responsibility for providing and processing medical services and the establishment of an internal market. However, many services, and antenatal care is an example, are semi-monopolies. The provider of these services might not be in too strong a bargaining position for funds (cost per patient) if there was no link between remuneration and some attempt to measure the value of the service in terms of outcome and consumer satisfaction.

Thus audit itself needs to be audited. A good example of this is Barrett's caesarean section audit (Barrett et al, 1989) in which five auditors reviewed the case notes of a random sample of emergency caesarean sections for fetal distress. The initial audit showed a wide inter-observer variation, all five auditors agreeing in only 20% of cases. Furthermore, when re-presented with the same case notes, a marked inconsistency with first-time decisions was observed; the cumulative inconsistency rate being one case in four. This study reinforces the point that audit must be preceded by a validation of the audit process itself.

There is one final value of audit which lies beyond the more straightforward benefits that may result from the direct educational and disciplining effects. This is a more nebulous but ironically possibly more important effect which results, not from the information provided by audit, but from the very process of audit itself. This is the famous Hawthorne effect, whereby in the very process of examining a human activity, that activity is changed. Thus audit has a symbolic component to it—it sends a signal to health professionals that their work is being monitored and that they are accountable to their patients.

SUMMARY

The obstetric record as initiated at the antenatal booking clinic essentially identifies the degree of risk engendered in that pregnancy so that consequent obstetric and paediatric management is tailored appropriately. Whether carried by the patient or based in the hospital with a summary carried by the patient (shared-care card), this record should be exhaustive, the emphasis being on quality, not quantity, of information recorded. To obviate human error in history-taking, patient management or record transcription, we believe on-line computerization of patient records with spin-off paperwork to be the only patient management system to fulfil the above criteria. User-friendly software can be designed with highly branching programmes which provide clinical action suggestions in high-risk cases. Various 'error traps' enhance the accuracy of information recorded. Such systems can be operated by medical and midwifery staff with minimal keyboard skills and are well accepted by patients and staff. Inexpensive and versatile micro-computer networks are excellent for such systems. The operational effects are discussed.

Audit means different things to different people and one's view on the subject depends on which definition is selected. Obstetricians are quick to take credit for instituting audit in the form of local and national data collection exercises, such as statistics on perinatal mortality, birthweight, etc. While these exercises certainly constitute observational studies, they cannot be used to make conclusions about the quality of care. There is no sound inference that can be made from a review of information contained in amalgamated databases of hospital statistics. Audit, as properly defined, hinges on inference: the inference that the quality of care was or was not of a high standard. Descriptive statistics, therefore, can be used to generate hypotheses but should not be used as a form of audit, at least not in obstetrics.

Auditing the quality of care involves a study of *process*. It therefore depends on the assumption that we know which practices maximize beneficial outcomes. This exercise is therefore only relevant when we have good evidence linking the process of care with these outcomes. In some cases the accepted standard against which the process of care can be compared is very obvious. In other cases, however, the accepted standard should itself be audited to ensure that it is based on sound evidence.

REFERENCES

Baird D (1976) In Walker J, MacGillivray I & MacNaughton MC (eds) *Combined Textbook of Obstetrics and Gynaecology*, 9th edn. Edinburgh: Livingstone.

Barrett JFR, Jarvis GJ, Macdonald HN, Buchan PC, Tyrell S & Lilford RJ (1989) *The Inconsistencies of Clinical Decisions revealed by an Obstetric Audit*. Proceedings of the British Congress of Obstetrics and Gynaecology, No. 89.

Brownbridge G, Herzmark G & Wall T (1985) Patient reactions to doctor's computer use in general practice consultations. *Social Science and Medicine* **20:** 47.

Brownbridge G, Lilford RJ & Tindale-Biscoe S (1988) Use of a computer to take booking histories in a hospital antenatal clinic. *Medical Care* **26:** 474–487.

Bulpitt CJ, Berlin LJ, Coles EC et al (1976) A randomized controlled trial of computer held medical records in hypertensive patients. *British Medical Journal* **i:** 677.

Chalmers I, Enkin M & Keirse MJNC (1989) Effective care in pregnancy and childbirth: a synopsis for guiding practice and research. In Chalmers I, Enkin M & Keirse MJNC (eds) p 1465. *Effective Care in Pregnancy and Childbirth*. Oxford: Oxford University Press.

Cruikshank PJ (1984) Patient satisfaction: is the computer a plus or a minus? *Computers in Medicine* **1:** 42.

Edwards LE, Barrada MI, Tatreau RW & Hakanson EY (1979) A simplified antepartum risk scoring system. *Obstetrics and Gynecology* **54:** 237.

Elbourne D, Richardson H, Chalmers I, Waterhouse I & Holt E (1987) The Newbury maternity care study: a randomized controlled trial to evaluate a policy of women holding their own obstetric records. *British Journal of Obstetrics and Gynaecology* **94**: 612–619.

Friedman RB, Huhta J & Cheung S (1978) An automated verbal medical history system. *Archives of Internal Medicine* **138**: 1359.

Gibbons PS, Pishotta RT, Hoawad AM, Lowensohn RI & Woo D (1982) The Obtile perinatal database. *Acta Obstetrica et Gynecologica Scandinavica Supplement* **109**: 51.

Gledhill VX, McPherson TA & Mackay IR (1970) The application of computers to medical research: a computer system for the storage and retrieval of medical records. *Australian Annals of Medicine* **19**: 16.

Gonzalez FA & Fox HE (1989) The development and implementation of a computerized on-line obstetric record. *British Journal of Obstetrics and Gynaecology* **96**: 1323.

Jelovsek F & Hammond W (1978) Formal error rate in a computerized obstetric record. *Methods of Information in Medicine* **17**: 151.

Körner report (1982) *Steering Group for Health Services Information. First Report to the Secretary of State.* London: HMSO.

Lilford RJ & Chard T (1984) The use of a small computer to provide action suggestions in the booking clinic. *Acta Obstetrica et Gynecologica Japonica* **36**: 119–125.

Lilford RJ, Bingham P, Fawdry R, Setchell M & Chard T (1983) The development of on-line history taking systems in antenatal care. *Methods of Information in Medicine* **22**: 189–197.

Lilford RJ, Chard T, Bingham P & Corrigan E (1985) Use of a microcomputer network for history taking in a prenatal clinic. *American Journal of Perinatology* **2**: 143–147.

Lovell A, Zander LI, James CE, Foot S, Sibden AV & Reynolds A (1987) The St Thomas's maternity case notes study: a randomized control trial to assess the effects of giving expectant mothers their own maternity case notes. *Pediatric and Perinatal Epidemiology* **1**: 57.

Lucas RW (1977) A study of patients' attitudes to computer interrogation. *International Journal of Man and Machine Studies* **9**: 69.

Malone-Lee J (1987) *The Development of a Software Package for Urodynamic Studies.* Proceedings of the International Continence Society, Bristol, UK.

Maresh M, Beard RW, Combe D et al (1982) Computerization of obstetric information using a microcomputer. *Acta Obstetrica et Gynecologica Scandinavica Supplement* **109**: 42.

Marg E, Crossman RFW, Goodeve PJ & Wakamatsu H (1972) An automated case history taker for eye examination. *American Journal of Optometry* **49**: 105.

Newcombe HB & Trimble BK (1975) Criteria for automatic record linkage. *Journal of Clinical Computing* **4**: 205.

RCOG (1982) *Report of Working Party on Antenatal and Antepartum Care* (1982) London: Royal College of Obstetricians and Gynaecologists.

Robinson DW, Walmsley GL, Horrocks JC et al (1975) Histories obtained by two-stage questionnaire with automated transcript in specialist gynaecological practice. *British Medical Journal* **iv**: 510.

Rosen MC, Sokol RJ & Chik L (1978) Use of computers in the labor and delivery suite: an overview. *American Journal of Obstetrics and Gynecology* **132**: 589.

Saunders M, Campbell S & White H (1982) Unique real-time method of obstetric data collection. Lecture notes in medical information. Proceedings of Dublin Conference.

Schuman SH, Curry HB, Braunstein ML et al (1975) Improving on doctor–patient communication. *Journal of Family Practice* **2**: 263.

Simmons AM & Miller OW (1971) Automated patient history-taking. *Hospitals* **45**: 56.

Slack WV (1971) Computer-based interviewing system dealing with non-verbal behaviour as well as keyboard responses. *Science* **171**: 84.

Sokol RJ & Chik C (1982) A perinatal database system for research and clinical care. *Acta Obstetrica et Gynecologica Scandinavica Supplement* **109**: 57.

Stead WW, Hammond WE & Estes EM (1977) Evaluation of an audio mode of the automated medical history. *Methods of Information in Medicine* **16**: 20.

Thomson AM & Barron SL (1980) A standard maternity information system. In Chalmers I & McIlwaine G (eds) *Perinatal Audit and Surveillance*. London: Royal College of Obstetricians and Gynaecologists.

Van Hemel OJS (1977) *An obstetric database: human factors, design and reliability*. Thesis for Doctor of Medicine, University of Amsterdam.

Index

Note: Page numbers of article titles are in **bold** type.